T0184548

In Clinical Practice

Taking a practical approach to clinical medicine, this series of smaller reference books is designed for the trainee physician, primary care physician, nurse practitioner and other general medical professionals to understand each topic covered. The coverage is comprehensive but concise and is designed to act as a primary reference tool for subjects across the field of medicine.

Tim Cross
Editor

Liver Disease in Clinical Practice

Second Edition

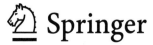 Springer

Editor
Tim Cross
Royal Liverpool University Hospital
Liverpool, UK

ISSN 2199-6652   ISSN 2199-6660   (electronic)
In Clinical Practice

ISBN 978-3-031-10011-6   ISBN 978-3-031-10012-3   (eBook)
https://doi.org/10.1007/978-3-031-10012-3

This Springer imprint is published by the registered company Springer Nature Switzerland AG
The registered company address is: Gewerbestrasse 11, 6330 Cham, Switzerland

I would like to dedicate this book to all keyworkers, hospital and healthcare workers who worked so tirelessly and selflessly during the global pandemic.

Preface

The first edition of *Liver Disease in Clinical Practice* was published in 2017. It was hoped to get a second edition out in 2020, but as many of us will only be too aware, the COVID-19 pandemic has had a significant impact on our lives and this has led to a significant delay in its publication.

There have been many developments since the last edition, and as a result, some chapters have been added and others have been omitted particularly where there were concerns about duplication. Thus, we have included new chapters on IgG4 disease, drug-induced liver disease and Fontan-associated liver disease (FALD). Given the nature of the series, the book is not intended to be a comprehensive textbook of all aspects of liver disease, and so we have omitted chapters on primary biliary cholangitis, primary sclerosing cholangitis, nutrition, end of life care and alcohol-related liver disease. It is hoped that the first edition will provide a framework and guide to help clinicians manage these conditions.

Given the rapidly changing landscape in information on COVID-19, a decision was made not to include this topic, as the concern would be the information would be out of date by the time of publication. I hope this will not be a disappointment.

I'd like to thank all the authors for the generosity in providing time to write these chapters and hope it has given an opportunity for trainee doctors and researchers to sharpen their writing skills. It is a reflection on the wonderful international nature of hepatology community that we have had contributors from Australia, Canada, the USA and the UK. Finally, I'd also like to thank the production team at

Springer, in particular Siva, for being so generous with their time and for being so patient in waiting for this edition to finally materialize.

Liverpool, UK   Tim Cross
January 2022

Contents

1 Assessment of Liver Function 1
Ioannis Papamargaritis and Cyril Sieberhagen

2 Acute Liver Failure 19
Gregory Packer and Brian J. Hogan

3 Drug-Induced Liver Injury 37
Edmond Atallah and Guruprasad P. Aithal

**4 Liver Decompensation and Acute on
Chronic Liver Failure** 57
R. Nathwani, N. Selvapatt, and A. Dhar

5 Portal Hypertension: Varices 81
Amardeep Khanna, Ashish Goel,
and Dhiraj Tripathi

6 Frailty and Sarcopenia in Cirrhosis 105
Osama Siddiqui, Sydney Olson, Avesh Thuluvath,
and Daniela Ladner

7 Non-alcoholic Fatty Liver Disease 127
David Koeckerling, Thomas Marjot,
and Jeremy Cobbold

8 Chronic Hepatitis B 151
Navjyot Hansi, Loey Lung-Yi Mak, Upkar Gill,
and Patrick Kennedy

9 Chronic Hepatitis C 177
Ruth Tunney, Martin Prince, and Varinder Athwal

10 Autoimmune Hepatitis and Overlap Syndromes 195
Kristel K. Leung and Gideon M. Hirschfield

11 IgG4-Related Hepato-Pancreato-Biliary Disease ... 223
Eoghan McNelis and Emma Culver

12 Hereditary Haemochromatosis................... 245
William J. H. Griffiths

13 Pregnancy and Liver Disease 261
Hamish M. Miller and Rachel H. Westbrook

14 The Orphan Liver Disease 287
Reenam Khan and Philip Newsome

15 Fontan-Associated Liver Disease (FALD) 307
Hera Asad, Tehreem P. Chaudhry, and Petra Jenkins

**16 Diagnosis and Management of Hepatocellular
Carcinoma** 327
Elizabeth Sweeney and Tim Cross

17 Liver Transplantation.......................... 355
Rohit Gupta and James O'Beirne

18 The Hepatological Curiosities................... 381
Charmaine Matthews and Tim Cross

Index.. 405

Contributors

Guruprasad P. Aithal, MB, BS, PhD, FRCP Nottingham Digestive Diseases Centre, School of Medicine, Queen's Medical Centre, University of Nottingham, Nottingham, UK

National Institute for Health Research (NIHR) Nottingham Biomedical Research Centre, Nottingham University Hospitals NHS Trust and the University of Nottingham, Nottingham, UK

Hera Asad Department of Gastroenterology and Hepatology, Royal Liverpool University Hospital, Liverpool, UK

Edmond Atallah Nottingham Digestive Diseases Centre, School of Medicine, Queen's Medical Centre, University of Nottingham, Nottingham, UK

National Institute for Health Research (NIHR) Nottingham Biomedical Research Centre, Nottingham University Hospitals NHS Trust and the University of Nottingham, Nottingham, UK

Varinder Athwal, MB, BS, MRCP, PhD Manchester University NHS Foundation Trust, Manchester, UK

Tehreem P. Chaudhry, MB, BS, BSc, MRCP Department of Gastroenterology and Hepatology, Royal Liverpool University Hospital, Liverpool, UK

Jeremy Cobbold, MA, MBBS, MRCP, PhD Department of Gastroenterology and Hepatology, Oxford University Hospitals NHS Foundation Trust, Oxford, UK

Tim Cross, BMedSci (hons), MD, FRCP Royal Liverpool University Hospital, Liverpool, UK

Emma Culver Experimental Medicine Division, Level 5, University of Oxford, John Radcliffe Hospital, Headington, UK

A. Dhar, PhD, MRCP Department of Hepatology, Imperial College London, London, UK

Upkar Gill Hepatologist, Immunobiology Centre QMUL, Blizard Institute, Barts and The London SMD, QMUL, London, UK

Ashish Goel Liver Unit, Queen Elizabeth Hospital Birmingham, University Hospitals Birmingham, Birmingham, UK

William J. H. Griffiths, PhD, FRCP Cambridge Liver Unit, Cambridge University Teaching Hospitals NHS Foundation Trust, Addenbrooke's Hospital, Cambridge, UK

Rohit Gupta Department of Hepatology, Sunshine Coast University Hospital, Birtinya, QLD, Australia

Navjyot Hansi Addenbrooke's Hospital, Cambridge, UK

Gideon M. Hirschfield, MA, MB, BChir, FRCP, PhD Division of Gastroenterology and Hepatology, Department of Medicine, Toronto Centre for Liver Disease, Toronto General Hospital, University Health Network, University of Toronto, Toronto, ON, Canada

Brian J. Hogan, BSc, MRCP, FEBTM, FFICM Institute of Liver Studies, King's College Hospital, London, UK

Petra Jenkins, MB, BS (Hons), MRCP Liverpool Heart and Chest Hospital, Liverpool, UK

Patrick Kennedy, MB BCh, BAO, BMedSci, MRCP, MD Translational Hepatology, Blizard Institute, Barts and The London SMD, QMUL, London, UK

Amardeep Khanna Liver Unit, Queen Elizabeth Hospital Birmingham, University Hospitals Birmingham, Birmingham, UK

David Koeckerling Medical Sciences Division, University of Oxford, Oxford, UK

Daniela Ladner, MD, MPH Northwestern University Transplant Outcomes Research Collaborative (NUTORC), Northwestern University Feinberg School of Medicine, Chicago, IL, USA

Kristel K. Leung Division of Gastroenterology and Hepatology, Department of Medicine, Toronto Centre for Liver Disease, University Health Network, University of Toronto, Toronto, ON, Canada

Loey Lung-Yi Mak Division of Gastroenterology & Hepatology, Blizard Institute, London, UK

Thomas Marjot Oxford Centre for Diabetes, Endocrinology and Metabolism, University of Oxford, Oxford, UK

Charmaine Matthews, MB ChB, MRCP(UK) Royal Liverpool University Hospital, Liverpool, UK

Eoghan McNelis Experimental Medicine Division, Level 5, University of Oxford, John Radcliffe Hospital, Headington, UK

Hamish M. Miller Sheila Sherlock Liver Centre, Royal Free Hospital, London, UK

R. Nathwani Department of Hepatology, Imperial College London, London, UK

Philip Newsome, PhD Institute of Biomedical Research, The Medical School, University of Birmingham, Birmingham, UK

James O'Beirne, MB, BS, MD, EDIC, FRCP, FRACP Department of Hepatology, Sunshine Coast University Hospital, Birtinya, QLD, Australia

Sydney Olson Northwestern University Transplant Outcomes Research Collaborative (NUTORC), Northwestern University Feinberg School of Medicine, Chicago, IL, USA

Gregory Packer Department of Critical Care Medicine, University Hospitals Birmingham, Birmingham, UK

Ioannis Papamargaritis Aintree University Hospital, Liverpool, UK

Martin Prince, MRCP, PhD Manchester University NHS Foundation Trust, Manchester, UK

N. Selvapatt Department of Hepatology, Imperial College London, London, UK

Osama Siddiqui Northwestern University Transplant Outcomes Research Collaborative (NUTORC), Northwestern University Feinberg School of Medicine, Chicago, IL, USA

Cyril Sieberhagen, MD, MRCP Aintree University Hospital, Liverpool, UK

Elizabeth Sweeney Royal Liverpool University Hospital, Liverpool, UK

Avesh Thuluvath, MD Northwestern University McGaw Medical Center, Chicago, IL, USA

Dhiraj Tripathi, MD, FRCP Liver Unit, Queen Elizabeth Hospital Birmingham, University Hospitals Birmingham, Birmingham, UK

Ruth Tunney North-West Deanery, Manchester, UK

Rachel H. Westbrook, PhD, MRCP Sheila Sherlock Liver Centre, Royal Free Hospital, London, UK

Chapter 1
Assessment of Liver Function

Ioannis Papamargaritis and Cyril Sieberhagen

Case Study

A 50-year-old man has been referred to the Liver Clinic by his GP following the discovery of a mildly elevated ALT on a routine blood test. The letter states that the patient "does not drink too much alcohol" and has "no obvious reason" to have deranged LFTs.

The blood tests done by his GP reveal:

Normal Full Blood Count and renal function.

Random blood glucose (8.5 mmol/L).

LFT's

Bilirubin 10 μmol/L (3–17 μmol/L).
Alanine aminotransferase (ALT) 115 IU/L (10–45 IU/L).
Alkaline phosphatase (ALP) 95 IU/L (30–105 IU/L).
Gamma glutamyl transpeptidase (GGT) 75 IU/L (15–40 IU/L).
Albumin 38 g/L (35–50 IU/L).
Prothrombin time 11.7 s (9–12.7 s).

I. Papamargaritis · C. Sieberhagen (✉)
Aintree University Hospital, Liverpool, UK
e-mail: i.papamargaritis1@nhs.net;
Cyril.sieberhagen@liverpoolft.nhs.uk

© Springer Nature Switzerland AG 2022   1
T. Cross (ed.), *Liver Disease in Clinical Practice*, In Clinical Practice, https://doi.org/10.1007/978-3-031-10012-3_1

Questions
1. Would you like any more information from the referral?
2. What is the differential diagnosis?
3. What additional tests should be done?
4. Which invasive and non-invasive investigations are you aware of to aid prognosis and guide subsequent management of liver disease?

An Overview of Anatomy and Functions of the Liver

The liver is the largest solid organ in the body weighing approximately 1600 grams in men and 1400 grams in women. It lies in the right upper quadrant of the abdomen with its upper border between the fifth and sixth ribs and its lower border along the right costal margin. 75% of hepatic blood flow is delivered by the portal vein while the hepatic artery provides 25% [1].

The liver is important in a wide variety of metabolic and immunological functions.

Metabolic

The liver is a central hub for carbohydrate, protein and lipid metabolism. It is responsible for glycogenolysis and gluconeogenesis and maintains plasma glucose levels via this pathway. Glucose homeostasis is reliant on the relative concentration of insulin and glucagon [1, 2].

The liver has diverse functions pertaining to protein metabolism including synthesis and degradation of amino acids and proteins including albumin, globulin and clotting factors. The production of ammonia from the deamination of amino acids and subsequent conversion to urea also happens almost exclusively in the liver, although there is some contribution from skeletal muscle [1, 2].

Cholesterol degradation and excretion is dependent on the liver. It performs lipogenesis; triglyceride production and the bulk of lipoproteins are synthesized in the liver. Bile production enables fat emulsification and absorption of fat soluble vitamins such as Vitamin A, D, E and K from the diet [2].

Immunologic

The liver is an important immunological site and acts as a sieve for vast amounts of pathogenic substances travelling via the portal vein from the intestine. Kupffer cells in the hepatic sinusoids have roles in phagocytosis, cytokine and chemokine release and activation of the hepatic stellate cells. Intrahepatic populations of lymphocytes, natural killer cells and dendritic cells also form part of the liver's defence mechanism [2].

Common Risk Factors for Deranged Liver Enzyme Tests

Alcohol

Assessment of alcohol intake is vital when considering causes for deranged liver function tests. This is done with open questions; but it is important to quantify the amount of alcohol consumed in units. Current UK guidelines set the maximum alcohol consumption at no more than 14 units per week for both men and women. A quick and easy guide to remember units:

1 unit: 1 single shot of spirits
1.5 units: 1 small glass of wine (125 mL)
2 units: 1 can of beer/lager/ale/cider or 1 medium glass of wine (175 mL)
3 units: 1 pint of beer/lager/ale/cider or 1 large glass of wine (250 mL)
9 units: 1 bottle of wine.

Metabolic Factors

Non-alcoholic fatty liver disease is on the rise and will soon be the most common cause for deranged liver enzymes. Metabolic risk factors including obesity, Type 2 Diabetes Mellitus, dyslipidaemia and hypertension should be taken into account when trying to identify the underlying cause for abnormal liver function test results.

Risk Factors for Viral Hepatitis

Always consider risk factors for viral hepatitis when investigating deranged liver function tests. These include:

Hepatitis A: Acquired through faecal-oral spread through contaminated food or water. Self-limiting illness and a vaccine is available.

Hepatitis B: Acquired through blood to blood contact, often through sexual contact, contaminated needles and perinatal transfer. Majority of infections will resolve spontaneously, but approximate 15% will acquire chronic infection. Vaccination is available.

Hepatitis C: Acquired through blood to blood contact, most often through injection drug use through contaminated needles, but can also be acquired less commonly through sexual contact and perinatal transfer. No vaccination available, but effective treatment results in cure.

Hepatitis D: Acquired as a superadded infection in the context of active Hepatitis B infection.

Hepatitis E: Acquired through faecal-oral spread through contaminated water. Can also be acquired via zoonotic spread especially undercooked pork products. Usually self-limiting, but can develop chronic disease in the immunosuppressed. No vaccine available.

Drug-Induced Liver Injury

Almost all available medications can cause a degree of liver enzymes derangement. New or recent medication along with the full list of patient's medications should be included in the history taking, paying specific attention to any antibiotic use in the previous 2–3 months.

Interpretation of Liver Function Tests

As the liver is a multifunctional organ, with an extensive amount of reserve and ability to regenerate, clinical features may not manifest until the liver is near the end-stage of the spectrum of severity. The term liver function tests (LFTs) includes tests of:

- synthetic function (albumin, prothrombin time),
- excretory function (bilirubin),
- underlying necroinflammation (serum aminotransferases: ALT and aspartate aminotransferase (AST)) and,
- cholestasis (ALP, GGT).

The interpretation of abnormal LFTs requires a systematic approach with regards to:

- Taking a complete history including family history and eliciting the relevant physical signs and risk factors.
- Recognizing the pattern of LFT abnormality (i.e. impaired synthetic function, hepatocellular injury – "hepatitic picture", cholestasis or a mixed picture).
- An awareness of the duration and severity of elevation of LFT abnormalities.

Initial Approach to Potential Liver Disease

According to the recently published British Society of Gastroenterology (BSG) guidance, the initial investigation of potential liver disease should include bilirubin, albumin, ALT, ALP, gGT and FBC if not performed in the last 12 months.

A strategy of simply repeating abnormal tests can only be justified where there is a high degree of certainty that the abnormality will resolve in response to an identified acute insult. In other cases, detection of the first abnormality should trigger investigation of the aetiology or repeat testing to assess progression or disease severity where there is a suspicion that the underlying cause may require urgent referral/admission.

Parenchymal Liver Screen

An **abdominal US** should be performed in all cases where the diagnosis is unclear in order to investigate the liver parenchyma in detail and exclude any obstructive causes.

"Full liver screen" is a loose term to describe a set of serum-based investigations to elucidate a cause of abnormal LFT's in the context of suspected chronic liver disease.

It consists of the following (Table 1.1):

TABLE 1.1 A typical "full liver screen"

Disease	Test
Chronic hepatitis B	Hepatitis B surface antigen
Chronic hepatitis C	Hepatitis C antibody Hepatitis C RNA (if antibody positive)
Autoimmune hepatitis	Anti-smooth muscle antibody Anti-nuclear antibody Anti-liver kidney microsomal antibody Immunoglobulin G
Primary biliary cholangitis	Antimitochondrial antibody Immunoglobulin M
Haemochromatosis	Ferritin Transferrin saturation (>45%) HFE genotype
Wilson's disease	Caeruloplasmin (normally low)
Alpha-1 antitrypsin deficiency	Alpha-1 antitrypsin level and phenotype (if level low)
Coeliac disease	Anti-TTG or Anti-endomysial antibody (if low IgA)

Tests of Hepatocellular Damage

Serum Aminotransferases (ALT and AST) [3, 4]

Alanine aminotransferase (ALT) and aspartate aminotransferase (AST) are intracellular enzymes that are released into plasma during hepatocellular injury and are used as a marker of hepatic inflammation or necrosis.

ALT is a liver specific enzyme located in the cytosol of hepatocytes. Persisting abnormality in ALT should encourage the clinician to seek a cause.

AST is in the liver cytosol and mitochondria, but also in cardiac and skeletal muscle, kidney, brain and pancreas. It is, therefore, less specific than ALT as damage to any of these organs result in a rise.

An elevated AST to ALT ratio, especially if AST is more than twice that of ALT, may signify alcohol related liver disease (ALD) [5] (about 70% of patients with ALD have a ratio > 2). In Non-alcoholic fatty liver disease (NAFLD) an AST/ALT ≥0.8 is thought to signify significant liver fibrosis (Ishak stage 3/6).

Table 1.2 summarizes the wide differential diagnosis of elevated serum aminotransferases and Fig. 1.1 suggests a diagnostic algorithm.

Alkaline Phosphatase (ALP)

ALP is an enzyme that is present in the liver, bone, intestine and placenta. Levels can rise if there is damage to any of these tissues. It is usually elevated to at least four times the upper limit of normal in patients with cholestasis. A simultaneous rise in GGT is a very sensitive indicator of hepatobiliary disease. If still in doubt, serum electrophoresis can be used to determine the ALP isoenzyme, especially if more than one cause for ALP elevation is suspected. An elevation of ALP can indicate either intrahepatic or extrahepatic biliary disease, and patients would require an ultrasound to investigate the biliary tree.

TABLE 1.2 Causes of elevated serum transaminases.

Degree of elevation	Cause
Mild (<100 iu/L)	Non-alcoholic fatty liver disease (NAFLD)
	Alcohol consumption
	Chronic viral hepatitis B or C
	Haemochromatosis
	Coeliac disease
	Non-hepatic (thyroid disease, haemolysis, myopathy, strenuous exercise) (AST elevation)
Moderate (100–350 iu/L)	As above, plus
	Alcoholic hepatitis
	Autoimmune hepatitis
	Acute biliary obstruction
	Budd-Chiari syndrome
	Wilson's disease
Major (>1000 iu/L)	Paracetamol poisoning
	Acute viral hepatitis
	Autoimmune hepatitis
	Ischaemic hepatitis
	Budd-Chiari syndrome

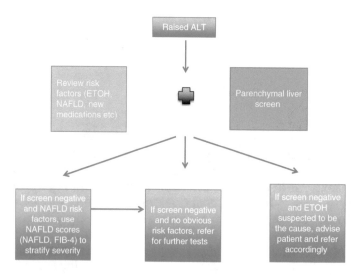

FIGURE 1.1 Diagnostic algorithm for elevated serum aminotransferases [6]

TABLE 1.3 Causes of elevated alkaline phosphatase in liver disease

Degree of elevation	Cause
Minor (<3× ULN)	All types of liver disease (hepatitis, cirrhosis, infiltrative diseases, sepsis, congestive cardiac failure)
Major (>3× ULN)	Biliary obstruction due to stones, pancreatic cancer, cholangiocarcinoma
	Liver malignancy/metastases
	Primary sclerosing cholangitis
	Primary biliary cholangitis
	Sepsis
	Cholestatic drug-induced liver injury (DILI)
	Sarcoidosis, amyloidosis

An isolated ALP elevation requires consideration of other conditions such as bone disorders, which include osteomalacia, Paget disease of the bone and bone metastases.

Low levels of ALP may occur in Wilson's disease and hypothyroidism. Table 1.3 shows causes of elevations in ALP and Fig. 1.2 proposes a diagnostic algorithm.

Isolated GGT Elevation

Apart from being a useful diagnostic marker for hepatobiliary diseases in association with ALP, GGT on its own can be elevated in many other conditions such as alcoholism, myocardial infarction, chronic obstructive pulmonary disease, renal failure, diabetes, obesity and pancreatic disease and is therefore often non-specific, thus investigation of an isolated GGT is not recommended.

Bilirubin

Understanding the physiology of bilirubin production and excretion within the digestive system is the key to recognizing the patterns of elevation.

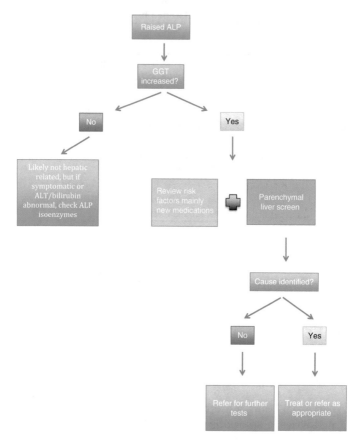

FIGURE 1.2 Diagnostic algorithm for elevated ALP [6]

Bilirubin is formed when haemoglobin is broken down within the reticulo-endothelial system in the liver, spleen and bone marrow. It is transported to the liver bound to albumin where it is conjugated into a water-soluble form. Conjugation facilitates its excretion into bile. Bile is then excreted via the common bile duct into the small bowel where it is reduced by gut bacteria into urobilinogen. Enterohepatic circulation enables reabsorption of the urobilinogen back into bile whilst a small proportion is excreted into urine and stool as stercobilinogen, giving stool its usual brown colour.

Hyperbilirubinaemia can either be predominantly uncon-jugated or conjugated. This measurement is most useful in determining at which level of bilirubin metabolism the pathology occurs. Unconjugated hyperbilirubinaemia is most commonly due to haemolysis and ineffective erythropoiesis whilst conjugated hyperbilirubinaemia usually reflects under-lying parenchymal liver disease or biliary obstruction (Table 1.4, Fig. 1.3).

TABLE 1.4 Causes of hyperbilirubinaemia [7]

Unconjugated	Conjugated
Increased bilirubin production • Haemolysis • Ineffective erythropoiesis (G6PD, thalassaemia, sickle cell disease) • Blood transfusion • Haematoma	Hepatocellular diseases • Viral hepatitis • Chronic autoimmune hepatitis • DILI • Alcoholic hepatitis • PBC • PSC
Hereditary disorders (impaired hepatic uptake or conjugation of bilirubin) • Gilbert syndrome (most common) • Criggler-Najjar syndrome	Infiltrative diseases • Tumours (primary, metastatic) • Infections (tuberculosis, parasites) Hereditary disorders • Dubin-Johnson syndrome • Rotor syndrome
Drugs • Rifampicin • Probenecid	Extrahepatic biliary obstructive disease • Cholangiocarcinoma • Pancreatic disease (cysts, carcinoma, chronic pancreatitis) • Cholecystitis • Choledocholithiasis Drugs • Allopurinol • Phenytoin • Anabolic steroids • Statins • Chlorpromazine • Herbal medications Sepsis Parenteral nutrition

Abbreviations: *DILI* drug-induced liver injury, *PBC* primary biliary cholangitis, *PSC* primary sclerosing cholangitis, *G6PD* Glucose-6-phosphate isomerase deficiency

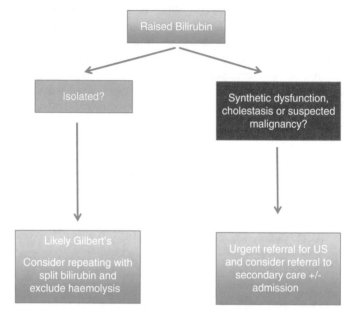

FIGURE 1.3 Algorithm for elevated bilirubin [6]

Test of Liver Synthetic Function

Prothrombin Time

The liver plays a significant role in haemostasis through production of coagulation factors (factor II, VII, IX, X), which are vitamin K dependent. Fat soluble vitamin K is dependent on bile salts for absorption. Conditions resulting in a reduction of bile salt production/excretion may therefore result in a prolongation of the prothrombin time. Administration of intravenous vitamin K will distinguish between true synthetic dysfunction and Vitamin K deficiency, resulting in correction of the PT in vitamin K deficiency and no effect in synthetic dysfunction.

The use of international normalized ratio (INR) minimizes variability in reporting of PT across different laboratories.

Albumin

Albumin is one of the major products of the liver. Hypoalbuminaemia in the context of liver disease suggest impaired synthetic function and provides information on prognosis. Due to its long half-life (17–30 days), low levels usually indicate chronic rather than acute liver dysfunction [8].

Causes of hypoalbuminaemia:

1. Decreased synthesis—severe liver disease, malnutrition, acute phase reaction, e.g., sepsis, surgery.
2. Plasma expansion—ascites, oedema.
3. Body losses—burns, protein losing enteropathy, nephrotic syndrome.
4. Increased catabolism—alcohol, malignancy, pregnancy.

Platelets

Thrombocytopaenia is quite common in chronic liver disease and is an indicator of advanced disease. The usual mechanisms are: decreased production, splenic sequestration and increased destruction. Decreased production is caused by bone marrow suppression (alcohol, iron overload, drugs) and by a reduction in thrombopoietin levels. Splenomegaly (as caused by portal hypertension in advanced liver injury) causes splenic sequestration. Platelet destruction is increased non-specifically in liver cirrhosis because of shear stress and fibrinolysis whereas in specific causes of autoimmune liver disease, immunologically mediated destruction of platelets occurs owing to antiplatelet immunoglobulin.

Liver Fibrosis

Chronic liver disease results in the development of fibrosis which subsequently progresses to cirrhosis. Cirrhosis may be complicated by portal hypertension, liver parenchymal failure and hepatocellular carcinoma. Although liver fibrosis was originally thought to be irreversible, there is now evidence that in certain disease processes it may be a dynamic process with the potential of significant regression [9].

Liver biopsy has historically been the gold standard for grading and assessing progression of liver fibrosis. Biopsy remains a useful way of assessing fibrosis, inflammation and also in identifying a second pathology where uncertainty exists with regards to the primary diagnosis. There are, however, significant limitations with liver biopsy being an invasive procedure with complications, sampling error given heterogenicity of the organ and inter-observer variability [10, 11].

Non-invasive methods of assessing liver fibrosis have now become popular including serological and radiological methods of assessment.

Serological testing has the advantage of high applicability and inter-laboratory reproducibility but is limited due to lack of liver specificity and so results can be influenced by other factors such patient co-morbidities. However, the use of FIB-4 or NAFLD fibrosis score, or ELF testing when NAFLD is suspected should be first line investigation in primary care. Depending on the results, a referral for elastography should be considered.

Radiological methods, such as transient elastography are becoming the modality of choice to ascertain the degree of fibrosis. It is quick, cost effective and reproducible and examines a significantly larger mass of liver tissue compared to liver biopsy. Interpretation of results should always take into account patient demographics, disease aetiology and laboratory parameters. The applicability however is limited in obese patients and has been shown to produce unreliable results. It can also not be performed in patients with ascites. Cholestasis, acute hepatitis, congestive cardiac failure, food and alcohol intake can increase liver stiffness and results need to be interpreted with caution in these circumstances [10–12].

Special Circumstances: Pregnancy [6]

Pregnancy results in a hyperdynamic circulation state, which has some similarities to the hyperdynamic state present in patients with decompensated chronic liver disease. On physical examination of a pregnant woman, it is not uncommon to see palmar erythema or multiple spider naevi.

There are also some physiological changes in LFTs which are given in Table 1.5. ALP is raised in third trimester due to placental production and foetal bone development. Alpha-fetoprotein (AFP) can also be raised as it is produced by the foetal liver.

TABLE 1.5 Physiological changes in blood markers during pregnancy

Blood marker	First trimester	Second trimester	Third trimester
ALT/AST	No change	No change	No change
Bilirubin	No change	No change	No change
ALP	No change	No change or increased	Increased up to fourfold
gGT	No change	No change	No change
Albumin	Decreased	Decreased	Decreased
Prothrombin time	No change	No change	No change
Platelets	No change	No change	No change

Answer to Question 1: History Clarification
The past medical history of the patient includes type 2 diabetes and hypertension. He is taking Metformin 500 mg BD and Amlodipine 5 mg OD. He has not had any over the counter medication, herbal remedies or new medications prescribed by the GP. He lives with his long-term partner, has not travelled abroad and does not have any tattoos. He has never had a blood transfusion in the past or injected drugs intravenously. He drinks a bottle of wine per week and denies drinking more than that in the past. His BMI is 31 kg/m^2.

Examination reveals an obese but otherwise well patient with no signs of chronic liver disease, no palpable hepatosplenomegaly and no evidence of decompensation, e.g. Jaundice, ascites, encephalopathy or bleeding.

Answer to Question 2
The differential diagnosis in this patient would include:

- Non-alcoholic fatty liver disease (NAFLD).
- Autoimmune hepatitis.
- Haemochromatosis.
- Chronic viral hepatitis (B or C).

He is at risk of NAFLD because he has diabetes, hypertension and an elevated BMI. The ALT and GGT are usually raised in NAFLD, although an elevation in ALP can also be seen. Ultrasound of the liver would reveal a fatty liver and features of portal hypertension (e.g. large spleen, ascites and reduced portal vein flow <20 cm/sec) may be present in the presence of cirrhosis.

Answer to Question 3
It is important to exclude other liver disorders before a diagnosis of NAFLD is made. The parenchymal liver screen is a fundamental component in the diagnostic approach. In this patient, his liver screen was unremarkable. Given the metabolic risk factors and negative parenchymal liver screen, the likely diagnosis is NAFLD. Assessment of any liver fibrosis would be important, ideally using non-invasive tests.

Answer to Question 4

Assessment of the presence of liver fibrosis has significant prognostic implications. Liver biopsy is an invasive option which provides valuable information, however, does have limitations.

Non-invasive options include:

Serological markers - This can be divided into direct and indirect biomarkers. Examples of indirect markers include the AST to platelet ratio index (APRI), FIB-4 score and NAFLD fibrosis score. Indirect markers available include procollagen type III amino-terminal peptide (PIIINP) and serum hyaluronic acid [10, 11].

Radiological markers - Transient elastography is an established tool to assess liver fibrosis non-invasively. It is applicable in a wide range of aetiologies and guides further management and informs the need to proceed to liver biopsy where appropriate.

References

1. Tortora GJ, Derrickson BH. Principles of anatomy and physiology. 12th ed. Hoboken: Wiley; 2008.
2. Nash K, Guha IN. Basic science. In: Hepatology: clinical cases uncovered. 1st ed. New York, NY: Wiley-Blackwell; 2011.
3. Dufour DR, Lott JA, Nolte FS, Gretch DR, Koff RS, Seeff LB. Diagnosis and monitoring of hepatic injury. II. Recommendations for use of laboratory tests in screening, diagnosis, and monitoring. Clin Chem. 2000;46(12):2050–68.
4. Limdi JK, Hyde GM. Evaluation of abnormal liver function tests. Postgrad Med J. 2003;79(932):307–12.
5. Cohen JA, Kaplan MM. The SGOT/SGPT ratio--an indicator of alcoholic liver disease. Dig Dis Sci. 1979;24(11):835–8.
6. Newsome PN, et al. Figure 1–3 adapted from Guidelines on the management of abnormal liver blood tests. Gut Jan. 2018;67(1):6–19.
7. Bloom S, et al. Table 4 adapted from Oxford Handbook of Gastroenterology and Hepatology. 2nd edition, December 2011.

8. Friedman LS, Keefe EB. Handbook of liver disease. 3rd ed. Philadelphia, PA: Elsevier Health Sciences; 2011.

9. Pellicoro A, Ramachandran P, Iredale JP. Reversibility of liver fibrosis. Fibrogenesis Tissue Repair. 2012;5(Suppl 1):S26.

10. Cui XW, Friedrich-Rust M, De Molo C, Ignee A, Schreiber-Dietrich D, Dietrich CF. Liver elastography, comments on EFSUMB elastography guidelines 2013. World J Gastroenterol. 2013;19(38):6329–47.

11. Ferraioli G, Filice C, Castera L, et al. WFUMB guidelines and recommendations for clinical use of ultrasound elastography: part 3: liver. Ultrasound Med Biol. 2015;41(5):1161–79.

12. Westbrook RH, Dusheiko G, Williamson C. Pregnancy and liver disease. J Hepatol. 2016;64(4):933–45. https://doi.org/10.1016/j.jhep.2015.11.030.

Chapter 2
Acute Liver Failure

Gregory Packer and Brian J. Hogan

Key Learning Points
- Recognition of the acute liver failure syndrome.
- Understanding of the role and limitations of prognostic criteria.
- Knowledge of initial resuscitative measures.
- Recognition of the common life-threatening complications specific to acute liver failure.
- Understanding of the specialist interventions available in a tertiary referral centre.

Chapter Review Questions

A 20-year-old female presents to her local Emergency Department having been found drowsy in her bedroom by a family member. Her mother states she is usually well and was last seen 2 days ago.

She looks very unwell. She has a Glasgow Coma Score of 8. Her saturations are 95% on air, she is tachypnoeic at 35 breaths per minute. She is tachycardic (140/min) and hypo-

G. Packer
Department of Critical Care Medicine, University Hospitals Birmingham, Birmingham, UK
e-mail: gregory.packer@uhb.nhs.uk

B. J. Hogan (✉)
Institute of Liver Studies, King's College Hospital, London, UK
e-mail: brianhogan@nhs.net

© Springer Nature Switzerland AG 2022   19
T. Cross (ed.), *Liver Disease in Clinical Practice*, In Clinical Practice, https://doi.org/10.1007/978-3-031-10012-3_2

tensive (90/30 mmHg). Her lactate is 12 mmol/L. Her blood glucose is 2 mmol/L.

She has an alanine aminotransferase (ALT) of 10,360 iU/L, a Bilirubin of 54 umol/L and an alkaline phosphatase (ALP) of 138 iU/L. Her white cell count is moderately elevated and her platelets slightly low at 90×10^9/L. Her international normalised ratio (INR) is 4.9.

The Emergency Department clinicians have called you, asking for medical input.

1. What is the most likely diagnosis?
2. What initial measures should be taken in the Emergency Department?
3. The ammonia level is reported as 230 umol/L, what is the resulting key concern and what measures can you take to mitigate this?

Introduction

Acute liver failure (ALF) is a clinical syndrome in which an acute insult provokes massive hepatocellular necrosis in the absence of pre-existing chronic liver disease.

ALF is characterised initially by jaundice, coagulopathy (INR > 1.5) and encephalopathy and can rapidly progress to a life-threatening multi-organ failure [1, 2].

Patients with a significant acute liver injury (a combination of jaundice and coagulopathy) should undergo regular assessment for deterioration or for the onset of hepatic encephalopathy.

Modern classifications are based upon time interval between development of jaundice and encephalopathy (Fig. 2.1) and give clues to likely causes and therefore prognosis (Table 2.1):

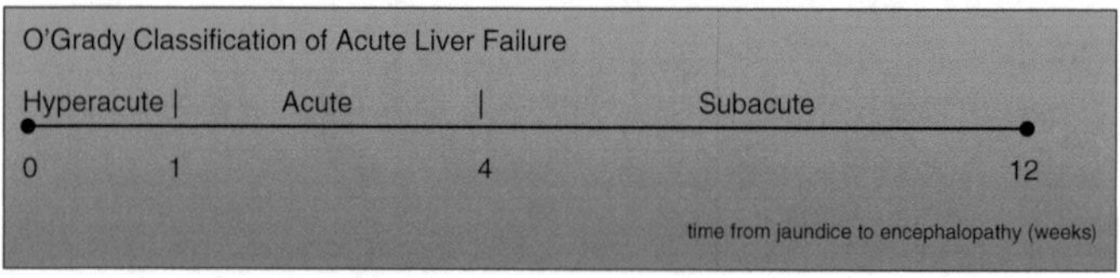

O'Grady Classification of Acute Liver Failure

Hyperacute | Acute | Subacute

0   1   4   12

time from jaundice to encephalopathy (weeks)

FIGURE 2.1 O'Grady classification as described by O'Grady et al. in 1993 [3]

TABLE 2.1 Summary of the more common causes of Acute Liver Failure

Cause		Presentation	Specific test(s)	Specific treatment(s)
Infectious/ Viral	Hepatotropic (A, B, D, E)	Hyperacute or Acute	Viral serology	Antivirals
	Nonhepatotropic (CMV, EBV, HSV1/2, VZV, dengue)	Viral prodrome		
Drugs	Paracetamol (acetaminophen)	Hyperacute	History, paracetamol levels	N-acetylcysteine
	Non-paracetamol (carbamazepine, cocaine, ecstasy, flucloxacillin, isoniazid, nitrofurantoin, sodium valproate, statins, Phenytoin, many others)	Hyperacute or acute	History, drug screen	Possible role for trial of corticosteroids
	Mushrooms (*Amanita phalloides*)	Diarrhoea	History, eosinophil count	Penicillin G
Cardiovascular	Ischaemic/hypoxic hepatitis	Hyperacute or acute	Clinical findings of shock, echocardiogram	Cardiovascular support
	Budd-Chiari syndrome	Acute or subacute	Imaging	TIPPS, revascularisation
	Portal venous thrombosis	Acute or subacute	Imaging	TIPPS, revascularisation

(continued)

TABLE 2.1 (continued)

Cause	Presentation	Specific test(s)	Specific treatment(s)
Autoimmune	Autoimmune hepatitis		Auto-antibodies and serum IgG levels	Possible role for trial of corticosteroids
Metabolic	Wilson's disease		Copper, caeruloplasmin, Kaiser-Fleischer rings, genetic testing	Chelation
Pregnancy-related	Acute fatty liver of pregnancy (AFLP) HELLP syndrome	Hyperacute or acute	Pregnancy test Imaging	Delivery
Others	Heat stroke Malignancy HLH Seronegative/indeterminate		Temperature Imaging/biopsy Ferritin, triglycerides, clinical scores	Cooling/rehydration Etoposide, dexamethasone, cyclosporine A

- Hyperacute liver failure is frequently caused by paracetamol or other drug toxicity and is the subtype with the highest rates of transplant free survival.
- Subacute liver failure is commonly associated with drug-induced liver injury or indeterminate (seronegative) hepatitis and generally has a worse prognosis.

Epidemiology

Acute liver failure is a rare syndrome, and the incidence and aetiologies vary globally, particularly between more and less economically developed countries:

- In more developed countries annual incidence is approximately 1–6 per million [4], the most common aetiology is paracetamol overdose and viral hepatitis is less common [5–7].
- In less developed countries annual incidence is higher (e.g. 63 per million in Thailand), viral hepatitis (particularly Hepatitis B) is the most common aetiology and paracetamol overdose is rarer [8].

There are a multitude of other potential rarer causes including inborn errors of metabolism.

Aetiology of ALF can be divided into:

- primary—due to direct liver-specific injury, e.g. viral hepatitis or paracetamol-overdose,
- secondary—due to systemic illness, e.g. hypoxic hepatitis or malignant infiltration.

Liver transplantation is only likely to be considered in primary aetiologies [1].

Prognosis

Prognosis in ALF has improved dramatically over the last 5 decades: approximately 75% of patients now surviving, and up to 60–72% without transplantation [5–7].

Likely reasons for this improvement are [1]:

- Improved living conditions in developing countries (reducing incidence of viral hepatitis).
- Public health interventions (e.g. some countries, including the UK, restrict the quantity of paracetamol that can be easily bought).
- Better recognition and initial management of ALF.
- More rapid referral and transfer to specialist centres.

Better survival outcomes without transplantation can paradoxically make decision-making about liver transplantation more difficult. Transplantation incurs major perioperative risks and the complications inherent in life-long immunosuppression. This is clearly better avoided if the patient will survive without transplantation [1]. There is also a societal cost to unnecessary transplantation, in that the donor liver will then be unavailable for another listed patient.

Prognostic criteria help identify those most at risk of death from ALF, and therefore those most likely to benefit from transplantation. The most widely used in UK clinical practice have historically been the Modified King's College Criteria (KCC) [9] (Table 2.2).

The specificity of the KCC is high, especially for paracetamol-induced ALF, at between 92 and 95%, however, the sensitivity is lower at 58–69% [10]. Put simply this means that if a patient meets the criteria they are highly likely to die without transplantation. However, rigidly applying the criteria alone risks transplanting a substantial group of patients who would survive without transplantation.

Some argue that better outcomes in ALF since the criteria were formulated mean they now lead to unnecessary trans-

TABLE 2.2 UK revised Criteria/Modified King's College Criteria for identifying a poor prognosis in ALF (currently used by the UK Organ Donor and Transplant Service, NHSBT) https://www.odt.nhs.uk/transplantation/liver/

Paracetamol-induced	Any of:
	• Arterial pH < 7.25 (despite 24 h of fluid resuscitation)
	• All three of:
	  – An international normalised ratio (INR) of greater than 6.5
	  – Serum creatinine of greater than 300 micromoles per litre
	  – Encephalopathy (of grade III or IV)
	• Serum lactate >4.0 mmol/L (despite 24 h of fluid resuscitation)

Non-paracetamol-induced	Favourable aetiologies (ecstasy/acute viral hepatitis) with encephalopathy: • INR > 6.5 (PT > 100S) or • Three of: INR > 3.5 (PT > 50S), age > 40 or < 10 years, bilirubin>300 µmol/L and J-E > 7 days Unfavourable aetiologies (idiosyncratic drug-induced, indeterminate) • INR >6.5, or • If hepatic encephalopathy is absent, then INR >2 and any two from the following: Age > 40 or < 10 years; INR >3.5 • If hepatic encephalopathy is present, then jaundice to encephalopathy time > 7 days; serum bilirubin >300 umol/L

plantation [11, 12]. In paracetamol-overdose in particular centres have recently reported 69% survival in those meeting the KCC [12].

For liver transplant listing in the UK Revised Criteria are now used. These more complex criteria better predict mortality than the KCC with a sensitivity of 92% and specificity of 80% [1, 12, 13].

Initial Resuscitation and Referral

Management of ALF is based upon rapid recognition of the syndrome, early resuscitation and commencement of appropriate organ support. Once the patient is initially stabilised, systematic investigations should be undertaken to diagnose or exclude likely causes.

N-acetylcysteine is highly effective in paracetamol-induced acute liver injury. Benefit may be seen in other aetiologies and its use is recommended in all aetiologies [1].

The potential severity of the organ failures seen in ALF mandates early and close collaboration between the initially admitting clinicians and local critical care services, and tertiary centre specialist hepatology, transplant surgery and specialist liver critical care teams.

Measures to avoid cerebral oedema with severely raised intracranial pressure and fatal brainstem herniation into the foramen magnum ("coning") must be considered early.

Patients with ALF can be expected to deteriorate rapidly so early liaison with specialist centres and critical care support with transfers (usually intubated) is highly recommended (Table 2.3).

TABLE 2.3 Initial Resuscitation in ALF

Initial assessments	Potential concerns	Initial actions
Airway	Inability to protect own airway (typically Glasgow coma score < 8)	Intubation
Breathing	Oxygen saturation < 94%	Supplemental oxygen
Circulation	Hypotension, clinical signs of shock, hyperlactataemia	Fluid resuscitation and advanced cardiovascular support

TABLE 2.3 (continued)

Initial assessments	Potential concerns	Initial actions
Disability	Hypoglycaemia Young patient Encephalopathy > grade 2 Hypercapnia	Supplemental parenteral glucose Early implementation of a neuroprotective strategy (see section below)
Exposure	Evidence of organ failure or encephalopathy Coagulopathy	Early broad-spectrum antibiotics and anti-fungal Consider an individualised strategy with point of care viscoelastic testing N-acetylcysteine infusion

Respiratory Support

Endotracheal intubation and invasive ventilation is required in high grade encephalopathy both to prevent aspiration and to maintain normocapnia as part of neuroprotection (alleviating the risk of hypercapnia-mediated cerebral vaso-dilation contributing to raised intracranial pressure).

As with other critically ill patients, those with ALF are at risk of developing pulmonary oedema, pneumonia and acute respiratory distress syndrome secondary to their multi-organ dysfunction and iatrogenic interventions [14].

Lung protective ventilation (with lower tidal volumes, higher positive end expiratory pressure [PEEP] and tolerance of hypercapnia) reduces the risk of ventilator-acquired lung injury but in ALF this must not be at the expense of neuroprotection (via hypercapnia or very high PEEP reducing cerebral venous drainage) [1, 15].

Cardiovascular Support

Fluid resuscitation is crucial in early management to restore circulating volume and adequate systemic perfusion. Resuscitation should be guided initially by close clinical assessment and the use of advanced haemodynamic monitoring is advisable.

Lactate as a prognostic marker in ALF is best considered once adequate fluid resuscitation has been completed [1]. Crystalloids (ideally buffered solutions) should be used [16]. Albumin containing solutions are commonly used but lack a convincing evidence base [17].

ALF typically progresses to a severe vasodilatory shock and, once hypovolaemia has been corrected, vasopressors are likely to be required. Noradrenaline is the mainstay vasopressor with vasopressin and steroids as potential adjuncts in refractory shock [18].

Neurological Support

Raised intracranial pressure (ICP) is now only seen in approximately 20% of patients with ALF. However once present mortality remains greater than 50% [1].

The likely pathological mechanism is a "dual hit":

- high blood ammonia leading to glutamine accumulation, astrocyte swelling and mitochondrial dysfunction,
- high levels of circulation inflammatory cytokines, as part of the severe systemic inflammatory response.

both leading to development of cerebral oedema.

The risk of severe intracranial hypertension is highest in:

- young patients (with little or no cerebral atrophy and so less space within the skull to accommodate cerebral oedema before intracranial hypertension occurs);
- hyperacute presentations;
- high grade encephalopathy;
- persistently elevated ammonia.

High arterial ammonia levels (>100 µmol/L) are associated with cerebral oedema and very high levels (>200 µmol/L) with spontaneous intracranial haemorrhage [19].

Invasive ICP monitoring is now rarely used in ALF in the UK as severe intracranial hypertension has become less common. Invasive ICP monitors are associated with a risk of iatrogenic intracranial haemorrhage (up to 4.2%) [1]. Reverse jugular venous catheters and transcranial doppler offer potential less invasive alternatives.

Neuroprotective measures should be instituted as standard in critically ill patients with ALF, especially in high risk subgroups:

- *Hypertonic sodium infusion (30% NaCl) to maintain serum sodium 145–150 mmol/L* (to limit osmotic shifts into the brain worsening cerebral oedema).
- *Early continuous renal replacement therapy to reduce ammonia < 100micromol/L* (with ultrafiltration rate up-titrated to achieve effective clearance [20]).
- Deep sedation.
- Minimise non-essential nursing interventions.
- Maintenance of normothermia/avoidance of hyperthermia.
- Head of bed elevation to 30°.
- Maintenance of normoxia.
- Maintenance of normocapnia.
- Maintenance of mean arterial pressure to achieve cerebral perfusion pressure 55–60 mmHg.
- Maintenance of normoglycaemia.

Coagulopathy Management

The apparent coagulopathy seen in ALF—prolonged prothrombin time—is often not reflected by impaired functional testing or in a greater likelihood of clinically significant bleeding [21]. ALF patients have a complex coagulation picture: most have a "balanced coagulopathy" with reduced pro- and anti-coagulant factors; some are even pro-thrombotic.

Thrombocytopaenia and low fibrinogen levels are generally a better marker of bleeding risk than prothrombin time [1].

Key points in managing apparent coagulopathy are:

- Do not administer FFP for perceived bleeding risk alone or for minor procedures (e.g. central line insertions).

    - This is clinically unnecessary and may confound prognostic criteria.

- Should major bleeding occur use functional testing if available (e.g. thromboelastography) to guide coagulopathy correction.
- Vitamin K should be administered, especially if poor nutrition is suspected—this will not confound prothrombin time abnormality due to acute liver failure.

Metabolic Support

Hypoglycaemia is a marker of severe ALF and requires close monitoring and intravenous correction. Low volume high concentration dextrose solutions are advisable to avoid cerebral oedema.

ALF is a highly catabolic state requiring careful attention to nutrition. Early nutrition specialist input and enteral feeding is therefore recommended [22]. In patients with high grade encephalopathy and high ammonia levels, protein administration may be restricted for 24–48 h to avoid elevating ammonia further.

Renal Support

Acute kidney injury requiring haemofiltration is common (>50%) in ALF and appears to reflect the degree of systemic illness. Early and continuous renal replacement therapy improves survival in hyperammonaemia and severe lactic acidosis [20].

Microbiological Considerations

Patients with ALF are relatively immunosuppressed and have very high risk of infection (historical rates of bacteraemia up to 80% and fungaemia 32%) [23]. Empirical treatment with broad-spectrum antibiotics and antifungals is recommended [24].

Liver Transplantation

The supportive measures outlined above are crucial and effective organ support may allow time for native liver regeneration to occur, particularly in hyperacute ALF. However, in the UK liver transplantation remains the definitive treatment for those meeting poor prognostic criteria and hence expected to die without transplantation. Internationally, as discussed in the Prognosis section, there is increasing interest in managing ALF (particularly paracetamol-induced) without transplantation [7, 12].

In the UK, liver transplantation only occurs in a small number of specialist centres with donor organs allocated via a national system. Transplantation decision-making occurs in a collaborative manner with surgical, hepatology, anaesthetic and critical care input and, in difficult cases, discussion amongst specialist centres.

Decisions around transplantation are multifactorial: the UKRC help identify those unlikely to survive without transplantation but donor livers are a scarce resource and an assessment must also be made of the patient's medical comorbidities, physiological reserve and ability to comply with the demands of life-long immunosuppression and medical follow-up. It is possible for an individual with severe psychiatric comorbidities, active intravenous drug use or similar concerns to be considered inappropriate for transplantation, even in ALF [13].

5-year survival rates for patients transplanted in the UK for ALF are 84% Survival worsens with older age (particularly >65 years) and greater severity of multi-organ failure prior to transplantation.

Early recognition and listing of patients for transplantation is vital as they can be expected to become more physiologically unstable with time. In rare cases it may even be decided to perform a total hepatectomy (to remove the inflammatory drive of having a large amount of necrotic hepatic tissue) whilst awaiting organ availability as a temporary last ditch stabilising measure.

Plasma Exchange

Plasma exchange (or plasmapheresis) is the removal of the patient's plasma and replacement with donor fresh frozen plasma. It removes many low and medium molecular weight molecules—specifically including pro-inflammatory cytokines. High volume plasma exchange refers to replacement of 15% of body weight with fresh frozen plasma.

A single RCT has demonstrated improved transplant-free survival, as well as improved haemodynamic and biochemical markers, compared to standard medical therapy only [25].

Extra-Corporeal Liver Support

Multiple extra-corporeal liver support (ECLS) systems have been trialled without evidence of benefit. The most promising device may be the molecular adsorbent recirculating system (MARS), which has been trialled as a bridging therapy to transplantation in ALF but without a survival benefit [26]. Whilst further systems are being developed and trialled currently ECLS remains a potential hope rather than a clinical option.

Clinical Pearls
1. ALF requires early recognition, early invasive organ support and early referral to a specialist centre.
2. Have a high suspicion for cerebral oedema, especially in younger people.

3. Early renal replacement therapy improves mortality and reduces risk of cerebral oedema.
4. Empirical antimicrobials should be started before evidence of infection.
5. Coagulopathy in ALF is complex – in the absence of major bleeding attempting correction with blood products is unnecessary and will confound prognostication.

Chapter Review Answers
1. This is acute liver failure. In the UK the most common aetiology is paracetamol overdose although other causes must also be considered and excluded.
2. Key early interventions include:

   (a) Consideration of intubation given her low GCS.
   (b) Fluid resuscitation and likely vasopressors.
   (c) Correction of hypoglycaemia.
   (d) Empirical N-acetylcysteine.
   (e) Empirical broad-spectrum antibiotics.
   (f) Referral to Intensive Care to facilitate the above.

3. The key concern in a young person with a high ammonia level and decreased consciousness is cerebral oedema. This is likely to become life-threatening unless aggressively controlled.

   Key interventions will include:

   (a) Invasive ventilation to avoid hypercapnia and maintain normoxia.
   (b) Early and continuous renal replacement therapy to clear ammonia.
   (c) Hypertonic saline to minimise fluid shifts into the brain.
   (d) Deep sedation/minimal touch nursing/keeping the bed head up 30 degrees.
   (e) Maintaining adequate cerebral perfusion pressure with vasopressors.
   (f) Early referral for specialist opinion, transfer and consideration of liver transplantation.

References

1. Jayalakshmi VT, Bernal W. Update on the management of acute liver failure. Curr Opin Crit Care. 2020;26(2):163–70. https://doi.org/10.1097/MCC.0000000000000697.
2. Trey C, Davidson CS. The management of fulminant hepatic failure. Prog Liver Dis. 1970;3:282–98.
3. O'Grady JG, Schalm SW, Williams R. Acute liver failure: redefining the syndromes. Lancet. 1993;342(8866):273–5.
4. Bower WA, Johns M, Margolis HS, Williams IT, Bell BP. Population-based surveillance for acute liver failure. Am J Gastroenterol. 2007;102(11):2459–63. https://doi.org/10.1111/j.1572-0241.2007.01388.x.
5. Bernal W, Hyyrylainen A, Gera A, et al. Lessons from lookback in acute liver failure? A single centre experience of 3300 patients. J Hepatol. 2013;59(1):74–80. https://doi.org/10.1016/j.jhep.2013.02.010.
6. Reuben A, Tillman H, Fontana RJ, et al. Outcomes in adults with acute liver failure between 1998 and 2013: an observational cohort study. Ann Intern Med. 2016;164(11):724–32. https://doi.org/10.7326/M15-2211.
7. Hey P, Hanrahan TP, Sinclair M, et al. Epidemiology and outcomes of acute liver failure in Australia. World J Hepatol. 2019;11(7):586–95. https://doi.org/10.4254/wjh.v11.i7.586.
8. Thanapirom K, Treeprasertsuk S, Soonthornworasiri N, et al. The incidence, etiologies, outcomes, and predictors of mortality of acute liver failure in Thailand: a population-base study. BMC Gastroenterol. 2019;19(1):18. https://doi.org/10.1186/s12876-019-0935-y.
9. Bernal W, Donaldson N, Wyncoll D, Wendon J. Blood lactate as an early predictor of outcome in paracetamol-induced acute liver failure: a cohort study. Lancet. 2002;359(9306):558–63. https://doi.org/10.1016/S0140-6736(02)07743-7.
10. O'Grady JG. Transplant in haste, repent at your leisure? Liver Transpl. 2015;21(5):570–1. https://doi.org/10.1002/lt.24124.
11. Gow PJ, Warrilow S, Lontos S, et al. Time to review the selection criteria for transplantation in paracetamol-induced fulminant hepatic failure? Liver Transpl. 2007;13(12):1762–3. https://doi.org/10.1002/lt.21301.
12. Porteous J, Cioccari L, Ancona P, et al. Outcome of acetaminophen-induced acute liver failure managed without intracranial pressure monitoring or transplantation. Liver Transpl. 2019;25(1):35–44. https://doi.org/10.1002/lt.25377.

13. Liver Advisory Group N. Liver transplantation: selection criteria and recipient registration policy pol 195/6. Zalewska A for liver advisory group on behalf of NHSBT 2017. www.odt.nhs.uk/pdf/liver_selection_policy.pdf. 2021

14. Baudouin SV, Howdle P, O'Grady JG, Webster NR. Acute lung injury in fulminant hepatic failure following paracetamol poisoning. Thorax. 1995;50(4):399–402.

15. Acute Respiratory Distress Syndrome Network, Brower RG, Matthay MA, et al. Ventilation with lower tidal volumes as compared with traditional tidal volumes for acute lung injury and the acute respiratory distress syndrome. N Engl J Med. 2000;342(18):1301–8. https://doi.org/10.1056/NEJM200005043421801.

16. Self WH, Semler MW, Wanderer JP, et al. Balanced crystalloids versus saline in noncritically ill adults. N Engl J Med. 2018;378(9):819–28. https://doi.org/10.1056/NEJMoa1711586.

17. Caironi P, Tognoni G, Masson S, et al. Albumin replacement in patients with severe sepsis or septic shock. N Engl J Med. 2014;370(15):1412–21. https://doi.org/10.1056/NEJMoa1305727.

18. Eefsen M, Dethloff T, Frederiksen HJ, Hauerberg J, Hansen BA, Larsen FS. Comparison of terlipressin and noradrenalin on cerebral perfusion, intracranial pressure and cerebral extracellular concentrations of lactate and pyruvate in patients with acute liver failure in need of inotropic support. J Hepatol. 2007;47(3):381–6. https://doi.org/10.1016/j.jhep.2007.04.015.

19. Bernal W, Hall C, Karvellas CJ, Auzinger G, Sizer E, Wendon J. Arterial ammonia and clinical risk factors for encephalopathy and intracranial hypertension in acute liver failure. Hepatology. 2007;46(6):1844–52. https://doi.org/10.1002/hep.21838.

20. Cardoso FS, Gottfried M, Tujios S, Olson JC, Karvellas CJ, US Acute Liver Failure Study Group. Continuous renal replacement therapy is associated with reduced serum ammonia levels and mortality in acute liver failure. Hepatology. 2018;67(2):711–20. https://doi.org/10.1002/hep.29488.

21. Habib M, Roberts LN, Patel RK, Wendon J, Bernal W, Arya R. Evidence of rebalanced coagulation in acute liver injury and acute liver failure as measured by thrombin generation. Liver Int. 2014;34(5):672–8. https://doi.org/10.1111/liv.12369.

22. Plauth M, Bernal W, Dasarathy S, et al. ESPEN guideline on clinical nutrition in liver disease. Clin Nutr. 2019;38(2):485–521. https://doi.org/10.1016/j.clnu.2018.12.022.

23. Karvellas CJ, Pink F, McPhail M, et al. Predictors of bacteraemia and mortality in patients with acute liver failure.

Intensive Care Med. 2009;35(8):1390–6. https://doi.org/10.1007/s00134-009-1472-x.

24. European Association for the Study of the Liver. Electronic address: easloffice@easloffice.eu, Clinical practice guidelines panel, Wendon J, et al. EASL Clinical Practical Guidelines on the management of acute (fulminant) liver failure. J Hepatol. 2017;66(5):1047–81. https://doi.org/10.1016/j.jhep.2016.12.003.

25. Larsen FS, Schmidt LE, Bernsmeier C, et al. High-volume plasma exchange in patients with acute liver failure: an open randomised controlled trial. J Hepatol. 2016;64(1):69–78. https://doi.org/10.1016/j.jhep.2015.08.018.

26. Saliba F, Camus C, Durand F, et al. Albumin dialysis with a noncell artificial liver support device in patients with acute liver failure: a randomized, controlled trial. Ann Intern Med. 2013;159(8):522–31. https://doi.org/10.7326/0003-4819-159-8-201310150-00005.

Chapter 3
Drug-Induced Liver Injury

Edmond Atallah and Guruprasad P. Aithal

Key Learning Points

1. Drug-induced liver injury should be considered in all presentations of acute liver injury as well as jaundice without evidence of biliary obstruction.
2. Liver biopsy and HLA genotyping can help clinical management by differentiating DILI from AIH and excluding DILI secondary to certain drugs.
3. High-quality evidence does not support empirical use of steroids to treat DILI unless in scenarios when auto-immune hepatitis cannot be excluded.
4. In cases of drug-induced AIH treated with corticosteroid therapy, withdrawal of immunosuppressive therapy does not lead to relapse of liver injury.

Chapter Review Questions

An 18-year-old male presents with jaundice. His medical history includes severe acne, for which he was treated with isotretinoin

E. Atallah · G. P. Aithal (✉)
Nottingham Digestive Diseases Centre, School of Medicine,
Queen's Medical Centre, University of Nottingham,
Nottingham, UK

National Institute for Health Research (NIHR) Nottingham
Biomedical Research Centre, Nottingham University Hospitals
NHS Trust and the University of Nottingham, Nottingham, UK
e-mail: Edmond.atallah@nottingham.ac.uk;
Guru.aithal@nottingham.ac.uk

© Springer Nature Switzerland AG 2022   37
T. Cross (ed.), *Liver Disease in Clinical Practice*, In Clinical
Practice, https://doi.org/10.1007/978-3-031-10012-3_3

(vitamin A) that was switched to minocycline 3 weeks ago due to lack of response. His liver profile showed alanine transaminase (ALT) 500 U/L, aspartate aminotransferase (AST) 300 U/L, alkaline phosphatase (ALP) 100 U/L, bilirubin 85 μmol/L, albumin 40 g/L, prothrombin time (PT) 12 s, antinuclear antibodies (ANA) positive (titre 1:400), smooth muscle antibodies (SMA) positive and immunoglobulin G (IgG) 18.3 g/L. An ultrasound abdomen was normal and his virology screen was negative.

Question 1 What is the most appropriate next step?

1. Monitor liver enzymes off minocycline.
2. Request a liver biopsy.
3. Request anti-soluble liver antigen (anti-SLA) antibodies.
4. Request genotyping for Wilson's disease.

Question 2 The patient underwent a liver biopsy which showed interface hepatitis with plasma cells and eosinophils. There was evidence of cholestasis with no established fibrosis. Based on the available evidence, what is the histological feature that favours DILI over idiopathic autoimmune hepatitis (AIH)?

1. Cholestasis canalicular.
2. Interface hepatitis.
3. Prominent portal plasma cells.
4. Prominent intra-acinar eosinophils.

Question 3 Following the liver biopsy, the patient was started on oral prednisolone 40 mg once daily, and minocycline was withheld. His liver enzymes improved, and his jaundice has resolved. However, his acne has flared. What will be the most appropriate next step in his management?

1. Restart his minocycline.
2. Start the patient on azathioprine.
3. Switch to oral budesonide.
4. Withdraw steroids with clinical follow-up.

Introduction and Epidemiology

- Idiosyncratic drug-induced liver injury (DILI) is an acute liver injury following exposure to a medication within the recommended dose range which is distinctive from liver injury caused by drug overdose, commonly associated with paracetamol.
- DILI usually occurs after a latency period that ranges from a few days to months post-exposure compared to a period from hours to days in liver injury due to overdose.
- It is the second most common reason for withdrawal of drugs from the market worldwide after licensing, accounting for 32% of drug withdrawals between 1975 and 2007 [1].
- From a prospective polulation-based study in Europe, its estimated crude incidence is 19 per 100,000 (95%CI, 15.4–23.3) [2]. Nonetheless, the incidence of DILI secondary to specific commonly used medications is significantly higher [2, 3]:

  – Amoxicillin-clavulanate (43 per 100,000; 95% CI 24–70).
  – Flucloxacillin (39 per 100,000; 95% CI 27–55).
  – Nitrofurantoin (73 per 100,000; 95% CI 20–187).
  – Infliximab (675 per 100,000; 95% CI 184–718).
  – Azathioprine (752 per 100,000; 95% CI, 205–1914).
  – Incidence may be higher in the elderly; DILI incidence in those aged >70 receiving consecutive prescriptions is 111 per 100,000 (95% CI, 71–164).

- DILI is a common cause of emergency admissions with jaundice after excluding biliary pathology. Following a large national audit in the UK of 881 consecutive patients admitted with jaundice, where a biliary obstruction was ruled out by imaging, idiosyncratic DILI was the second most common cause of liver injury (15% of cases) after alcoholic liver disease [4].

Risk Factors Associated with DILI

- Although idiosyncratic DILI is clearly distinguishable from overdose hepatotoxicity, serious DILI occurs more frequently with medications taken in a daily dose of >50–100 mg compared to lower doses with a significant association between daily dose and acute liver failure, live transplantation and death [1].
- Prolonged duration of exposure to certain medications (co-amoxiclav and flucloxacillin) has been associated with an increased risk of developing a liver injury.
- Multiple genetic risk factors have been associated with susceptibility to DILI. While candidate gene studies have demonstrated an association between allelic variants in genes coding for drug metabolising enzymes and transporters, DILI due to over 15 currently used drugs have been associated with human leukocyte system (HLA) alleles.

Pathogenesis

- Multiple concurrent and sequential actions are involved in the development of idiosyncratic DILI and determine the severity of the liver injury and its manifestations (Fig. 3.1).
- The main upstream events include drug-specific pathways induced by drugs or their metabolites. Multiple genetic and environmental factors influence the expression and activities of proteins involved in drug disposition and determine the formation of reactive metabolites that induce the production of excessive reactive oxygen species leading to lipid peroxidation and cellular death. Furthermore, dysregulation of the antioxidant pathways in the cells might promote exacerbation of DILI [1].
- Downstream events include an innate immune response that determines the progression and severity of DILI by promoting or inhibiting the inflammatory process.

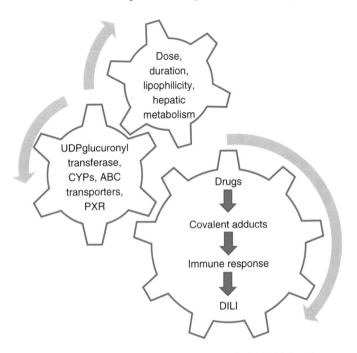

FIGURE 3.1 Risk factors and events associated with DILI pathogenesis. Abbreviations: *CYPs* cytochrome P450 enzymes, *UDP-glucuronosyltransferase* uridine diphospho glucuronosyltransferase, *PXR* pregnane xenobiotic-sensing receptor, *ABC* ATP-binding cassette family

• Adaptive immunity has been shown to have an important role in the pathogenesis of DILI. Drug metabolite adducts are recognised by the immune system through antigen-presenting cells in conjunction with major histocompatibility complex molecules (MHC). Multiple genome-wide association studies have demonstrated that the human leukocyte system (HLA) plays a significant role in increasing or decreasing susceptibility to DILI. HLA genotypes associated with DILI are thought to increase the specificity of the peptide-binding groove for the drug or drug-peptide complex, enhancing the presentation of these molecules as antigens to T-cells and causing immunological destruction of hepatocytes [1].

Case Definitions and Phenotypes of Idiosyncratic DILI

Thresholds to define DILI were defined in 2011 as follows:

1. More than or equal to five-fold elevation above the upper limit of normal (ULN) for ALT OR
2. More than or equal to two-fold elevation for ALP after ruling out a bone pathology OR
3. More than or equal to three-fold elevation in ALT and simultaneous elevation of bilirubin exceeding two-fold.

Patterns of DILI

The pattern of DILI is based on the earliest identified liver chemistry elevations (ALT and ALP in particular) above the upper limit of normality (ULN) that fit DILI criteria and defined using R-value where $R = (ALT/ULN)/(ALP/ULN)$. There are three patterns of DILI: hepatocellular ($R \geq 5$), cholestatic ($R \leq 2$) and mixed ($R > 2$ and < 5). Drugs associated with specific patterns and phenotypes are summarised in Table 3.1.

TABLE 3.1 Drugs associated with specific phenotypes of drug-induced liver disease

Phenotype	Drugs associated with phenotype
Acute hepatocellular pattern of DILI	• NSAIDs: diclofenac, naproxen, nimesulide, piroxicam • Anaesthetics: enflurane, halothane, isoflurane • Antimicrobials: ketoconazole, terbinafine, tetracyclines; anti-tuberculosis drugs such as isoniazid, pyrazinamide, rifampicin; anti-HIV agents such as didanosine, nevirapine, zidovudine • Neuropsychotropics: tricyclics (most), fluoxetine, paroxetine, sertraline; illegal compounds such as cocaine and ecstasy • Anti-epileptics: carbamazepine, phenytoin, valproate • Cardiovascular drugs: bezafibrate, captopril, enalapril, lisinopril, lovastatin, simvastatin, ticlopidine • Antineoplastics: cyclophosphamide, cisplatin, doxorubicin • Others: herbal remedies
Acute cholestatic pattern of DILI	• Hormonal preparations: androgens, anabolic steroids, oral contraceptives, tamoxifen • Antimicrobials: clindamycin, co-amoxiclav, co-trimoxazole, erythromycin, flucloxacillin, troleandomycin • Analgesics/anti-inflammatory drugs: gold salts, sulindac Neuropsychiatric drugs: carbamazepine, chlorpromazine, tricyclic antidepressants • Immunosuppressants: azathioprine, ciclosporin • Others: allopurinol

(continued)

TABLE 3.1 (continued)

Phenotype	Drugs associated with phenotype
Mixed pattern of DILI	Carbamazepine, lamotrigine, phenytoin and sulfonamides
Autoimmune hepatitis	Minocycline, nitrofurantoin, diclofenac, indometacin, statins, infliximab, halothane, herbal medicine (germander), methyldopa
Checkpoint inhibitor-induced liver injury (ChILI)	• Anti-CTLA-4: ipilimumab • Anti-PD-1: pembrolizumab, nivolumab • Anti-PD- L1: atezolizumab, avelumab, durvalumab
Drug reaction with eosinophilia and systemic symptoms (DRESS)	Allopurinol, carbamazepine, dapsone, lamotrigine, nevirapine, phenobarbitone, phenytoin and sulfonamide
Drug-associated fatty liver disease	Amiodarone, 5-fluorouracil, irinotecan, methotrexate, tamoxifen
Acute fatty liver (microvesicular steatosis)	Amiodarone, didanosine, stavudine
Nodular regenerative hyperplasia	Azathioprine, bleomycin, busulfan, oxaliplatin, 6-thioguanine
Vanishing bile duct (ductopenic) syndrome	Amoxicillin–clavulanate, azathioprine, carbamazepine, chlorpromazine, co-trimoxazole, erythromycin, flucloxacillin, phenytoin, terbinafine
Secondary sclerosing cholangitis	Amiodarone, amoxicillin–clavulanate, atorvastatin, infliximab, 6-mercaptopurine, venlafaxine
Hepatocellular adenoma or carcinoma	Contraceptive steroids, danazol and androgens

Hepatocellular DILI

- Acute hepatocellular DILI is the most common manifestation of DILI, with a remarkable increase of ALT alone or associated with a modest rise in ALP with R ≥ 5 [5, 6].
- Liver histology usually shows changes of non-specific acute hepatitis and eosinophilia may be seen; viral hepatitis is the main differential diagnosis. It is an important cause of acute liver failure, accounting for 10–15% of ALF cases in the USA and Europe [7, 8].

Cholestatic DILI

- It is characterised by an elevation in ALP and GGT levels and usually associated with symptoms of pruritus and jaundice, hence reduced quality of life.
- Liver histological features are bile duct injury and cholestasis in small bile canaliculi. In rare cases with prolonged jaundice and gradual loss of intrahepatic bile ducts, they progress to vanishing bile duct syndrome which may evolve to liver failure requiring liver transplant or death [9].
- Bland cholestasis is a distinctive phenotype characterised by prolonged jaundice with pruritis with minimal to moderate elevation of liver enzymes. It is typically caused by oestrogens and oral contraceptives in women and anabolic steroids in men. Liver biopsy usually illustrates bland cholestasis with minor inflammatory changes and hepatocellular necrosis. Despite its prolonged course, it usually has a good prognosis, rarely leading to liver failure or death [10].

Specific Phenotypes of DILI

Drug-Induced Autoimmune Hepatitis

- It is a clinically challenging phenotype that has been described following exposure to certain medications (for example, nitrofurantoin and minocycline) after a long latency period of up to 2 years [11].

- It has also been described with α-methyldopa, diclofenac, herbal supplements, infliximab, adalimumab and statins. It is associated with biochemical and/or histological features that are indistinguishable from AIH, including the presence of anti-nuclear antibodies, hyper-gammaglobulinemia and interface hepatitis with plasma cells on histology.

Checkpoint Inhibitor-Induced Liver Injury (ChILI)

- Hepatitis secondary to checkpoint inhibitors has emerged as a distinctive entity following the remarkable expansion of the therapeutic role of checkpoint inhibitors as treatment for several malignancies.
- Its incidence varies according to the treatment regimen, 1–4% in programmed cell death 1 inhibitor (anti-PD-1), 4–9% in cytotoxic T lymphocyte-associated protein 4 inhibitor (anti-CTLA-4) and 18% in patients treated with a combination of anti-PD-1 and anti-CTLA-4 [12].
- The pattern of liver injury is heterogeneous, with cholestatic liver injury being the least common.
- Histological characteristics of ChILI are different from DILI due to other drugs and AIH. Although there are no specific histological features of ChILI, some histological characteristics described include granulomas and central endotheliitis (caused by anti-CTL A-4 therapy) and lobular hepatitis (caused by anti- PD-1 or anti P.D.- L1 therapy) [11].

Causality Assessment

1. The Roussel Uclaf Causality Assessment Method (RUCAM) is the only validated scale and the most common diagnostic tool used in investigations related to DILI [13].
2. It is a scoring system based on multiple domains related to the pattern of DILI (hepatocellular versus cholestatic/mixed). The domains of assessment include:

(a) Time to onset of DILI from the beginning of the drug/herb.
(b) The course of DILI after cessation of the drug/herb.
(c) Risk factors (alcohol and age).
(d) Concomitant drug(s)/herb(s) in addition to suspected causative agent.
(e) Exclusion of alternative aetiology of liver injury.
(f) Previous reports of hepatotoxicity in relation to the suspected drug/herb.
(g) Response to (unintentional) re-exposure.

3. Total score and resulting causality grading: ≤ 0, excluded; 1–2, unlikely; 3–5, possible; 6–8, probable; and ≥ 9, highly probable.

4. RUCAM scale after clinical suspicion of DILI can standardise and support the assessment. However, blind application of this diagnostic tool is not sufficient to attribute causality and can lead to biased conclusions. Therefore, clinical judgement remains the mainstay of DILI diagnosis.

Severity of DILI

- DILI can progress to acute liver failure (ALF), accounting for 7–15% of total ALF cases [1].
- The degree of elevation of liver enzymes does not accurately reflect the severity of the liver injury or predict clinical outcome. However, elevated conjugated bilirubin indicates an adverse prognosis. Mortality/ liver transplant rates exceed 10% in DILI patients with hepatocellular injury and jaundice [5, 6].
- The outcome is worse when acute liver failure develops in DILI than that in paracetamol overdose. Patients developing features of acute liver failure (jaundice, encephalopathy, ascites and coagulopathy) should be referred urgently to a liver transplant centre.

Stepwise Approach to Clinical Diagnosis of DILI

- DILI can mimic any acute or chronic liver injury, and the first step of diagnosis is the physician's clinical suspicion in any liver injury following exposure to prescribed medication or over the counter medications, including herbal and dietary supplements.
- Determining the onset of liver injury after exposure (latency), course of reaction after withholding medication (de-challenge), recurrence on re-exposure (rechallenge), time to resolution and knowledge about the hepatotoxic potentials of the suspected drug are crucial to establishing a temporal relationship with the suspected agent.
- Time to onset of DILI differ significantly between drugs; although most DILI cases occur within 3 months of exposure to a drug, apparent clinical DILI can arise following a prolonged period of drug exposure or after cessation of the drugs as with amoxicillin-clavulanate and flucloxacillin [11].
- The exclusion of alternative diagnoses is crucial, as illustrated in the proposed algorithm (Fig. 3.2). Every patient with suspected DILI should have abdominal imaging to rule out biliary obstruction or focal lesions, a virology screen including hepatitis E (HEV RNA), EBV and CMV and an autoimmune screen. In patients with cancer or who are immunosuppressed, viral PCR need to be considered.

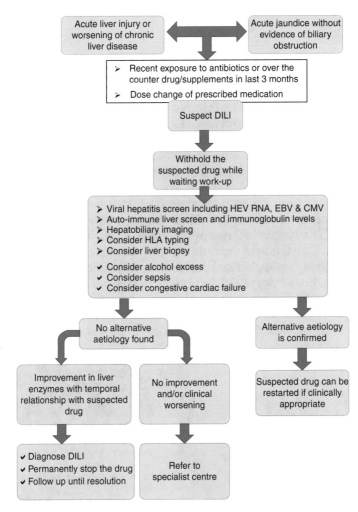

FIGURE 3.2 Proposed algorithm to suspect, diagnose and manage idiosyncratic drug-induced liver injury (DILI)

Role of Liver Biopsy

DILI can cause any pattern of liver pathology, although certain histological features are particularly suggestive of drug-induced aetiology. An evaluation of histological characteristics of idiopathic AIH and DILI revealed that eosinophilic infiltration, which is usually regarded as a feature of drug reaction, was not useful to differentiate both aetiologies and was more prominent in AIH [14]. In fact, the presence of canalicular cholestasis favoured DILI in all patterns of liver injuries, whereas rosette formation, portal plasma cells, severe portal inflammation and the presence of fibrosis favoured AIH. Moreover, some histological characteristics have been associated with clinical severity. The degree of necrosis, fibrosis stage, microvesicular steatosis, panacinar steatosis, cholangiolar cholestasis, ductular reaction, neutrophils and portal venopathy were all associated with the severity of DILI whereas the presence of granulomas and eosinophils were more likely to be present in milder cases [15]. Figures 3.3 and 3.4 illustrate portal and lobular changes in severe hepatocellular DILI secondary to zanubrutinib [16].

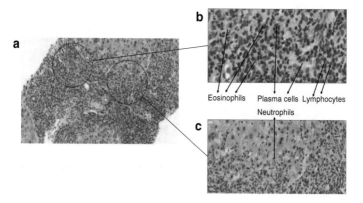

FIGURE 3.3 Histopathological changes of portal tracts in zanubrutinib-induced liver injury [16]. (**a**) Prominent portal and interface inflammation; (**b**) High-power imaging showing inflamed portal tracts with lymphocytes, plasma cells, neutrophils and eosinophils. (**c**) Inflammation at the interface with neutrophil infiltration

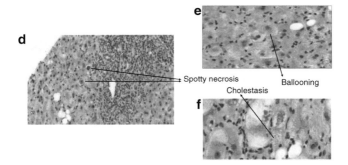

FIGURE 3.4 Histopathological changes of liver lobules in zanubrutinib-induced liver injury [16]. Lobular inflammation with spotty necrosis (**d**), ballooning (**e**) and cholestasis (**f**)

Hence, the benefits of a liver biopsy should be weighed against the risks and its limitations. Liver biopsy is justified when:

- Autoimmune hepatitis is one of the differential diagnoses in consideration.
- Incomplete or no biochemical resolution after discontinuation of the drug.
- Atypical clinical/laboratory features.
- Liver injury related to checkpoint inhibitors to inform specific treatment.

Role of Pharmacogenetic Testing

- Performance characteristics of HLA alleles as a diagnostic test in patients with DILI are comparable to those of auto-antibodies and immunoglobulin profiles that are routinely performed in clinical practice for cases with acute liver injury [17].
- Pharmacogenetic testing might be helpful in the following clinical scenarios:

- **HLA- DRB1*0301** or **DRB1*0401** could be an adjunct in the differential diagnosis of DILI versus AIH; international AIH diagnostic criteria attributes additional scores for carriage of one of these alleles.
- **HLA-B*5701** allele increases the risk of DILI following exposure to flucloxacillin 80-fold. 85% of those who develop DILI carry HLA-B*5701 compared to 6% of the general population. In clinical practice, this can be used to support the diagnosis as well as to rule out flucloxacillin-induced DILI with a negative predive value over 95% in challenging cases where DILI is one of the differential diagnoses [1].
- **HLA-DRB1*1501** can help the clinical management of acute liver injury cases with recent exposure to amoxicillin/clavulanate to differentiate DILI from seronegative hepatitis by providing supportive (though not conclusive) evidence for the diagnosis of DILI.

Management

- The most critical step is timely recognition of liver injury and withdrawal of the suspected drug. In most cases, DILI improves after the withdrawal of the culprit drug.
- Empirical treatment with corticosteroids is not advisable, except when DILI with autoimmune features cannot be confidently differentiated from AIH. Checkpoint inhibitor-induced liver injury has been widely treated with steroids. This is based on the obvious assumption that immune mechanisms underlie its pathogenesis. However, there is emerging evidence that indicates that the liver injury in subgroups of these patients resolves without immunosuppression. On the other hand, there is no high-quality evidence to support a specific dose or regimen of immunosuppression so far [18].
- In the event that steroids are initiated when distinguishing between DILI and AIH is unclear, withdrawing

immunosuppression once the injury completely resolves should be considered. Seventy per cent or more of patients with idiopathic AIH relapse over the 4-year follow-up without immunosuppression [19].

- Rechallenge of medications adjudicated as causative agent is not recommended, with 30% of cases developing recurrent DILI, which is associated with jaundice in 64%, hospitalisation in 52% and deaths in 13% of cases [20]. However, in certain cases, such as with the first-line anti-tuberculosis treatment regime, reintroduction of drugs after DILI has resolved are justified as the benefits of reintroduction outweigh the risks [1].

Chapter Review Answers

Question 1. What is the most appropriate next step?
1. Monitor liver enzymes off minocycline.
2. **Request a liver biopsy.**
3. Request anti-soluble liver antigen (anti-SLA) antibodies.
4. Request genotyping for Wilson's disease.

Answer
- The correct answer is option 2. The patient developed an acute liver injury with jaundice three weeks after starting minocycline, so drug-induced liver injury should be suspected, and the drug should be withheld as the first step. However, the differential diagnoses include AIH; therefore, a liver biopsy is indicated. Withdrawal of minocycline is an essential step, but just monitoring of liver enzymes may delay treatment (if it were to be AIH) and be misleading as AIH is known to have marked fluctuation and may appear to resolve, leading to presumption of DILI. Anti-SLA antibodies are positive in a small minority of patients with AIH, and this test is indicated when seronegative AIH is suspected. Wilson's disease can present acutely, but in this patient, serological markers are suggestive of acute immune mediated liver injury, so Wilson's disease genotyping is not necessary.

Question 2. The patient underwent a liver biopsy which showed interface hepatitis with plasma cells and eosinophils. There was evidence of cholestasis with no established fibrosis. Based on the available evidence, what is the histological feature that favours DILI over idiopathic autoimmune hepatitis (AIH)?

1. **Cholestasis canalicular.**
2. Interface hepatitis.
3. Prominent portal plasma cells.
4. Prominent intra-acinar eosinophils.

Answer

- The correct answer is option 1 (cholestasis canalicular), which favours a diagnosis of DILI over AIH based on a standardised histological evaluation of well-characterised DILI cases compared to AIH [14]. Options 3 and 4 (prominent portal plasma cells and intra-acinar eosinophils) were significantly associated with AIH compared to DILI. Interface hepatitis was not a feature that distinguished DILI from AIH.

Question 3. Following the liver biopsy, the patient was started on oral prednisolone 40 mg once daily, and minocycline was withheld. His liver enzymes improved, and his jaundice has resolved. However, his acne has flared.What will be the most appropriate next step in his management?

1. Restart his minocycline.
2. Start the patient on azathioprine.
3. Switch to oral budesonide.
4. **Withdraw steroids with clinical follow-up.**

Answer

- Based on history, investigations and causality assessment, the diagnosis is minocycline-induced liver injury which is well described to present with autoimmune features. The patient's liver enzymes and jaundice resolved after withdrawing minocycline and immunosuppression with steroids. There is no indication to start long-term immunosuppression (azathioprine) as the offending agent has been removed and the liver injury has resolved. It is safe to taper down his steroids with clinical follow-up as most cases with AIH relapse within the first year, while a small number relapse between 2 and 4 years. It is not recommended to rechallenge with minocycline due to high risk of morbidity and mortality from further liver injury.

References

1. Aithal GP. Drug-induced liver injury. Medicine. 2015;43(10):590–3.
2. Björnsson E, Bergmann O, Björnsson H, Kvaran R, Olafsson S. Incidence, presentation, and outcomes in patients with drug-induced liver injury in the general population of Iceland. Gastroenterology. 2013;144(7):1419–25.
3. Wing K, Bhaskaran K, Pealing L, Root A, Smeeth L, van Staa TP, et al. Quantification of the risk of liver injury associated with flucloxacillin: a UK population-based cohort study. J Antimicrob Chemother. 2017;72(9):2636–46.
4. Donaghy L, Barry FJ, Hunter JG, Stableforth W, Murray IA, Palmer J, et al. Clinical and laboratory features and natural history of seronegative hepatitis in a nontransplant centre. Eur J Gastroenterol Hepatol. 2013;25(10):1159–64.
5. Andrade RJ, Lucena MI, Fernandez MC, Pelaez G, Pachkoria K, Garcia-Ruiz E, et al. Drug-induced liver injury: an analysis of 461 incidences submitted to the Spanish registry over a 10-year period. Gastroenterology. 2005;129(2):512–21.
6. Chalasani N, Bonkovsky HL, Fontana R, Lee W, Stolz A, Talwalkar J, et al. Features and outcomes of 899 patients with drug-induced liver injury: the DILIN prospective study. Gastroenterology. 2015;148(7):1340–52. e7
7. Reuben A, Koch DG, Lee WM, Acute Liver Failure Study Group. Drug-induced acute liver failure: results of a U.S. multicenter, prospective study. Hepatology. 2010;52(6):2065–76.
8. Wei G, Bergquist A, Broome U, Lindgren S, Wallerstedt S, Almer S, et al. Acute liver failure in Sweden: etiology and outcome. J Intern Med. 2007;262(3):393–401.
9. Hoofnagle JH, Bjornsson ES. Drug-induced liver injury - types and phenotypes. N Engl J Med. 2019;381(3):264–73.
10. Robles-Diaz M, Gonzalez-Jimenez A, Medina-Caliz I, Stephens C, Garcia-Cortes M, Garcia-Munoz B, et al. Distinct phenotype of hepatotoxicity associated with illicit use of anabolic androgenic steroids. Aliment Pharmacol Ther. 2015;41(1):116–25.

11. Andrade RJ, Chalasani N, Björnsson ES, Suzuki A, Kullak-Ublick GA, Watkins PB, et al. Drug-induced liver injury. Nat Rev Dis Primers. 2019;5(1):58.
12. De Martin E, Michot JM, Papouin B, Champiat S, Mateus C, Lambotte O, et al. Characterisation of liver injury induced by cancer immunotherapy using immune checkpoint inhibitors. J Hepatol. 2018;68(6):1181–90.
13. Danan G, Teschke R. RUCAM in drug and herb induced liver injury: the update. Int J Mol Sci. 2015;17(1):14.
14. Suzuki A, Brunt EM, Kleiner DE, Miquel R, Smyrk TC, Andrade RJ, et al. The use of liver biopsy evaluation in discrimination of idiopathic autoimmune hepatitis versus drug-induced liver injury. Hepatology. 2011;54(3):931–9.
15. Kleiner DE, Chalasani NP, Lee WM, Fontana RJ, Bonkovsky HL, Watkins PB, et al. Hepatic histological findings in suspected drug-induced liver injury: systematic evaluation and clinical associations. Hepatology. 2014;59(2):661–70.
16. Atallah E, Wijayasiri P, Cianci N, Abdullah K, Mukherjee A, Aithal GP. Zanubrutinib-induced liver injury: a case report and literature review. BMC Gastroenterol. 2021;21(1):244.
17. Kaliyaperumal K, Grove JI, Delahay RM, Griffiths WJH, Duckworth A, Aithal GP. Pharmacogenomics of drug-induced liver injury (DILI): molecular biology to clinical applications. J Hepatol. 2018;69(4):948–57.
18. De Martin E, Michot JM, Rosmorduc O, Guettier C, Samuel D. Liver toxicity as a limiting factor to the increasing use of immune checkpoint inhibitors. JHEP Rep. 2020;2(6):100170.
19. Björnsson ES, Bergmann O, Jonasson JG, Grondal G, Gudbjornsson B, Olafsson S. Drug-induced autoimmune hepatitis: response to corticosteroids and lack of relapse after cessation of steroids. Clin Gastroenterol Hepatol. 2017;15(10):1635–6.
20. Hunt CM. Mitochondrial and immunoallergic injury increase risk of positive drug rechallenge after drug-induced liver injury: a systematic review. Hepatology. 2010;52(6):2216–22.

Chapter 4
Liver Decompensation and Acute on Chronic Liver Failure

R. Nathwani, N. Selvapatt, and A. Dhar

Key Learning Points
- ACLF is an increasingly recognized syndrome.
- It has a high mortality rate of 50% at 90 days.
- The pathogenesis of ACLF is multifactorial.
- Treatment and prevention of sepsis is a key determinant to survival.
- Cardiac dysfunction is increasingly recognized in ACLF.

Case Study
A 45-year-old man presents to Accident and Emergency with a 1 week history of progressive painless jaundice and fatigue. He consumes 40 units of alcohol per week but otherwise there are no relevant features to his past medical, medication, and family histories. At admission his temperature is 37.8 °C; he is icteric with a distended abdomen, spider naevi, and caput medusa. Initial bloods: WCC 15, Ne 11, Haemoglobin 14 g/dL, Platelets 80 × 10⁹/L, INR 1.9, Na 131 mmol/L,

R. Nathwani · N. Selvapatt · A. Dhar (✉)
Department of Hepatology, Imperial College London, London, UK
e-mail: rooshi.nathwani@nhs.net; nowlan.selvapatt@nhs.net; ameet.dhar1@nhs.net

© Springer Nature Switzerland AG 2022   57
T. Cross (ed.), *Liver Disease in Clinical Practice*, In Clinical Practice, https://doi.org/10.1007/978-3-031-10012-3_4

K 3.7 mmol/L, Cr 101 µmol/L, Ur 4.2, ALT<5 IU/L, AST 39 IU/L, bilirubin 125 µmol/L, Alkaline phosphatase 99 IU/L, Albumin 26 g/dL, CRP 22.

1. Which immediate management steps would you institute?

   (a) Intravenous fluid, FFP, and platelets, septic screen including blood cultures and ascitic tap, antibiotics, bd 20% HAS.
   (b) i.v. fluid, septic screen including blood cultures and ascitic tap, antibiotics, b.d. 20% HAS, 10 mg iv vitamin K, 2 mg terlipressin, ultrasound liver with Dopplers and urgent OGD to exclude variceal bleeding, 30 mg b.d. lactulose.
   (c) i.v. fluid, septic screen including blood cultures and ascitic tap, antibiotics, 10 mg iv vitamin K.
   (d) Fluid resuscitation with clotting products with target Plts >100 and INR <1.5, septic screen including blood cultures and ascitic tap, antibiotics, b.d. 20% HAS, and start 40 mg prednisolone for treatment of alcoholic hepatitis.

2. Within the first 12 h of admission in the Acute Assessment Unit he de-saturates and requires oxygen with FiO2 of 35% to maintain saturations >92%, and since admission he has passed between 5 and 15 mL of urine per hour. The next course of action should be.

   (a) Repeat chest X-ray, central, and arterial line, low dose noradrenaline and discussion with local transplant centre,
   (b) ABG, fluid challenge, central venous monitoring, referral to ITU,
   (c) ABG, fluid challenge, central venous monitoring, referral to local transplant centre,
   (d) 1 mg terlipressin, 20% HAS, ascitic drain insertion, referral to ITU.

3. 3 days after admission, septic screen yields no positive cultures; he is apyrexial on iv tazosin. He has required ITU admission for haemofiltration and non-invasive ventilation; he has developed mild confusion with liver flap but maintains GCS 15. Bloods: WCC 9, Ne 6, haemoglobin 13 g/dL, Platelets 70×10^9, INR 2.8, Na 128 mmol/L, K 4.2 mmol/L, Creatinine 110 μmol/L, Ur 3.8 mmol/L, ALT<5 IU/L, AST 45 IU/L, bilirubin 205 μmol/L, Alkaline phosphatase 99 IU/L, Albumin 32 g/dL, CRP <5. Next management steps should be:

   (a) Transjugular liver biopsy, prednisolone, referral to local liver transplant centre;
   (b) Transjugular liver biopsy, pentoxifylline, referral to local liver transplant centre;
   (c) Prednisolone and pentoxifylline, referral to local liver transplant centre;
   (d) Transjugular liver biopsy, prednisolone, discussion with patient and next of kin to establish clear ceilings of care.

Introduction

Liver decompensation can present as an acute event or as a chronic progression of underlying cirrhosis in the presence of portal hypertension. The most common features include presence of varices, ascites, jaundice, and encephalopathy.

Acute-on-chronic liver failure (ACLF) is a clinically important syndrome, characterized by an acute decompensation of established liver disease with development of organ failure. Observed in between 24% and 40% of hospitalized cirrhotics, ACLF is associated with a 28-day mortality of 33.9% [1–3]. A key difference in this syndrome compared to chronic decompensation of liver disease is its characteristic rapid evolution. Furthermore, there is greater chance of reversibility in patients with ACLF when early aggressive medical therapy is initiated.

In keeping ACLF being an emerging clinical entity, defining this syndrome has proven challenging. A recent consensus amongst hepatologists defines ACLF as *a syndrome in patients with chronic liver disease with or without previously diagnosed cirrhosis, which is characterized by acute hepatic decompensation resulting in liver failure (jaundice and prolongation of the INR (International Normalized Ratio) and one or more extrahepatic organ failures. This syndrome is associated with increased mortality within a period of 28 days and up to 3 months from onset* [1].

ACLF and Prognostication Models

Prognosis of patients with acute decompensation events were largely based on liver scoring systems such Child-Turcotte-Pugh score or model for end-stage liver disease score (MELD) or general organ failure scores such as Sequential Organ Failure Assessment score (SOFA) and Acute Physiology and Chronic Health Evaluation (APACHE) II.

However, more recently various condition specific scoring systems have been devised, incorporating features of organ failure scoring systems including the CLIF-C Organ Failure score, to predict the prognosis for patients with ACLF. These include the CLIF-C ACLF score (https://www.efclif.com/scientific-activity/score-calculators/clif-c-aclf) for ACLF and the CLIF-C AD score in patients with acute decompensation without ACLF (https://www.efclif.com/scientific-activity/score-calculators/clif-c-ad) [4].

The severity of ACLF is graded from 0 to 3, with 28-day mortality risk increasing with severity, summarized in Table 4.1 [1].

TABLE 4.1 Diagnostic criteria and grading of ACLF and associated 28-day mortality

| | ACLF Grade | | | |
	ACLF 0	ACLF 1	ACLF 2	ACLF 3
Definition	• No organ failure • Single organ failure + serum creatinine <132.6 umol/L and no HE • Patients with HE + serum creatinine <132.6 umol/L	• Renal failure • Single liver, coagulation, circulatory, or respiratory failure + serum creatinine 132.6–168.0 umol/L and/or grade 1 or grade 2 HE • HE + serum creatinine 132.6–168.0 umol/L	• Two organ failures	• Three organ failures or more
28-day mortality	4.7%	22.1%	32.0%	76.7%

Pathogenesis of Acute-on-Chronic Liver Failure

Whilst the exact mechanisms of action are still to be determined, impaired immune regulation and systemic inflammation are characteristic hallmarks for this syndrome [5]. Figure 4.1 outlines the postulated pathogenesis of acute-on-chronic liver failure (ACLF). Precipitating events of ACLF include bacterial infection and alcoholism in the West and exacerbation of hepatitis B, followed by bacterial infection and alcoholism in the East [6]. Persons with cirrhosis often have demonstrably impaired cardiac, adrenal, and renal function. Furthermore, vascular alterations secondary to portal

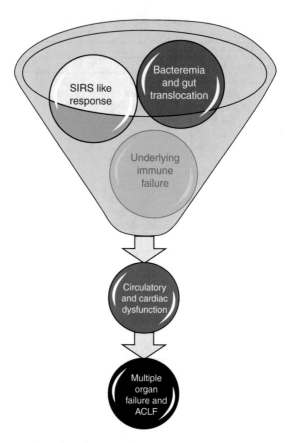

FIGURE 4.1 Postulated pathogenesis of acute on chronic liver failure

hypertension can predispose to the rapid evolution of multiple organ dysfunction.

Cirrhosis related small bowel bacterial overgrowth, impaired immunity, and increased intestinal permeability led to increased bacterial translocation into the portal circulation and mesenteric lymphatics which have impaired elimination. Porto-systemic collaterals vascular supply and shunting result in higher activation of liver immune compartments and subsequent SIRS response. Systemic immune dysfunction associated with cirrhosis confers poorer pathogen clearance and increased susceptibility to infection. The SIRS response in addition to pre-existing and inadequate cardiac, adrenal, and vasomotor responses exacerbate underlying circulatory dysfunction leading to multiple organ failure and ultimately increased mortality.

1. "The Gut-Liver-Immune axis"

    Patients with cirrhosis are at increased risk of bacterial translocation due to increased small bowel bacterial overgrowth (SIBO), and permeability due to loss of cellular tight junctions, decreased bile acids and immunological alterations, e.g. decreased IgA and increased inflammatory cytokines [5]. Increased gut derived bacteria in the portal and lymphatic circulation is postulated to be a key driver of systemic inflammatory responses.

    Numerous defects in innate immune responses (such as impaired white cell response and liver synthesis of antimicrobial proteins) have been demonstrated and are believed to confer inferior clearance of infections in ACLF [5].

    Portal hypertension results in splanchnic vasodilation and increased flow into the portal circulation [5]. Hepatic inflammation in cirrhosis results in increased intrahepatic vascular resistance and consequently arterio-venous shunting. The combination of increased gut translocation increased intrahepatic vascular resistance and portal hypertension facilitates systemic translocation of gut-derived organisms. This is thought to alter hepatic perfusion activating resident Kupffer cells which trigger systemic inflammatory responses.

2. Circulatory dysfunction

    Circulatory dysfunction is both systemic (macrocirculatory) and intrahepatic (microcirculatory):

    (a) *Systemic circulatory dysfunction in ACLF:* patients with ACLF display an exacerbation of the hyperdynamic circulation that persists in patients with advanced cirrhosis. Here there are both peripheral and splanchnic arterial vasodilatation resulting in a reduction in systemic mean arterial pressure, renal hypoperfusion and further deterioration in end organ function.

(b) *Intrahepatic microcirculatory dysfunction:* Activation of hepatic stellate cells leads to vasoconstriction and a reduction in sinusoidal perfusion and ischaemia, inflammation and further exacerbation in portal hypertension and splanchnic arterial vasodilatation.

Inflammatory responses to bacterial translocation trigger a further exacerbation in circulatory dysfunction in patients with ACLF culminating in organ hypoperfusion. This results in activation of homeostatic compensatory mechanisms, such as renin-angiotensin axis, that serve to maintain peripheral circulating volume and organ perfusion to the vital organs.

3. Cardiac dysfunction (cirrhotic cardiomyopathy)

Cirrhotic cardiomyopathy is defined as chronic cardiac dysfunction in patients with cirrhosis, characterized by blunted contractile responsiveness to stress, and/or altered diastolic relaxation with electrophysiological abnormalities in the absence of other known cardiac disease. It is observed in 40–50% of cirrhotic patients. Cardiac abnormalities detected in cirrhotic patients with cardiac dysfunction include; (a) diastolic dysfunction (E:A ratio < 1), electromechanical uncoupling (prolonged QTc interval), and (b) systolic dysfunction (elevated β natriuretic peptide; BNP) and impaired chronotropic responses to pharmacological/physiological stress. This may contribute to the development of renal dysfunction in patients with decompensated cirrhosis [6].

4. Renal failure

Renal impairment, whether related to acute kidney injury (AKI) or hepatorenal syndrome (HRS), is a very common complication of cirrhosis. The causes of renal failure in cirrhotic patients presenting with or developing renal failure (defined as an increase in serum creatinine of ≥ 26.4 μmol/L in less than 48 h, or by a 50% increase in baseline serum creatinine in <7 days of hospitalization) include infection (46%), hypovolaemia (32%), hepatorenal syndrome (13%), parenchymal nephropathy (9%) and drug-induced (7.5%) [6, 7].

The probability of development of HRS at 1 year is 20% and 50% at 3–5 years [8]. The most recent definition of hepatorenal syndrome (HRS) as: *renal failure in a patient with advanced liver disease in the absence of an identifiable cause of renal failure.* The pathophysiology of HRS is complex but can be summarized into four main categories:

(a) *Hyperdynamic circulation*: reduction in central arterial blood volume/mean arterial pressure due to reduction in systemic vascular resistance (SVR) and splanchnic vasodilatation.
(b) *Activation of sympathetic nervous (SNS) and renin-angiotensin-aldosterone systems*: Activation of homeostatic counter-regulatory pathways in response to a reduction in central circulating volume (described above) results in renal arterial vasoconstriction.
(c) *Renal vasoconstrictor/vasodilator imbalance*: reductions in renal blood flow and glomerular filtration rate (GFR) due to increased production of vasoactive substances (e.g. NO, ET-1, leukotrienes, thromboxane A2).
(d) *Cardiorenal dysfunction*: blunted cardiac contractile and chronotropic responsiveness to physiological stress (e.g. sepsis/vasodilatation) leads to further reductions in renal perfusion.

5. Adrenal dysfunction (Hepatoadrenal dysfunction)

Adrenal insufficiency related to liver disease is relatively common. Clinical symptoms such as weakness, fatigue, dizziness, gastrointestinal complaints and hyponatraemia, are generally non-specific and often experienced in persons with cirrhosis anyway.

The pathophysiology is incompletely understood but shares distinct similarities to adrenal insufficiency described in septic shock. It is likely to be multifactorial due to reduced sterol precursor production in cirrhosis, structural adrenal damage, hormonal dysregulation, adrenal hypoperfusion and impaired hepatic cortisol clearance and corticosteroid secretion in ACLF.

Principles of Management of Liver Decompensation

General Approach to Management

Figure 4.2 provides some guidance for basic goals of management in persons presenting with evidence of acute decompensation of liver disease. Prompt assessment and identification of precipitating factors (e.g. sepsis) is essential as well as provision of early and appropriately intensive therapy as organ dysfunction can evolve rapidly.

Specific liver related complications of decompensation include variceal haemorrhage, ascites, encephalopathy. All patients with known liver disease with acute medical issues should be assessed and screened for evidence of these complications. Close monitoring for evidence of emerging organ dysfunction and prompt escalation of care and institution of appropriate treatment is paramount. Decisive management requires early consideration of higher dependency or intensive care and hepatology transplant centre input.

Variceal Haemorrhage

Variceal haemorrhage is a serious complication with a significant risk of mortality. The immediate goal is for resuscitation to achieve haemodynamic stability aiming for a target Hb of 70–90 g/L and avoiding over transfusion. In persons with decompensated cirrhosis survival outcomes are significantly better in those who are transfused when the haemoglobin is lower than 70 g/L compared to when transfusion was initiated below 90 g/dL [9]. This is likely to be related to permissively lowering portal pressures by reducing circulating volumes. Terlipressin 2 mg tds, a splanchnic and systemic vasoconstrictor,

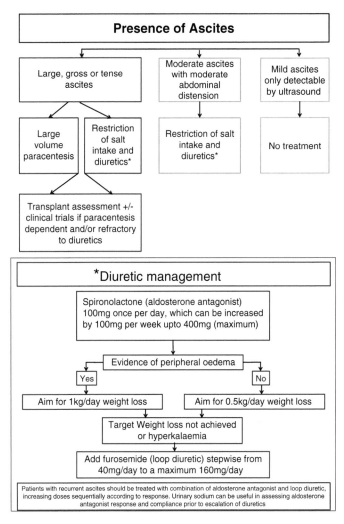

FIGURE 4.2 Decision making algorithm for assessment of complications associated with liver decompensation and ACLF with guidance of parameters for care escalation

should be administered to reduce portal pressures when variceal haemorrhage is suspected. A baseline ECG and close monitoring for evidence of ischaemia is essential. It should be used with caution in persons with significant cardiac disease or peripheral vascular disease and octreotide can be used as an alternative in these situations. Correction of clotting abnormalities is essential.

Infection is associated with failure to control bleeding and a higher incidence of early variceal re-bleeding. Therefore, empirical broad-spectrum antimicrobial agents (e.g. third generation cephalosporin's, piperacillin/tazobactam) are routinely administered in patients presenting with variceal bleeding for up to 7 days. Prophylactic antibiotics in patients presenting with acute variceal bleed, is associated with a reduction in mortality and incidence of bacterial infections [10]. To ensure prompt resuscitation two peripheral cannulas should be placed.

Following successful resuscitation or in the event of instability despite resuscitation early endoscopy should be performed, ideally under general anaesthetic, and treatment with band ligation or sclerotherapy where indicated. In the event of unsuccessful or incomplete therapy, a Sengstaken-Blakemore tube can be inserted as a temporary measure to control bleeding. In the event of uncontrolled bleeding where haemostasis cannot be achieved despite endoscopic intervention then transjugular intrahepatic porto-systemic shunts (TIPS) should be considered. Early pre-emptive TIPS insertion has been suggested in a select group of patients with cirrhosis however, this needs further exploration through clinical trials.

Ascites

The presence of ascites is indicative of a poor prognosis with 50% 2-year mortality. Diagnostic paracentesis should be performed in all patients with new onset ascites and all hospitalized patient admitted with complications of cirrhosis. Samples for leucocyte (neutrophil) count and microbiological culture should be performed to exclude bacterial peritonitis. A diagnosis of spontaneous bacterial peritonitis (SBP) can be made based on an ascitic neutrophil count of >250/mm^3. Most common causative organisms of SBP are gram-negative aerobic bacteria such as E.coli and therefore treatment should be with antibiotics with good gram negative cover as per local polices [8].

An ascitic fluid protein concentration of <15 g/L confers an increased risk of developing SBP and a serum-ascites albumin gradient (SAAG) can help diagnostically if the cause of ascites is not clearly related to cirrhosis (Table 4.2). Where the SAAG is greater than or equal to 11 g/L ascites can be ascribed to portal hypertension with 97% accuracy [8].

Figure 4.3 *provides an outline for management of patients with ascites. In the presence large volume ascites, particularly if evidence of respiratory compromise, then paracentesis should be considered with concomitant plasma expansion with infusion of albumin. During in-patient admission moderate restriction of salt intake, directed by a dietician can be beneficial. There is rarely a role for fluid restriction. Use of diuretics, particularly aldosterone antagonists such as spironolactone is very effective in management of chronic ascites, however in the acute setting if there is any concern about current or potential deterioration of renal function or serum sodium then they should be temporarily discontinued. In the presence of severe hyponatraemia (<120 mmol/L), progressive renal failure, worsening hepatic encephalopathy or severe muscle cramps then diuretics should be discontinued* [8].

TABLE 4.2 Causes of ascites as per serum-ascites albumin gradient

SAAG ≥11 g/L	SAAG <11 g/L
Cirrhosis	Peritoneal carcinomatosis
Alcoholic hepatitis	Tuberculous peritonitis
Congestive heart failure	Fungal and parasitic infections
Budd-Chiari syndrome	Pancreatitis
Portal vein thrombosis	Serositis
Idiopathic portal fibrosis	Nephrotic syndrome

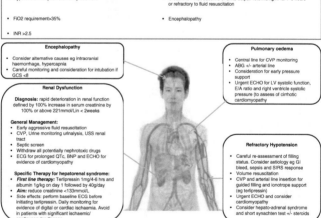

Evidence of Liver Decompensation
(jaundice, encephalopathy, ascites, renal impairment, GI haemorrhage)

ACLF
Evidence of extra hepatic organ failure*

Initial Management

1) Screen for Sepsis (blood, urine, ascitic fluid, sputum, stool, radiographs)
2) Low threshold for antibiotics (CRP and WCC may not be significantly raised)
3) Fluid resuscitation (crystalloid, colloid, albumin, blood)
4) Review nephrotoxic and hepatotoxic drugs
5) Ultrasound to assess space occupying lesions, vasculature, ascites
6) Correct clotting (if evidence of bleeding)
7) Early dietician review (low threshold for nasogastric tube/entral feeding)
8) Careful consideration of parameters for discussion with specialist services (ITU, local and regional hepatology specialists*

Alcoholic Hepatitis
Score using Maddrey's DF
Consider prednisolone if DF>32 +/- histological evidence and not high risk for sepsis or active GI bleeding

Upper GI haemorrhage
Volume resuscitation
Terlipressin 2mg iv qds
Prophylactic broad spectrum antibiotics
Target Hb 8-9 g/L
OGD immediately after resuscitation

Ascites
Diagnostic Ascitic tap for SBP (coagulopathy not a contraindication)
Consider drainage if tense ascites with evidence of respiratory compromise

Encephalopathy
Consider precipitants (sepsis, drugs, bowel opening)
Aim for 2x bowel motions per day:
Lactulose 15mls bd starting dose
Phosphate enemas as required

*Guidance parameters for escalation of care for High Dependency or Intensive Care Management:
Decompensation with evidence of organ failure with one or more of:

• Hypotension despite volume replacement
• Creatinine >1.5x baseline or urine output <0.5mls/kg/hr for > 6 hours or refractory to fluid resuscitation
• FiO2 requirement>35%
• Encephalopathy
• INR >2.5

Encephalopathy
• Consider alternative causes eg intracranial haemorrhage, hypercapnia
• Careful monitoring and consideration for intubation if GCS <8

Renal Dysfunction
Diagnosis: rapid deterioration in renal function defined by 100% increase in serum creatinine by 100% in or above 221mmol/Lin < 2weeks

General Management:
• Early aggressive fluid resuscitation
• CVP, Urine monitoring urinalysis, USS renal tract
• Septic screen
• Withdraw all potentially nephrotoxic drugs
• ECG for prolonged QTc, BNP and ECHO for evidence of cardiomyopathy

Specific Therapy for hepatorenal syndrome:
• *First line therapy:* Terlipressin 1mg/4-6 hrs and albumin 1g/kg on day 1 followed by 40g/day
• *Aim:* reduce creatinine <133mmol/L
• Side effects: perform baseline ECG before initiating terlipressin. Daily monitoring for evidence of digital or cardiac ischaemia. Avoid in patients with significant ischaemic/cardiovascular disease

Pulmonary oedema
• Central line for CVP monitoring
• ABG +/- arterial line
• Consideration for early pressure support
• Urgent ECHO for LV systolic function, E/A ratio and right ventricle systolic pressure (to assess of cirrhotic cardiomyopathy

Refractory Hypotension
• Careful re-assessment of filling status. Consider aetiology eg GI bleed, sepsis and SIRS response
• Volume resuscitation
• CVP and arterial line insertion for guided filling and ionotrope support (eg terlipressin)
• Urgent ECHO and consider cardiomyopathy
• Consider hepato-adrenal syndrome and short synachten test +/- steroids

FIGURE 4.3 An empirical guide for management of ascites and considerations for escalation of therapies based on EASL guidelines [8]

Encephalopathy

Hepatic encephalopathy is a brain dysfunction caused by liver insufficiency and/or perihepatic shunting, manifesting as a wide spectrum of neurological or psychiatric abnormalities ranging from subclinical alterations to coma. The West Haven classification systemic is often used in clinical practice to grade the severity of hepatic encephalopathy. Broadly speaking, hepatic encephalopathy can be considered "Covert" which tends to be episodic, subclinical, and often spontaneous. "Overt" encephalopathy tends to be recurrent or persistent with more obvious clinical manifestations. In the acute scenario treatment is focused on treating sepsis, removing precipitants (most commonly medications and drugs) and addressing nutrition. Lactulose is generally the initial treatment, due to assumed prebiotic effects and laxative effect which aids ammonia excretion. The addition of phosphate enemas may be required to aid bowel opening especially if there is evidence of distally impacted stool. In patients where lactulose has had a lack of response and who are opening their bowels at least twice per day then second line options include i.v. L-ornithine L-aspartate. Probiotics, albumin, neomycin, and metronidazole have also been trialed. To date there is no evidence to support rifaximin in the acute setting, however, it is indicated as an adjunct to lactulose for the treatment of chronic, recurrent encephalopathy. Rifaximin is well tolerated and has a good safety profile with minimal side effects experienced [11].

Alcoholic Hepatitis

Alcoholic hepatitis is a specific entity that describes the manifestation of an acute hepatitis characterized by jaundice and liver failure following a history of prolonged heavy alcohol ingestion. The severity of alcoholic hepatitis can be defined by Maddrey's discriminant function >32 or a Glasgow alcoholic hepatitis score ≥9.

In up to 80% of cases alcoholic hepatitis superimposes on underlying cirrhosis. Clinically differentiating decompensation in a person with alcohol related liver disease and acute alcoholic hepatitis can pose a diagnostic challenge. In this scenario, consideration should be placed on obtaining a liver biopsy for histological confirmation. Histological hallmarks of alcoholic hepatitis include:

- Neutrophil infiltrate.
- Mallory-Denk bodies and hepatocyte ballooning.
- Lobular inflammation.

Relatively few effective and safe treatments are available for alcoholic hepatitis. Prednisolone with or without N-Acetylcysteine confers short term benefit up until 28 days [12, 13]. Furthermore, in those who steroid treatment is initiated, response guided treatment should be provided by calculating the 7-day Lille score (www.lillemodel.com/score.asp). Using calculations based on age, albumin, creatinine, PT and bilirubin at baseline and day 7 scores above 0.45 are associated with inferior responses and marked decrease in 6-month survival. Prior to commencement of steroids, it is vital that a full septic screen is performed, and any evidence of infection is addressed. Use of steroids following appropriate treatment of underlying sepsis is safe. However, if sepsis is suspected during steroid treatment, steroids should be discontinued whilst antibiotic therapy is ongoing. Steroids should be avoided in persons with active GI haemorrhage. Early liver transplantation for acute alcoholic hepatitis has been demonstrated to be efficacious in well selected cases, although remains available in a limited number of countries [14].

Infections and Sepsis

Bacterial infections are the leading cause morbidity/mortality in cirrhotic patients. The presence of sepsis in patients with cirrhosis increases the mortality rate by 50% and the commonest sites of primary infection include spontaneous bacterial peritonitis (SBP), urinary and chest sepsis. With widespread use of antimicrobial agents, Clostridium difficile infection is emerging as a significant cause of morbidity and increased mortality in hospitalized cirrhotic patients. Importantly, 30–50% infections are "culture negative", defined by clinical/radiological evidence of infection in the absence of overt microbiological positive cultures. These infections are thought to arise as a consequence of systemic translocation of gut-derived bacteria.

Renal Failure and Hepatorenal Syndrome

Acute kidney injury is a common feature of presentation in patients with ACLF and requires careful management with fluid resuscitation and plasma expanders with monitoring of response of urine output and central venous pressures, where appropriate.

HRS can be classified into the following categories:

- *Type 1*: rapidly progressive impairment in renal function as defined by a 100% increase in serum creatinine from baseline or/above 221 μmol/L in less than 2 weeks. Median survival of 4 weeks.
- *Type 2*: patients with refractory ascites stable or slowly progressive impairment in renal function not meeting the above criteria. Median survival of 6 months.

Sepsis is one of the commonest triggers of HRS probably through activation of SIRS responses and worsening of circulatory dysfunction/central hypovolaemia. In addition to treatment of the underlying trigger for the acute decompensation episode (e.g. sepsis), administration of a volume expander (albumin 1 g/kg on day 1 followed by 40 g/day) and a splanchnic/systemic vasoconstrictor (terlipressin 1 mg/4–6 h and increased to a maximum of 2 mg/4–6) are indicated in order to improve circulatory dysfunction and renal perfusion. Predictors of response to terlipressin/albumin therapy include earlier onset renal failure (creatinine <381 μmol/L), lower severity of liver dysfunction (Bilirubin <117 μmol/L; MELD<28) and a sustained increase in mean arterial pressure >5 mmHg from the initiation of treatment to day 3. Ischaemic side effects related to terlipressin have been reported in 10% patients (digital, mesenteric, coronary ischaemia, cardiac arrhythmias) and should be avoided in patients with significant ischaemic/cardiovascular disease. Alternatives therapeutic agents that have also shown to be of benefit in treatment of HRS include midodrine/octreotide and noadrenaline/albumin; although these are less established compared to the current standards of care [8]. The use of albumin outside of defined indications such as SBP and HRS is controversial and remains unclear, albeit in hospitalized patients there does not seem to be a clinical or survival benefit [15, 16].

Adrenal Failure

At least half of patients with ACLF have concomitant adrenal insufficiency in ACLF and is a marker of severity of disease. A number of studies show that hydrocortisone administration, at doses of 200 mg/day, reduces vasopressor requirements and severity of organ failure in ACLF patients with septic shock. In patients with ACLF, sepsis and unresponsiveness to fluid- or vasopressor therapy, use of steroids should therefore be considered. Screening can be performed with an early morning cortisol but a short synacthen test is required for diagnostic confirmation.

Coagulopathy

In patients with compensated cirrhosis, protein synthesis of both pro-coagulant (factors I, II, V, VII, IX, XI) and anti-coagulant factors (protein C, anti-thrombin) are concomitantly reduced. Acute insults such as sepsis alter the fine balance of endogenous pro-coagulants and anti-coagulants. Overall, even in the context of prolonged prothrombin times bleeding diathesis is not necessarily more likely and in fact thromboembolic events in these scenarios are common.

Platelet dysfunction occurs in cirrhosis due to splenic sequestration and reduced hepatic thrombopoietin production. Elevated circulating levels of Von Willebrand factor detected in cirrhotic patients may compensate for the reduction in platelet numbers and function. Nevertheless, current clinical guidelines recommend that in hospitalized patients with cirrhosis who are actively bleeding or undergoing invasive procedures (e.g. biopsy, paracentesis) platelet transfusions are indicated in those with counts below $50 \times 10^9/L$ [17].

There are limitations of standard tests used at present assess coagulopathy in current clinical care. Prothrombin time (INR) is a quick and inexpensive test. Its main limitation is that it does not measure the extent of pro-coagulant activity and hence the overall coagulation status of patients. The sole use of prothrombin time as a marker of bleeding risk can result in over-transfusion of clotting products.

More appropriate tests should aim to assess haemostasis as a whole. Thrombin elastography (TEG) has been utilized widely in intra-operative settings and critical care settings and is a more complete marker of coagulation and bleeding risk. It is increasingly being used to guide correction of coagulation in all cirrhotics, with or without ACLF however, further work is required to assess its validity.

Summary

Liver decompensation, in particular ACLF, is an increasingly recognized clinical entity. Sepsis is a key precipitant of systemic inflammatory responses and multiple organ failures. Admitting physicians need to carefully assess and manage effective resuscitation, hepatic, and extra hepatic complications. These patients unfortunately have high short-term mortality and therefore early diagnosis and intensive management are a necessity for optimal care. In early stages of ACLF liver transplantation has demonstrated survival of

72–92% but in more advanced cases this drops to as low as 44% ([18–20]. Further work is ongoing to understand a future role and utility of liver transplantation in patients with ACLF which will require better understanding of patient selection and prognostication models.

Case Study Answers

A 45-year-old man presents to Accident and Emergency with a 1 week history of progressive painless jaundice and fatigue. He consumes 40 units of alcohol per week but otherwise there are no relevant features to his past medical, medication, and family histories. At admission his temperature is 37.8 °C; he is icteric with a distended abdomen, spider naevi, and caput medusa. Initial bloods: WCC 15, Ne 11, Haemoglobin 14 g/dL, Platelets 80 × 10⁹/L, INR 1.9, Na 131 mmol/L, K 3.7 mmol/L, Cr 101 µmol/L, Ur 4.2, ALT<5 IU/L, AST 39 IU/L, bilirubin 125 µmol/L, Alkaline phosphatase 99 IU/L, Albumin 26 g/dL, CRP 22.

1. Which immediate management steps would you institute?

   (c) **i.v. fluid, septic screen including blood cultures and ascitic tap, antibiotics, 10 mg iv vitamin K.**

   The initial goal for management in this situation is resuscitation and early diagnosis and treatment of sepsis. There is evidence of renal dysfunction and circulatory volume expansion is required with salt containing fluids. There is no evidence of active GI bleeding, and whilst an ultrasound is indicated this should happen after appropriate resuscitation and treatment.

2. Within the first 12 h of admission in the Acute Assessment Unit he de-saturates and requires oxygen with FiO_2 of 35% to maintain saturations >92%, and since admission he has passed between 5 and 15 mL of urine per hour. The next course of action should be.

   (b) **ABG, fluid challenge, central venous monitoring, referral to ITU.**

An arterial blood gas will accurately define oxygenation and may support requirements for escalation of ventilation. Lactate is also useful in guiding end organ perfusion. This patient may require both respiratory and renal support in a level 2 or 3 setting and early discussion with ITU is essential to ensure proactive and aggressive management.

3. 3 days after admission, septic screen yields no positive cultures; he is apyrexial on iv tazosin. He has required ITU admission for haemofiltration and non-invasive ventilation, he has developed mild confusion with liver flap but maintains GCS 15. Bloods: WCC 9, Ne 6, haemoglobin 13 g/dL, Platelets 70×10^9, INR 2.8, Na 128 mmol/L, K 4.2 mmol/L, Creatinine 110 µmol/L, Ur 3.8 mmol/L, ALT<5 IU/L, AST 45 IU/L, bilirubin 205 µmol/L, Alkaline phosphatase 99 IU/L, Albumin 32 g/dL, CRP <5. Next management steps should be:

(d) **Transjugular liver biopsy, prednisolone, discussion with patient and next of kin to establish clear ceilings of care.**

The clinical presentation and biochemistry is suggestive of an underlying alcoholic hepatitis and a liver biopsy may help with confirming diagnosis prior to commencement of steroids for treatment. This patient is demonstrating evidence of progressive liver failure, and has respiratory, renal and cognitive impairment. He may benefit from management at a tertiary hepatology centre. At this time juncture he is an unlikely candidate for liver transplantation. Whilst recovery with careful management is the goal, his predicament is severe. Clear discussions are needed to explain the severity of this illness and prognosis. The patient's wishes should incorporated within decision making regarding ceilings of care and be re-visited depending on clinical progression.

References

1. Moreau R, et al. Acute-on-chronic liver failure is a distinct syndrome that develops in patients with acute decompensation of cirrhosis. Gastroenterology. 2013;144(7):1426–37.
2. Jalan R, et al. Acute-on chronic liver failure. J Hepatol. 2012;57(6):1336–48.
3. Hernaez R, et al. Acute-on-chronic liver failure. Gut. 2017;66(66):541–53.
4. Jalan R, et al. The CLIF consortium acute decompensation score (CLIF-C ads) for prognosis of hospitalised cirrhotic patients without acute-on-chronic liver failure. J Hepatol. 2015;62(4):831–40.
5. Selvapatt N, et al. Understanding infection susceptibility in patients with acute-on-chronic liver failure. Intensive Care Med. 2014;40(9):1363–6.
6. European Association for the Study of the Liver. Electronic address: easloffice@easloffice.eu, European Association for the Study of the Liver. EASL guidelines, EASL clinical practice guidelines for the management of patients with decompensated cirrhosis. J Hepatol. 2018;69(2):406–60. https://doi.org/10.1016/j.jhep.2018.03.024.
7. Martin-Lhall M, et al. Prognostic importance of the cause of renal failure in patients with cirrhosis. Gastroenterology. 2011;140(2):488–96.
8. European Association for the Study of the Liver. EASL guidelines, EASL clinical practice guidelines on the management of ascites, spontaneous bacterial peritonitis, and hepatorenal syndrome in cirrhosis. J Hepatol. 2010;53(3):397–417.
9. Villanueva C, et al. Transfusion strategies for acute upper gastrointestinal bleeding. N Engl J Med. 2013;368:11–21.
10. Chavez-Tapia NC, et al. Antibiotic prophylaxis for cirrhotic patients with upper gastrointestinal bleeding. Cochrane Database Syst Rev. 2010;2010(9):CD002907.
11. EASL guidelines, EASL clinical practice guidelines on hepatic encephalopathy in chronic liver disease: 2014 practice guideline by the EASL and AASLD. J Hepatol. 2014;60(2):715–35.
12. Thursz MR, et al. Prednisolone or pentoxifylline for alcoholic hepatitis. N Engl J Med. 2015;372(17):1619–28.
13. Nguyen-Khac E, et al. Glucocorticoids plus N-acetylcysteine in severe alcoholic hepatitis. N Engl J Med. 2011;365:1781–9.

14. Mathurin P. Early liver transplantation for acute alcoholic hepatitis: We can't say. J Hepatol. 2021;75:718–22.
15. Caraceni P, et al. Long-term albumin administration in decompensated cirrhosis (ANSWER): an open-label randomized trial. Lancet. 2018;391(10138):2417–29.
16. China L, et al. A randomized trial of albumin infusion in hospitalized patients with cirrhosis. N Engl J Med. 2021;384:808–17.
17. Northup P, et al. Coagulation in liver disease: a guide for the clinician. Clin Gastroenterol Hepatol. 2013;11:1064–74.
18. Moon DB, et al. Adult living donor liver transplantation for acute-on-chronic liver failure in high-model for end-stage liver disease score patients. Am J Transplant. 2017;17:1833–42.
19. Thuluvath PJ, et al. Liver transplantation in patients with multiple organ failures: feasibility and outcomes. J Hepatol. 2018;69:1047–56.
20. Sundaram V, et al. Factors associated with survival of patients with severe acute-on-chronic liver failure before and after liver transplantation. Gastroenterology. 2019;156(5):1381–1391.e3.

Chapter 5
Portal Hypertension: Varices

Amardeep Khanna, Ashish Goel, and Dhiraj Tripathi

Key Learning Points
- Patients with cirrhosis should be screened for varices.
- A new entity has been proposed called compensated advanced chronic liver disease (cACLD) to show that severe fibrosis and cirrhosis in asymptomatic patients are a continuous spectrum and difficult to distinguish on clinical grounds alone.
- Liver stiffness measurement (LSM) in combination with platelet count has been validated to identify patients with cACLD, who are low risk of developing varices needing treatment and hence can avoid gastroscopy for varices screening.
- Hepatic venous pressure gradient (HVPG) measurement is the gold-standard method to assess the presence of portal hypertension.
- Patient with medium to large varices that have not bled require primary prophylaxis with non-selective beta-blockers or variceal band ligation.

A. Khanna · A. Goel · D. Tripathi (✉)
Liver Unit, Queen Elizabeth Hospital Birmingham, University Hospitals Birmingham, Birmingham, UK
e-mail: Dhiraj.Tripathi@uhb.nhs.uk; d.tripathi@bham.ac.uk

© Springer Nature Switzerland AG 2022
T. Cross (ed.), *Liver Disease in Clinical Practice*, In Clinical Practice, https://doi.org/10.1007/978-3-031-10012-3_5

- Variceal haemorrhage should be suspected in any patient with signs of chronic liver disease presenting with haematemesis or melaena.
- Patients presenting with an acute variceal haemorrhage should be resuscitated appropriately and vasoactive drugs and antibiotics commenced before early endoscopic therapies.
- Patients with variceal haemorrhage who are haemodynamically stable benefit from a restrictive transfusion policy, with a target haemoglobin of 70–80 g/dL.
- Transjugular intrahepatic portosystemic-stent shunts (TIPSS) has a role as salvage therapy for failure of endoscopies therapies, and early TIPSS normally within 72 h of acute variceal bleeding in selected cases should be considered.
- Patients that have recovered from an episode of acute variceal bleeding require secondary prophylaxis with combination of non-selective beta-blockers and band ligation to prevent re-bleeding. TIPSS can be considered in failure of secondary prophylaxis.

Clinical Case

A 38-year-old man presented to emergency department with few weeks history of worsening jaundice, increasing abdominal distension, and 1 week of intermittent black tarry stools and coffee ground vomiting. He consumed over 30 units of alcohol per day.

On examination, pulse was 110 bpm, blood pressure 138/78 mm Hg, and respiratory rate 16 bpm and oxygen saturations 97% on room air. GCS 15/15. There were stigmata of chronic liver disease, with grade 2 ascites. Digital rectal examination (DRE) confirmed melaena.

Blood tests were performed and results as follows:

Haemoglobin 68 g/dL.
White cell count 26.7 × 10^3/mm^3.
Bilirubin 176 μmol/L.

Creatinine 72 μmol/L.
Urea 7.0 mmol/L.
Albumin 24 mmol/L.
INR 1.8.
Platelets 251 10^9/L.

Following resuscitation with colloid and blood transfusion, antibiotics and terlipressin, endoscopy showed three grade 1–2 varices, with stigmata of recent bleed and portal hypertensive gastropathy. Two bands were applied to the oesophageal varices. Diagnostic ascitic tap ruled out SBP, and ascites was drained. On day 8 of hospital stay he was discharged on propranolol 40 mg BD and spironolactone 100 mg OD. However, he failed to attend his follow-up outpatient appointments for banding of varices and was readmitted 5 months later following a seizure. He complained of abdominal pain and continued to consume 15–20 units of alcohol per day. His HR was 110 bpm and blood pressure 89/56 mmHg on admission.

Blood tests showed:

Haemoglobin 73 g/dL.
White cell count 11×10^3/mm^3.
Platelets 46×10^9/L.
Creatinine 70 μmol/L.
Urea 6.5 mmol/L.
Bilirubin 46 μmol/L.
Albumin 27 mmol/L.
INR 2.2.

Diagnostic ascitic tap confirmed SBP (PMN 290 cells/mm^3). He was treated with IV fluids, blood transfusion, terlipressin, and antibiotics. His propranolol was suspended. Gastroscopy under general anaesthesia showed three grade 2–3 oesophageal varices with red sign and altered blood in lower oesophagus, and portal hypertensive gastropathy. Five bands were applied to the oesophageal varices. Ultrasound showed cirrhotic liver, patent portal vein, 15 cm splenomegaly, and mild ascites. His Child Pugh score was C12 and MELD score was 21. With concerns regarding high risk of re-bleeding and poor compliance to medication and EBL therapy, planned covered TIPSS was done on day 3 (final portal pressure gradient 7 mmHg). Post-TIPSS period was complicated with hepatic encephalopathy responsive to lactulose and rifaximin, and pneumonia. He was discharged on day 16 of the admission with haemoglobin of 102 g/L. On follow-up he remained abstinent, with no further episodes of decompensation and hepatic encephalopathy was well controlled.

Pathophysiology of Portal Hypertension

Classification of Portal Hypertension

Portal pressure is measured using hepatic venous pressure gradient (HVPG). HVPG is measured as a pressure gradient between wedged and free Hepatic Vein Pressure, therefore an estimate of pressure gradient across portal vein and inferior vena cava. Portal hypertension is defined as a portal pressure of greater than 6 mm Hg, and clinically significant portal hypertension (CSPH) is defined as a portal pressure of ≥ 10 mm Hg [1]. The hepatic venous pressure gradient (HVPG) remains the gold standard for deriving portal pressure in sinusoidal portal hypertension. The causes of portal hypertension can be classified at sinusoidal level (pre-, intra-, post-sinusoid) (see Table 5.1). There is a normal pressure gradient across the sinusoid of 3 mm Hg which allows for flow from the portal to the hepatic venous systems. Patients who have a pre-sinusoidal cause of portal hypertension (e.g. portal vein thrombosis) will have a normal sinusoid pressure, but those who have a sinusoidal cause of portal hypertension (e.g. cirrhosis) will have a high sinusoid pressure, and this is reflected as a high wedged hepatic vein pressure on trans-

TABLE 5.1 Common causes of portal hypertension classified by site

Site of portal hypertension	Cause
Pre-sinusoidal	
Extra-hepatic	Portal vein thrombosis
	Splenic vein thrombosis
	Extrinsic compression of portal vein
Intra-hepatic	Idiopathic non-cirrhotic portal hypertension (INCPH)
	Schistosomiasis
	Primary biliary cholangitis
	Sarcoidosis
Sinusoidal	Cirrhosis
	Alcoholic hepatitis
Post-sinusoidal	Budd Chiari syndrome
	Veno-occlusive disease
	Inferior vena caval obstruction
	Constrictive pericarditis

jugular hepatic pressure studies. The clinical course of cirrhosis is determined by combination of progressive worsening of portal hypertension, systemic inflammation activation, and bacterial translocation. In a multistate model ACLD has been classified from Stage 0 to Stage 6, defined by degree of portal hypertension. Compensated cirrhosis encompasses stages 0–2, while the development of variceal bleeding, ascites, or hepatic encephalopathy (alone or in combination) heralds' decompensation (see Table 5.2) [2].

TABLE 5.2 Multistate model of cirrhosis classification and clinical outcomes

State	HVPG grading	Clinical presentation	Outcome
0	LSM 15–20 kPa Or HVPG 5–10 mmHg	No varices, moderate portal hypertension (MPH)	Compensated
1	LSM >20 kPa Or HVPG >10 mmHg	No varices, CSPH	
2	CSPH	Varices	
3	CSPH	Variceal bleed	Decompensated
4	CSPH	First non-bleeding decompensation	
5	CSPH	Second decompensation event	
6	CSPH	Late decompensation-refractory ascites, persistent portosystemic encephalopathy or jaundice, infections, renal or another organ failure	ACLF or death

Portal Hypertension Due to Cirrhosis

Both, increases in resistance to portal inflow and increases in portal inflow itself, contributes to portal hypertension in cirrhosis [3]. The incremental progressive collateral shunting of portal blood flow into systemic circulation creates a true "steal" phenomenon. As a result, arterial steal from systemic circulation into splanchnic arterial system and venous steal from portal vein inflow of liver to porto-systemic collateral occurs. In advance cases flow in portal vein may become reversed [3].

Increased resistance to portal inflow: Distortion of normal liver architecture with increasing fibrosis leading to septation and nodule formation, results in increased resistance to flow. This is enhanced by hepatic stellate cells, which contract within the normal liver, change phenotype as fibrosis develops, and contract further.

In addition to the structural (and fixed) element described above, there is a more modifiable dynamic component to the portal resistance contributed by a variety of vasoactive molecules. In health, liver responds to both vasoconstricting and vasodilating substances, but with cirrhosis progression, both its response, and the balance of these substances change. Nitric Oxide (NO) is a vasodilator and is an important regulator of vascular resistance in the liver. In cirrhosis its production is reduced, and the liver's response to NO is impaired. The endothelin's, a group of vasoconstrictors show increased levels in cirrhosis, and the fibrotic liver is more sensitive to their vasoconstrictive effects. These combined changes lead to increased dynamic liver resistance to portal blood flow.

Increase in portal inflow: Splanchnic vasodilation, mediated by NO (extra-hepatic production increases in cirrhosis), and sGC-PKG signalling, and other vasoactive mediators, contributes to hyperdynamic circulation manifested as increased cardiac output and heart rate, with a decreased systemic vascular resistance and a low arterial blood pressure. This leads to greater blood flow through the portal vein, which in the presence of increased resistance, contributes to portal hypertension. Splenic congestion and opening of porto-systemic collaterals are other contributing factors to increased portal inflow.

With increasing hepatic resistance and flow diverted through the opened collaterals, liver perfusion becomes erratic and depends increasingly on hepatic arterial flow. This can result in continued liver injury due to hepatic ischemia.

Cirrhosis is now increasingly identified as pro-thrombotic state where there is coagulation imbalance and use of anticoagulation has been shown to reduce hepatic fibrosis and portal hypertension suggesting its role in pathogenesis. Further gut-derived bacterial induced inflammation has been postulated to stimulate fibrogenesis by stimulating hepatic stellate and Kupffer cells.

Development of Varices

The opening up of portosystemic collaterals is a hallmark of portal hypertension. These collaterals are usually present in lower oesophagus, stomach, rectum, umbilical region, and the retroperitoneum. With increasing portal pressure, these pre-existing connections are re-perfused and dilated (with possible contribution of neo-angiogenesis), leading to increased shunting of blood. This can be marked in the splenic or renal veins.

At the gastro-oesophageal junction, the venous blood flow from the oesophagus drains into the left gastric vein, which drains into the portal vein. Therefore, according to Laplace's law: as the portal pressure increases, the pressure in these collateral veins increases, forming dilated and tortuous veins in the oesophagus and stomach. Over time, the increased pressure reduces the wall thickness and increases the wall tension leading to rupture.

Gastro-oesophageal varices develop when the portal pressure is greater than 10 mm Hg, and the risk of rupture increases when pressure is greater than 12 mm Hg. The risk of rupture, and subsequent bleeding, is related to the pressure and flow within the varix, the size of the varix and the wall thickness. However, gastric veins can bleed at lower pressure due to their increased diameter and wall tension. The risk of variceal haemorrhage increases with severity of liver disease and presence of high risk stigmata of red wale signs (vessels on the variceal wall) at endoscopy predicts haemorrhage [4].

Varices are present in 44% of patients at 10 years following diagnosis of cirrhosis and 53% at 20 years [5]. Presence of varices is related to the severity of liver disease, with 85% of those with Childs C cirrhosis having varices as compared to 40% in Childs A stage. Varices develop, and grow at a rate of 8% per year, with a 1-year rate for first variceal haemorrhage of 7% and recurrent variceal of haemorrhage of up to 60%.

Manifestations of Varices

Varices are usually asymptomatic unless they bleed and patients may have clinical signs of portal hypertension on examination such as splenomegaly, ascites, and spider naevi.

Availability of better pharmacological treatments, including antibiotics and vasoconstrictors, improved endoscopic care, and advances in intensive care management [6], have improved the overall management of these patients. Although mortality from variceal haemorrhage has decreased (from 42% in 1980), it remains high at ~20%.

Diagnosis of Varices

Although, barium swallow may occasionally pick large varices and CT may show collateral vessels, upper GI endoscopy remains the gold standard for diagnosis of gastro-oesophageal varices.

UGI endoscopy also helps in estimation of size of oesophageal varices which is an important determinant of the risk of bleeding. It can be either graded as large (>5 mm in diameter) or small (<5 mm in diameter); or as grade 1 (small, straight varices that can be depressed with insufflation), grade 2 (tortuous varices that occupy less than ½ of oesophageal lumen), and grade 3 (occupy more than ½ of lumen) [7]. UGI endoscopy can also identify high risk signs for bleeding-red weal, cherry red spot and haematocystic spot.

Liver stiffness measurement (LSM), as measured by transient elastography (TE) has allowed identification of patients with compensated advanced chronic liver (cACLD) who are at risk of developing CSPH [8]. LSM using TE, measure on two separate days in a fasting state is sufficient to suspect cACLD in a asymptomatic patient with known cause or risk factor for chronic liver disease and warrants a referral to specialist centre for further work up. HVPG is the gold standard to assess presence of CSPH. In virus related cACLD TE > 20–25 kPa on two separate occasions in fasting state are sufficient to rule-in CSPH. LSM, spleen size, platelets, or a combination, have been subject to investigation to non-invasively assess whether a patient is at risk of developing varices, and thus warrants an endoscopy. cACLD patients who meet favourable Baveno VI criteria, with LSM <20 kPa with platelet count >150,000/mm^3 have low risk of developing varices needing treatment and can avoid screening gastroscopy. They should be followed up with yearly LSM and platelet count and gastroscopy performed if LSM is increasing or platelets are falling [9]. Although Baveno VI criteria have good sensitivity, the specificity is poor with up to 60% of patients having an unnecessary endoscopy if they meet unfavourable criteria. Moreover, facilities for LSM is not widely available in many smaller centres in the UK in contrast to diagnostic gastroscopy.

Surveillance of Varices

Current UK guidelines recommend that all patients with cirrhosis should have a screening endoscopy at the time of diagnosis. In compensated patients with ongoing liver injury repeat endoscopy should be performed at 2 years for those without varices and 1-year interval for those with small varices on index endoscopy. The recommended interval is 3 years and 2 years; for those without varices and those with small varices, respectively, if the aetiological factor has been removed [10]. Patients who are commenced on pharmaco-

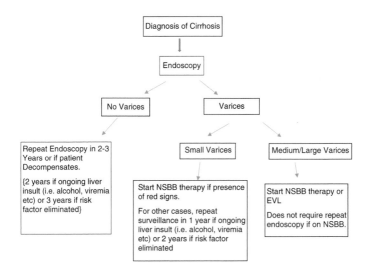

FIGURE 5.1 Algorithm for Diagnosis of Varices and Primary Prevention of Haemorrhage

logical treatment for varices as primary prophylaxis do not require surveillance endoscopy [9]. The time interval between surveillance endoscopies should be modified if there are changes in the underlying cause of cirrhosis, and its effect on cirrhosis progression, such as abstinence in alcoholic liver disease or the clearance of viral hepatitis. Similarly, when patients decompensate, repeat endoscopy should be offered unless patients are already on primary prophylaxis (see Fig. 5.1).

Treatment

Treatment to Prevent Development of Varices

There is currently no evidence for any treatment that prevents the development of varices in cirrhosis. Successful management of the aetiological factor (lifestyle modification and weight reduction with diet and exercise, abstinence of alcohol, viral suppression with newer anti-viral therapies) may improve both liver structure and function, translating in to reduced portal pressure. HVPG change of 10% or more is considered significant and is an acceptable surrogate of clinical outcomes in cirrhotic patients. A careful consideration should be given to managing co-morbidities such as diabetes, hypertension; pulmonary, cardiovascular, and renal disease. Portal hypertension leads to impaired gut motility, decreased nutrition absorption, and enteral protein loss. Management of malnutrition and sarcopenia has also been shown to impact the development of cirrhosis related complications and overall survival.

Non-selective beta blockade (NSBB) reduces portal pressure by 15–20% on average by decreasing portal venous inflow by splanchnic vasoconstriction. Despite this, they do not prevent the development of varices and currently there is no evidence to support their use in prevention of varices development. Up to few years ago evidence related mostly to propranolol and nadolol. More recently studies have shown carvedilol at a low dose (12.5 mg/day) to be more effective than propranolol in reducing HVPG, with lesser side effects compared to higher doses [11–13]. A study by Schwarzer et al., in 72 patients with Child A-C cirrhosis who underwent serial HVPG measurement showed a >/= 10% reduction in HVPG-response in 76% participants with low dose carvedilol (6.25–12.5 mg daily). Tolerability in those with advance disease with ascites was a concern due to side effect of hypotension [14].

Prophylactic Treatment to Prevent First Variceal Haemorrhage

Pharmacological treatment with non-selective beta-blockers or endoscopic band ligation both reduce the risk of bleeding from varices.

Risk of bleeding is related to the size of the varices, and the greatest benefit in prevention of bleeding is in patients with large varices (grade II and II varices) or small varices with red signs, and such patients should be started on primary prevention therapy. Patients with small varices without red signs do not require immediate commencement of treatment, and a surveillance endoscopy in 1 year may be performed. A randomized placebo-controlled UK trial is presently investigating carvedilol in primary prevention of small oesophageal varices (NCT03776955).

NSBB, such as propranolol, nadolol or carvedilol, have all been studied in primary prophylaxis of variceal haemorrhage and have been shown to reduce the rate of variceal haemorrhage by 40–50%. The choice of drug depends on local preferences, and usually in the UK propranolol or carvedilol are first line therapies [12].

NSBB reduce portal pressure through blocking $\beta1$- and $\beta2$-adrengic receptors in the heart and splanchnic circulation, respectively. This results in a reduction in cardiac output and an increase in splanchnic vasoconstriction which leads to reduced portal blood flow. Carvedilol also has vasodilator effects through $\alpha1$ receptor blockade which reduces intrahepatic resistance.

Most patients tolerate NSBB quite well, but up to 20% of patients discontinue treatment due to side effects. It is important to titrate up to the optimal dose as described in Table 5.3.

Once patients are commenced on NSBB, they do not require routine repeat endoscopy. Consideration should be given to temporarily stopping NSBB if patients develop hypotension and renal failure in the context of spontaneous bacterial peritonitis, but otherwise, NSBB therapy should continue indefinitely. If NSBBs are stopped endoscopic band ligation (EBL) should be performed.

Band ligation works by causing necrosis and fibrosis of the varix when a rubber band is placed on it. Bands should be placed within 5 cm of the gastro-oesophageal junction. Band ligation should be repeated at 2–4 weeks intervals until varices are obliterated.

Medium and large varices should be treated with either NSBB or EBL depending upon local resources and expertise,

TABLE 5.3 Drugs used in the management of oesophageal varices

Drug	Dose	Indications	Cautions
Propranolol	40 mg BD initially and titrate to dose maximum of 320 mg, or until HR of <50–55 bpm achieved	Primary and secondary prophylaxis	Contraindications of NSBB include severe COPD, peripheral vascular disease, heart block, heart failure Consideration to temporarily stop NSBB therapy when patients diagnosed with spontaneous bacterial peritonitis, renal impairment, or hypotension
Carvedilol	6.25 mg OD for 1 week and then increased to 12.5 mg if tolerated, or once HR <50–55 bpm achieved	Primary prophylaxis and consider in secondary prophylaxis	
Terlipressin	2 mg IV stat, then 1-2 mg every 4–6 h until haemostasis achieved, or for 3–5 days	Acute bleeding	Caution in ischaemic heart disease, peripheral vascular disease, epilepsy Terlipressin can cause hyponatraemia Other side effects include abdominal pain and diarrhoea
Octreotide	50 mcg bolus IV initially, followed by 50 mcg/h IV infusion until haemostasis achieved or for 3–5 days	Acute bleeding	Minor side effects include vomiting and diarrhoea

TABLE 5.3 (continued)

Drug	Dose	Indications	Cautions
Somatostatin	250 mcg bolus IV initially, followed by 250 mcg/h IV infusion for 3–5 days	Acute bleeding	Minor side effects include abdominal pain and diarrhoea

patient preference, characteristics, and contraindications. Although banding has been shown to have lower rates of bleeding than NSBB in a Cochrane meta-analysis, there is some evidence that carvedilol may have a similar or better efficacy than EBL. More study of carvedilol is necessary and a randomized control trial of carvedilol vs EBL in primary prevention of patients with medium to large varices (ISRCTN73887615) is presently recruiting.

In patients with large gastric varices alone, NSBB can be considered. Cyanoacrylate has been shown to be superior to NSBB in primary prevention of large gastroesophageal varices type 2 and isolated gastric varices type 1 in a single small randomized controlled trial. Further study is necessary before change in clinical practice.

Treatment of Variceal Haemorrhage

Variceal haemorrhage is associated with a mortality of 20%, and mortality increases with the severity of liver disease. It requires a co-ordinated management approach and early suspicion when patients with liver disease or possible liver disease present with haematemesis, coffee ground vomiting, melaena or rectal bleeding. Patients should be monitored closely for the development of renal failure, pneumonia, and encephalopathy. Following an episode of variceal haemorrhage like any decompensating event in a cirrhotic patient, consideration for formal liver transplant assessment is advised in eligible patients.

The goals of treatment are to stop the bleeding, prevent early re-bleeding and to prevent recurrent bleeding. Variceal haemorrhage is often a precipitant for other decompensating events such as encephalopathy or spontaneous bacterial peritonitis. Key points in the management of variceal haemorrhage are summarized in information Box 5.1.

Box 5.1 Key Points in Variceal Haemorrhage Management

- Resuscitation—Airway management including intubation if needed, High Flow Oxygen.
- Intravenous Access and commence terlipressin or alternative, antibiotics, and fluids or blood transfusion to maintain Hb of 70–80 g/dL in haemodynamically stable patients.
- Gastroscopy as soon as possible, but within 24 h.
- If evidence of Variceal Bleeding:

    – Endoscopic Band Ligation of Oesophageal Varices.
    – Cryanoacrylate or Thrombin Injection of Gastric Varices.

- If Bleeding Controlled:

    – Continue Terlipressin and Antibiotics for 5 days and then commence Secondary Prophylaxis with NSBB and continue banding programme until obliterated.

- Failure to Control Bleeding, or ReBleeding:

    – Balloon Tamponade or removable oesophageal stents.
    – TIPSS insertion if patent portal vein.

- Consider early TIPS if Childs C cirrhosis (C10–13) or MELD ≥19 with bleeding from oesophageal or gastric varices (GOV 1 and 2)within 72 h of initial bleed.

Medical Therapy

Resuscitation with volume replacement is key to ensure adequate organ perfusion, and colloids or crystalloids including normal saline should be used.

Careful assessment of the patient's airway should be performed, and intubation is required in cases of massive haemorrhage, or when the patient is at risk of aspiration, or has impaired consciousness due to hepatic encephalopathy. Endoscopic therapy can also be considerably facilitated in an intubated patient. Thus, an early liaison with anaesthesia is essential.

Once variceal haemorrhage is suspected, patients should be commenced on a vasoactive drug, such as terlipressin. Caution is required in patients with Ischemic heart disease, chronic renal failure, over 70s, pregnant women and breast-feeding mothers. Terlipressin is also described to cause hyponatremia and hence sodium levels should be carefully monitored. If terlipressin is unavailable or contraindicated, somatostatin or octreotide can be used. Vasoactive drugs should be used in combination with endoscopic therapy for up to 5 days.

In patients with advanced liver disease, bleeding from peptic ulcer disease is also common, so intravenous proton pump inhibitor therapy may also be considered. However, if there are no signs of peptic ulcer disease at endoscopy, proton pump inhibitors can be stopped.

A restrictive blood transfusion policy is superior to a liberal one, and unless the patient has significant cardiovascular disease (concern of precipitating cardiac, mesenteric, or peripheral limb ischaemia) or is haemodynamically unstable, the transfusion target should be to achieve a haemoglobin of 70–80 mg/dL [15].

Consideration should only be given to platelet transfusion when platelets are <50 x 10^9/L and there is active bleeding. A case by case decision is advised, if there is failure to control bleeding, for correction of coagulopathy with fresh frozen plasma.

Patients should be commenced on broad spectrum antibiotics for 5–7 days, in accordance with local guidelines, and this has been shown to increase survival [16, 17]. Patient risk factors and local antimicrobial susceptibility patterns should be considered to determine first line therapy for variceal haemorrhage prophylaxis. Intravenous Ceftriaxone should be considered in patients with advanced cirrhosis in settings with high prevalence of quinolone-resistant bacteria infections.

Episodic hepatic encephalopathy should be treated with lactulose, dose-titrated to aim 2–3 loose stools per day [17].

Endoscopic Variceal Ligation

Endoscopy should be performed as soon as the patient has been resuscitated in cases of massive haemorrhage, and all patients with variceal haemorrhage should have an endoscopy within 24 h. The use of pro-kinetic drugs, such as erythromycin, prior to endoscopy can improve endoscopic views. Caution should be taken with erythromycin in those with prolonged QT interval. Patients with altered consciousness should have airway protection before performing endoscopy. All patients with acute variceal haemorrhage should be considered for intensive care or other well monitored units.

Band ligation of oesophageal varices should be performed if there is active haemorrhage seen from a varix, if there are stigmata of recent bleeding (nipple sign, cherry red spots) or if there is no other source of bleeding found at endoscopy. Ligation can cause banding ulcers, which typically bleed a few days later. Occasionally, patients can develop oesophageal structuring after banding.

If endoscopy is not successful, balloon tamponade using a Linton, or Sengstaken Blackmore tube can act as a temporary bridge to definitive therapy. There is growing evidence for the use of removable expanding oesophageal stents. After 24 h of tamponade and vasoconstrictive therapy, bleeding may have stopped, and options include repeat endoscopy for banding, or TIPSS insertion. Balloon tamponade has been associated with oesophageal perforation, and if left inflated for longer than 24 h, there is an increased risk of mucosal necrosis. Balloon tamponade and removable oesophageal stents should only be placed by those that have sufficient training and experience.

All patients should have an ultrasound to check portal vein patency.

Failure of First Line Therapy

Early re-bleeding is defined as fresh haematemesis within 5 days of an initial bleeding episode that is associated with hypovolaemic shock and a 3 g drop in haemoglobin [16, 18].

If re-bleeding is severe or persistent despite combination of pharmacological and endoscopic therapy, salvage PTFE-covered TIPSS is likely to be the best option.

TIPSS Placement

TIPSS reduces portal pressure by shunting portal blood to the hepatic vein. Generally, TIPSS are placed by an interventional radiologist, and modern PTFE covered stents have vastly superior patency to uncovered stents. Up to 30% of patients develop hepatic encephalopathy after TIPSS, and this is treated as for other causes of encephalopathy, but rarely the stent may need to be modified to reduce its diameter or even occluded. Other complications of TIPSS placement include liver failure, TIPSS stenosis and thrombosis, infection, and cardiac complications.

The indications for TIPSS in acute variceal bleeding include salvage therapy where first line therapy has failed, and in selected high-risk patients where initial therapy has been successful (early TIPSS within 72 h of initial bleed). Salvage TIPSS is not recommended where Child Pugh score is >13. Early TIPSS can be considered in Childs C cirrhosis

(C10–13) or MELD ≥19 with bleeding from oesophageal or gastric varices (GOV 1 and 2) [19]. Further study is necessary to assess the benefit of early TIPSS in less advanced cirrhosis and in the presence of active bleeding at endoscopy.

Shunt surgery, or splenectomy in those with left sided portal hypertension, if there is local surgical expertise, can be considered in patients who cannot have a TIPSS for technical reasons, e.g. portal vein thrombosis.

Secondary Prophylaxis

Following a variceal haemorrhage, from day 5 onwards, patients should have combination of NSBB and endoscopic variceal ligation every 2–4 weeks until all varices are obliterated. At that point, repeat endoscopy should be performed in 3 months, then 6 months, and any further varices ligated.

Beta blocker therapy should also be commenced as evidence shows that a dual strategy of band ligation and beta blocker therapy are superior in preventing re-bleeding than either therapy alone. It is clear NSBB is key to successful secondary prophylaxis (propranolol or nodalol), although in a patient with refractory ascites should be used cautiously and stopped if patients develop systolic blood pressure of <90 mmHg, hyponatremia (Na <130 mEq/L) or acute kidney injury. Re-initiation of NSBB starting at low dose and gradual re-titration should be considered once these parameters have settled. Evidence is scarce to recommend the use of carvedilol in prevention of re-bleeding. A suitable candidate who continues to be intolerant of NSBB should be assessed for TIPSS placement. TIPSS can also be considered where a patient rebleeds despite optimal secondary prophylaxis.

For patients with portal hypertensive gastropathy, NSBB remains first line therapy to prevent recurrent bleed. Those with transfusion dependent PHG despite iron, and where NSBB therapy is ineffective or not tolerated should be considered for TIPSS.

Gastric Varices

Gastric varices are graded by the Sarin classification depending on location: Gastroesophageal varices (GOV) type 1 and 2, which are continuous with oesophageal varices; and Isolated Gastric varices (IGV) type 1 and 2 [20]. GOV1 are 2–5 cm below the gastroesophageal junction, while GOV2 are in the cardia and fundus. IGV1 occur in the fundus and IGV2 occur in gastric body, antrum, or pylorus.

Similarly, to oesophageal varices, the risk of bleeding is related to the size of the varix, presence of red spots, and the severity of underlying liver disease; however, IGV1 varices are the most likely to bleed. Gastric variceal haemorrhage is more severe than oesophageal and carries a higher risk of mortality.

Gastric varices (GOV2, IGV1, IGV2) should be injected with tissue adhesives, such as cyanoacrylate or histoacryl glue if there are signs of active bleeding [10]. Distal embolization is a complication of glue. Human thrombin has been used in a small number of studies and shows promise for the treatment of gastric varices. Using endoscopic ultrasound to guide injection may be of assistance in selected cases, particularly GOV2.

In patients with gastric varices, repeat glue, or human thrombin injection, at the same endoscopy intervals as band ligation is recommended, even though there is not the same evidence base.

Questions
1. How to define clinically significant portal hypertension?

   Answer: HVPG is gold standard for measuring the portal pressure. Normal portal pressures measure <5–6 mm Hg. Clinically significant portal hypertension is defined by portal pressures of >10 mm Hg.

2. When should a Hepatitis C patient with small varices without signs of significant risk of bleeding in whom SVR has been achieved, have a repeat endoscopy?

Answer: In patients with small varices without high risk stigmata in whom risk factor has been controlled (in this case viral suppression and sustained SVR), should have follow up endoscopy in 2 years' time.

3. When to consider stopping NSBB in patients with refractory ascites?

Answer: Patient with refractory ascites who are on beta blockers, consider stopping beta blockers temporarily or permanently when either systolic BP is <90 mm Hg, Hyponatremia of <130 mEq/L and/or presence of acute renal failure.

4. When should early TIPSS placement be considered?

Answer: In patients with Childs C cirrhosis (C10–13) or MELD ≥19 with bleeding from oesophageal or gastric varices (GOV 1 and 2) within 72 h of initial bleed.

References

1. Ripoll C, Groszmann R, Garcia-Tsao G, Grace N, Burroughs A, Planas R, et al. Hepatic venous pressure gradient predicts clinical decompensation in patients with compensated cirrhosis. Gastroenterology. 2007;133(2):481–8.
2. D'Amico G, Morabito A, D'Amico M, Pasta L, Malizia G, Rebora P, et al. Clinical states of cirrhosis and competing risks. J Hepatol. 2018;68(3):563–76.
3. Newby D, Hayes P. Hyperdynamic circulation in liver cirrhosis: not peripheral vasodilatation but 'splanchnic steal'. QJM. 2002;95(12):827–30.
4. La Mura V, Garcia-Guix M, Berzigotti A, Abraldes JG, García-Pagán JC, Villanueva C, et al. A new prognostic algorithm based on stage of cirrhosis and HVPG to improve risk-stratification after variceal bleeding. Hepatology. 2020;72(4):1353–65.
5. D'amico G, Pasta L, Morabito A, D'Amico M, Caltagirone M, Malizia G, et al. Competing risks and prognostic stages of cirrhosis: a 25-year inception cohort study of 494 patients. Aliment Pharmacol Ther. 2014;39(10):1180–93.

6. Carbonell N, Pauwels A, Serfaty L, Fourdan O, Lévy VG, Poupon R. Improved survival after variceal bleeding in patients with cirrhosis over the past two decades. Hepatology. 2004;40(3):652–9.
7. Fateen W, Ragunath K, White J, Khanna A, Coletta M, Samuel S, et al. Validation of the AASLD recommendations for classification of oesophageal varices in clinical practice. Liver Int. 2020;40(4):905–12.
8. Barr RG, Wilson SR, Rubens D, Garcia-Tsao G, Ferraioli G. Update to the Society of Radiologists in ultrasound liver elastography consensus statement. Radiology. 2020;296(2):263–74.
9. De Franchis R. Expanding consensus in portal hypertension: report of the Baveno VI consensus workshop: stratifying risk and individualizing care for portal hypertension. J Hepatol. 2015;63(3):743–52.
10. Tripathi D, Stanley AJ, Hayes PC, Patch D, Millson C, Mehrzad H, et al. UK guidelines on the management of variceal haemorrhage in cirrhotic patients. Gut. 2015;64(11):1680–704.
11. Li T, Ke W, Sun P, Chen X, Belgaumkar A, Huang Y, et al. Carvedilol for portal hypertension in cirrhosis: systematic review with meta-analysis. BMJ Open. 2016;6(5):e010902.
12. Tripathi D. Drugs used in therapy of portal hypertension. Clin Liver Dis (Hoboken). 2012;1(5):136–8.
13. Tripathi D, Stanley A. Editorial: optimal dose of carvedilol in portal hypertension… nearly there. Aliment Pharmacol Ther. 2018;47(9):1328–9. https://doi.org/10.1111/apt.14607.
14. Schwarzer R, Kivaranovic D, Paternostro R, Mandorfer M, Reiberger T, Trauner M, et al. Carvedilol for reducing portal pressure in primary prophylaxis of variceal bleeding: a dose-response study. Aliment Pharmacol Ther. 2018;47(8):1162–9.
15. Villanueva C, Colomo A, Bosch A, Concepción M, Hernandez-Gea V, Aracil C, et al. Transfusion strategies for acute upper gastrointestinal bleeding. N Engl J Med. 2013;368(1):11–21.
16. Hou MC, Lin HC, Liu TT, Kuo BIT, Lee FY, Chang FY, et al. Antibiotic prophylaxis after endoscopic therapy prevents rebleeding in acute variceal hemorrhage: a randomized trial. Hepatology. 2004;39(3):746–53.
17. European Association for the Study of the Liver. EASL clinical practice guidelines for the management of patients with decompensated cirrhosis. J Hepatol. 2018;69(2):406–60.

18. Ahn SY, Park SY, Tak WY, Lee YR, Kang EJ, Park JG, et al. Prospective validation of Baveno V definitions and criteria for failure to control bleeding in portal hypertension. Hepatology. 2015;61(3):1033–40.
19. Tripathi D, Stanley AJ, Hayes PC, Travis S, Armstrong MJ, Tsochatzis EA, et al. Transjugular intrahepatic portosystemic stent-shunt in the management of portal hypertension. Gut. 2020;69(7):1173–92.
20. Sarin SK, Lahoti D, Saxena SP, Murthy NS, Makwana UK. Prevalence, classification and natural history of gastric varices: a long-term follow-up study in 568 portal hypertension patients. Hepatology. 1992;16(6):1343–9.

Chapter 6
Frailty and Sarcopenia in Cirrhosis

Osama Siddiqui, Sydney Olson, Avesh Thuluvath, and Daniela Ladner

Key Learning Points
- Frailty is a syndrome of "decreased physiologic reserve" which leads to a decreased ability to function and adapt to acute stressors.
- Frailty is associated with declines across multiple organ systems (e.g. skeletal muscle loss, immune dysfunction), and increased risk of hospitalization, disability, and death.
- Sarcopenia describes progressive generalized loss of skeletal muscle mass and may be thought of as a precursor or subdomain of the broader functional decline seen in patients with frailty.

O. Siddiqui · S. Olson · D. Ladner (✉)
Northwestern University Transplant Outcomes Research
Collaborative (NUTORC), Northwestern University Feinberg
School of Medicine, Chicago, IL, USA
e-mail: Osama.siddiqui@northwestern.edu;
Sydney.olson@northwestern.edu; dladner@nm.org

A. Thuluvath
Northwestern University McGaw Medical Center,
Chicago, IL, USA
e-mail: Avesh.thuluvath@nortwestern.edu

© Springer Nature Switzerland AG 2022
T. Cross (ed.), *Liver Disease in Clinical Practice*, In Clinical
Practice, https://doi.org/10.1007/978-3-031-10012-3_6

- Although hyperammonemia and myostatin upregulation are known to be key drivers of skeletal muscle loss, dysfunction across multiple organ systems likely contributes to the progressive disability and depletion of physiologic reserve seen in frailty.
- The prevalence of frailty (17–49%) and sarcopenia (22–70%) varies across studies due to the variety of measures used (e.g. Karnofsky Performance Status, Fried Frailty Index, Liver Frailty Index, CT muscle mass measurement).
- It is especially important to assess frailty and sarcopenia in liver transplant patients as both are associated with an approximately twofold increased risk of waitlist mortality and have been shown to provide prognostic value beyond MELD scores.
- A nationally standardized process for assessing frailty and/or sarcopenia is needed for these valuable metrics to be incorporated into the management of patients with cirrhosis.

Chapter Review Questions

1. **Are frailty and sarcopenia are the same thing?**

   (a) Yes.
   (b) No.

2. **Which of the following is a key driver of sarcopenia in liver cirrhosis?**

   (a) Hyperglycemia.
   (b) Hyperammonemia.
   (c) Hyperuricemia.
   (d) Lactic acidosis.

3. **Frailty and sarcopenia are associated with a roughly _____ times increased risk of liver transplant waitlist mortality.**

   (a) 2
   (b) 4
   (c) 6
   (d) 8

Introduction

Originally described in the field of geriatrics, frailty is a syndrome of "decreased physiologic reserve" which leads to progressive disability and a decreased ability to adapt to acute illness. The syndrome is associated with declines across multiple organ systems (e.g. skeletal muscle loss, immune dysfunction), and increased risk of hospitalization, disability, and death [1]. For example, a frail person may develop sepsis due to a minor infection (e.g. urinary tract infection) rather than demonstrating a self-limiting course. Similarly, frail patients may have difficulty with activities of daily living and a higher risk of falls due to skeletal muscle loss. Although frailty was originally associated with aging, it is now known to be prevalent in chronic disease. Medical conditions such as renal failure and liver cirrhosis cause dysfunction across multiple organs and may accelerate the age-related depletion of physiologic reserve [2, 3].

Frailty is present in up to 49% of patients with liver cirrhosis and is associated with increased morbidity and mortality [3]. Cirrhosis (replacement of hepatocytes with scar tissue) has many etiologies (viral hepatitis, alcoholic steatohepatitis, etc.) and can lead to complications across multiple organ systems [4, 5]. Most patients with cirrhosis have compensated disease, but once they develop complications such as gastrointestinal variceal bleeding, ascites, and hepatic encephalopathy, their disease has progressed to "decompensated" cirrhosis [5]. These acute decompensating events can be life threatening, especially in those patients with cirrhosis who are frail. Frail patients lack the "physiologic reserve" present in healthy people to adequately respond to acute illness and decompensating events, and are therefore at increased risk of hospitalization and death [3]. Furthermore, frailty is associated with decreased quality of life and increased risk of depression in patients with cirrhosis [3].

Frailty is often discussed in conjunction with the term sarcopenia ("poverty of flesh," Greek). Sarcopenia is a progressive generalized loss of skeletal muscle mass that occurs with aging and chronic disease. It is an overlapping but distinct concept from frailty. For example, patients with decreased muscle mass may still have normal physical function and quality of life [6]. Although the exact relationship between sarcopenia and frailty remains controversial, loss of skeletal muscle mass may be thought of as a precursor or subdomain of the broader functional decline seen in patients with frailty [7]. Nevertheless, just like frailty, sarcopenia is associated with increased mortality in cirrhosis [8]. Studies directly comparing the relationship between sarcopenia and frailty, and their predictive power in cirrhosis are limited [9]. Therefore, frailty and sarcopenia are currently assessed independently rather than using one as a surrogate for the other.

Frailty and sarcopenia are emerging as important prognostic indicators in patients with cirrhosis. The Model for End-Stage Liver Disease (MELD) score is currently used to predict 3-month mortality in cirrhosis, particularly for liver transplant allocation. However, the prognostic value of the MELD score is limited by the fact that it is calculated based solely on four lab values (creatinine, bilirubin, INR, and sodium) [10]. Therefore, measures of frailty and sarcopenia can provide additional prognostic value by taking the overall health and "physiologic reserve" of patients into account. Patients who are frail or sarcopenic have a roughly twofold increased risk of mortality than their non-frail counterparts. Furthermore, models that combine the MELD score with measures of frailty [11] or sarcopenia [12] have been shown to have significantly improved predictive value. Therefore, it is important to consider frailty and sarcopenia in the care of cirrhosis patients, especially those awaiting transplant. A brief overview of the pathophysiology, measurement, and clinical implications of frailty and sarcopenia is presented below.

Pathophysiology of Frailty and Sarcopenia

The exact cause of frailty and sarcopenia in chronic liver disease remains unknown and the pathophysiology is not completely understood. Although hyperammonemia and

TABLE 6.1 The Pathophysiology of Frailty

Organ system	Pathophysiologic changes
Immune system	Chronic low-grade inflammation (high IL-6, CRP, TNF-a, neutrophils, macrophages) Dysfunctional immune activation leads to increased susceptibility to infection
Endocrine	Low levels of anabolic signals (growth hormone, IGF-1, vitamin D, testosterone, estradiol, DHEAS)
Skeletal muscle	Increased protein metabolism Loss of myocytes High levels of myostatin (due to hyperammonemia) inhibit muscle growth [13]
Nervous system	Impaired mitochondria, protein transport, and synaptic function Loss of high metabolic demand neurons
Gut microbiome	Decreased *Faecalibacterium prausnitzii* (known to have anti-inflammatory effects in the gut)

Adapted from Van Jacobs 2019 [3]

myostatin upregulation are known to be key drivers of skeletal muscle loss, dysfunction across multiple organ systems likely contributes to the overall depletion of "physiologic reserve" and functional capacity seen in patients with frailty [3, 13]. Some pathophysiologic changes associated with frailty in liver cirrhosis are summarized in Table 6.1.

Measuring Frailty and Its Clinical Impact

A variety of methods have been developed to measure frailty and sarcopenia in patients with cirrhosis. The prevalence of frailty (17–49%) [3] and sarcopenia (22–70%) [14] varies across studies depending on the measures and diagnostic thresholds used. However, regardless of measurement methodology, frailty and sarcopenia are associated with a roughly twofold increased risk of mortality in patients with cirrhosis.

The main features, predictive value, strengths, and limitations of some commonly used measures of frailty and sarcopenia are summarized below.

Karnofsky Performance Status (KPS)

The Karnofsky Performance Status (KPS) scale was originally developed in 1949 to assess patients with cancer in terms of their potential to benefit from chemotherapy. Later on, KPS scores were validated for use in patients with cirrhosis. KPS scores range from 0 to 100 and are assigned based on a physician's subjective assessment of a patient's ability to perform activities of daily living (Table 6.2). KPS scores can be further divided into four categories for risk stratification. These categories correspond to the Eastern Cooperative Oncology Group (ECOG) performance status which is also widely used in cancer trials. Cirrhosis patients with KPS scores of 10–30 (category 4) have an almost two-fold increased risk of mortality 3 months after listing for liver transplant (Table 6.2) [15]. KPS scores combined with MELD and age (AUC = 0.74) provide a superior prediction of 3-month mortality than MELD alone (AUC = 0.67) in patients with cirrhosis after hospital discharge [16]. Lower KPS scores are also associated with increased risk of graft failure and mortality after liver transplant [17].

Although the predictive value of KPS scores has been studied extensively in multiple clinical settings, their subjective nature is a major limitation. KPS scores have variable interobserver reliability [18] and correlate poorly with actual physical activity [19]. Furthermore, KPS scores are vulnerable to bias especially if used in high stakes settings. The Scientific Registry of Transplant Recipients (SRTR) discontinued the use of KPS scores for risk adjustment of transplant center outcomes due to concerns over their use to "game the system." [20] KPS scores reported to the United Network for Organ Sharing (UNOS) have also been shown to vary with factors such as UNOS region, center size, and market compe-

TABLE 6.2 Karnofsky Performance Status

Criteria	Score	KPS category	ECOG class	3-month waitlist mortality by KPS category	Adjusted hazard ratio [95% CI] for mortality by KPS category
Normal no complaints; no evidence of disease	100	KPS 1	0	18%	1.00 [reference]
Able to carry on normal activity; minor signs or symptoms of disease	90		1		
Normal activity with effort; some signs or symptoms of disease	80				
Cares for self; unable to carry on normal activity or to do active work	70	KPS 2	2	27%	1.21 [1.14–1.30]
Requires occasional assistance, but is able to care for most of his personal needs	60				

(continued)

TABLE 6.2 (continued)

Criteria	Score	KPS category	ECOG class	3-month waitlist mortality by KPS category	Adjusted hazard ratio [95% CI] for mortality by KPS category
Requires considerable assistance and frequent medical care	50	KPS 3	3	44%	1.45 [1.34–1.57]
Disabled; requires special care and assistance	40				
Severely disabled; hospital admission is indicated although death not imminent	30	KPS 4	4	85%	1.97 [1.81–2.16]
Very sick; hospital admission necessary; active supportive treatment necessary	20				
Moribund; fatal processes progressing rapidly	10				
Dead	0				

tition [18]. Therefore, more objective scales such as the Liver Frailty Index may provide a more valid and reliable measure of frailty in the clinical setting.

Fried Frailty Index (FFI)

The Fried Frailty Index (FFI) was originally developed in the field of geriatrics [1] but has also been used to study frailty in cirrhosis. FFI scores range from 0 to 5, and are determined based on a combination of objective (weight loss, 15 foot walk time, hand grip strength) and self-reported criteria (exhaustion, activity level) (Table 6.3). Based on their scores, patients are classified as **not frail** (0), **pre-frail** (1–2), or **frail** (3–5). Patients with cirrhosis classified as frail according to FFI have a significantly increased risk of hospitalization (58% vs. 36%, $p < 0.001$) [21] and mortality (22% vs. 10%, $p = 0.03$) [22] compared to their non-frail counterparts over 1 year. The association of FFI scores with hospitalization (IRR = 1.10, 95% CI 1.06–1.15, $p < 0.001$) [21] and mortality (HR = 1.45, 95% CI 1.04–2.02, $p = 0.03$) [22] remains significant even after adjusting for MELD score.

Although FFI scores have been shown to have predictive value in cirrhosis, they have some major limitations. The self-reported physical activity and exhaustion components are subjective and may not be accurate, especially in patients with hepatic encephalopathy. Furthermore, fluid retention in cirrhosis makes it challenging to accurately assess changes in body mass. The Fried Frailty Index provided an initial proof of concept of the predictive value of frailty in patients with cirrhosis. However, its utility in patients with cirrhosis remains limited since it was originally intended for use in the geriatric population. Therefore, frailty measures designed specifically for patients with cirrhosis have been developed.

TABLE 6.3 Fried Frailty Index

	Criteria	Measurement	Score
Objective	Unintentional weight loss	Unintentional weight loss of >10 pounds or ≥5% of body weight in the past year	0 = unintentional weight loss <5% and <10 lb.; or intentional weight loss 1 = unintentional weight loss ≥5% or ≥10 lb

	15 ft. walk time	Time to walk 15 feet compared to gender/height specific cutoffs
		Male:
		  Height ≤ 173 cm: ≥7 s
		  Height > 173 cm: ≥6 s
		Female:
		  Height ≤ 159 cm: ≥7 s
		  Height > 159 cm ≥6 s
			0 = 15 ft. walk time below gender/height-specific cutoff
			1 = 15 ft. walk speed above gender/height-specific cutoff

	Hand grip strength	Maximum handgrip strength in kilograms (kg) measured using a dynamometer compared to gender/BMI specific cutoffs
		Male:
		  BMI ≤24 with ≤29 kg
		  BMI 24.1–26 with ≤30 kg
		  BMI 26.1–28 with ≤30 kg
		  BMI >28 with ≤32 kg
		Female:
		  BMI ≤23 with ≤17 kg
		  BMI 23.1–26 with ≤173 kg
		  BMI 26.1–29 with ≤18 kg
		  BMI >29 with ≤21 kg
			0 = hand grip strength above gender/BMI-specific cutoff
			1 = hand grip strength below gender/BMI-specific cutoff

| Subjective | Activity level | Energy expenditure calculated from self-report of moderately strenuous physical activities[a] compared to gender specific cutoffs
Male: <383 kilocalories per week
Female: <270 kilocalories per week | 0 = calorie expenditure above gender-specific cutoff
1 = calorie expenditure below gender-specific cut points |
| | Exhaustion | Self-reported exhaustion based on 2 survey items from the CES-D scale[b]
The following two statements are read. (a) I felt that everything I did was an effort; (b) I could not get going. The question is asked "how often in the last week did you feel this way?"
0 = rarely or none of the time (<1 day), 1 = some or a little of the time (1–2 days), 2 = a moderate amount of the time (3–4 days), or 3 = most of the time | 0 = patient answered 0 or 1
1 = patient answered 2 or 3 |

Adapted from Van Jacobs 2019 [3] and Fried et al. 2001 [1]

[a]Walking, chores (moderately strenuous), mowing the lawn, raking, gardening, hiking, jogging, biking, exercise cycling, dancing, aerobics, bowling, golf, singles tennis, doubles tennis, racquetball, calisthenics, swimming (based on a short version of the Minnesota Leisure Time Activity questionnaire)

[b]Center for Epidemiology Studies Depression Scale

Liver Frailty Index (LFI)

The Liver Frailty Index (LFI) was developed by combining components of different frailty scales used in geriatrics (FFI, activities of daily living, etc.) to create a model that best predicted mortality in patients with cirrhosis listed for transplant [23]. LFI is calculated based on hand grip strength, chair stands, and balance with scores ranging from 1 to 7 (Table 6.4). Patients are classified as **robust** (<3.2), **pre-frail** (3.2–4.4), or **frail** (≥4.5) based on their LFI score. Patients with cirrhosis classified as frail by LFI have a roughly two-fold higher risk

Table 6.4 Liver Frailty Index

Criteria	Measurement	Score
Hand grip strength	Maximum grip strength in dominant hand measured using a dynamometer Measured in kilograms (average of three trials, adjusted for sex)	LFI score = (−0.330 × sex-adjusted grip strength) + (−2.529 × number of chair stands per second) + (−0.040 × balance time) + 6
Chair stands	Time (in seconds) to stand from seated position with arms folded across chest	
Balance	Maximum time (up to 10 s per position) a subject can maintain balance in three positions (feet side-to-side, semi-tandem, tandem)	

A calculator and detailed instructions are available at https://liver-frailtyindex.ucsf.edu/

of mortality than their non-frail counterparts at 6 months (14.8% vs. 6.5%), and 1 year (25.2% vs. 11.4%) after listing for transplant [24]. The association between LFI score and waitlist mortality remains significant after adjustment for MELD-Na, age, sex, and BMI (subhazard ratio: 1.92, 95% CI: 1.38–2.67, $p < 0.001$) [24]. Furthermore, the combination of LFI and MELD-Na (AUC = 0.79) is a superior predictor of waitlist mortality at 3 months than MELD-Na alone (AUC = 0.73) [11].

The objective nature, high interrater reliability [25], and predictive value of the Liver Frailty Index make it a promising candidate for guiding care. In the future, LFI scores may be considered as a factor for organ allocation in liver transplant. However, LFI scores are still vulnerable to variations based on patient effort and test administration which makes them less objective than MELD scores or imaging-derived sarcopenia measurements. Furthermore, LFI scores have largely been studied in outpatient liver transplant clinics, and their predictive value in other clinical settings, such as hospitalized patients, remains unclear [11, 23, 24]. The relationship of LFI scores with actual physical activity, quality of life, and post-transplant outcomes also requires further investigation.

CT Muscle Measurement

Measurement of skeletal muscle mass via Computerized Tomography (CT) is commonly used to diagnose sarcopenia in patients with cirrhosis. Most studies measure total cross-sectional muscle area at L3/L4 or psoas muscle area. The area is then usually normalized by patient height and compared to standardized cutoffs for sarcopenia. The standards and cutoffs vary across studies (Table 6.5) [14]. As a result, there is wide variation in the reported prevalence of sarcopenia in cirrhosis which ranges from 22% to 70% [14]. Nevertheless, in a recent meta-analysis, patients with cirrhosis defined as sarcopenic by the Skeletal Muscle Index had an

TABLE 6.5 CT muscle mass measurement

Muscles measured	Standardized index	Calculation	Common cutoff values
All muscles in cross section at L3/L4	Skeletal muscle index	Total muscle surface area in cross section (cm^2) divided by square of patient height (m^2)	Female: 38.5 cm^2/m^2 Male: 52.4 cm^2/m^2
Psoas muscle	Psoas muscle index	Psoas muscle surface area (cm^2) divided by square of patient height (m^2)	Variable by study
	Total psoas area	Sex-specific tertiles	Variable by study

almost 2 times higher risk of waitlist mortality compared to their non-sarcopenic counterparts (pooled hazard ratio = 1.72, 95% CI = 0.99–3.00, p = 0.05) [14]. For context, one of the studies in the meta-analysis reported a 1-year waitlist mortality rate of 37% and 21% for sarcopenic and non-sarcopenic patients respectively [14]. Despite the heterogeneity in measurement protocols, adding sarcopenia to MELD scores has been shown to significantly improve predictive value [12].

The objective nature and emerging predictive value of CT muscle mass measurements make them prime candidates to guide care and potentially graft allocation. However, a few caveats need to be addressed before widespread clinical implementation. As discussed previously, a standardized protocol for quantifying muscle mass with consistent criteria for sarcopenia is yet to be developed. Furthermore, the correlation between muscle mass assessed by CT and clinical tests of physical function remains unclear [6, 26]. Further research is needed to understand whether sarcopenia can be used as a surrogate measure for frailty, and how its predictive value compares to that of functional measures such as the Liver Frailty Index.

Frailty Interventions and the Future

Both pharmacologic and non-pharmacologic interventions are currently being developed to mitigate the impact of frailty and sarcopenia in cirrhosis. Exercise programs have been shown to improve some measures of muscle strength, physical function, and quality of life in patients with cirrhosis [27]. Similarly, a handful of basic science and translational studies suggest that amino acid formulas [28], ammonia lowering drugs, myostatin inhibitors, IGF-1 analogs, testosterone supplements, and stem cell transfusion [29] may help improve frailty and sarcopenia [30]. However, research in this area is still in its infancy and the feasibility, clinical impact, and risks of such interventions remain to be determined.

With all this information in mind, there is a clear role for greater incorporation of frailty and sarcopenia measurements into managing patients with cirrhosis. Looking to the future, frailty metrics are likely to be incorporated into (1) identifying transplant candidates who would benefit from frailty focused pre-habilitation [27], (2) advising organ allocation either formally through adding frailty as a variable in the UNOS priority list [11, 12] or informally through guiding clinicians' choice to accept or reject marginal grafts which may have worse outcomes in patients with frailty [31], and (3) shaping post-transplant follow-up and physical therapy regimens to more aggressively target patients vulnerable to complications due to frailty [27]. However, as expressed in a recent expert opinion statement by the American Society of Transplantation (AST), "there is no single frailty tool that has emerged in the literature as suitable for evaluation of patients with cirrhosis in all clinical scenarios (outpatient vs. inpatient; transplant vs. nontransplant) [32]." Therefore, a nationally accepted standardized method for assessing frailty and sarcopenia is needed before these valuable measurements can be universally incorporated into the management of patients with cirrhosis.

Summary

Originally described in the field of geriatrics, frailty is a syndrome of "decreased physiologic reserve" which leads to progressive disability and a decreased ability to adapt to stressors. Frailty is associated with declines across multiple organ systems (e.g. skeletal muscle loss, immune dysfunction), and increased risk of hospitalization, disability, and death. Although frailty was originally associated with aging, it is now known to be prevalent in chronic diseases such as renal failure and cirrhosis. Sarcopenia is characterized by a progressive generalized loss of skeletal muscle mass and may be thought of as a precursor or subdomain of the broader functional decline seen patients with frailty. Although the pathophysiology of frailty and sarcopenia is incompletely understood, hyperammonemia and myostatin upregulation are thought to play a key role in skeletal muscle loss. The prevalence of frailty (17–49%) and sarcopenia (22–70%) varies across studies depending on the measures and diagnostic thresholds used.

A variety of clinical tools have been developed to measure frailty and sarcopenia in patients with cirrhosis. Some commonly studied tools include the Karnofsky Performance Status (KPS), Fried Frailty Index (FFI), Liver Frailty Index (LFI), and CT muscle mass measurement. Each measure has its pros and cons, and more research is needed to compare their predictive value. Regardless of measurement methodology, frailty and sarcopenia are associated with a roughly twofold increased risk of mortality in cirrhosis. The association is slightly attenuated but remains significant after adjusting for MELD score. This is especially important to consider when evaluating patients with cirrhosis for transplant as the combination of MELD and frailty scores is a superior predictor of waitlist mortality than MELD scores alone. Going forward, exercise programs and pharmacologic interventions targeting frailty and sarcopenia are being studied to improve outcomes in cirrhosis and transplant. However, as expressed in a recent expert opinion statement by the American Society of Transplantation (AST), "there is no single frailty tool that has emerged in the literature as suitable for evaluation of patients with cirrhosis in all clinical scenarios (outpatient vs. inpatient; transplant vs. nontransplant)." Therefore, a nationally standardized process for assessing frailty and/or sarcopenia is needed for these valuable metrics to be incorporated into the management of patients with cirrhosis.

Chapter Review Answers
1. **Are frailty and sarcopenia are the same thing?**

   (a) Yes.
   (b) No.

   - No

   Frailty is a syndrome of decreased physiologic reserve in which declines across multiple organ systems lead to progressive disability and a decreased ability to adapt to acute illness. In contrast, sarcopenia involves a progressive generalized loss of skeletal muscle mass and may be thought of as a precursor or subdomain of the broader functional decline seen in patients with frailty.

2. **Which of the following is a key driver of sarcopenia in liver cirrhosis?**

   (a) Hypoglycemia.
   (b) Hyperammonemia.
   (c) Hyperuricemia.
   (d) Lactic acidosis.

   - B

   Hyperammonemia is thought to be a key driver of sarcopenia in liver cirrhosis due to its upregulation of myostatin which inhibits muscle growth

3. **Frailty and sarcopenia are associated with a roughly _____ times increased risk of liver transplant waitlist mortality.**

   (a) 2
   (b) 4

(c) 6
(d) 8

- A

  Although the prevalence of frailty and sarcopenia varies with measurement methodology, most studies
  show a roughly two-fold increased risk of mortality
  in liver cirrhosis patients listed for transplant.

References

1. Fried LP, Tangen CM, Walston J, et al. Frailty in older adults: evidence for a phenotype. J Gerontol A Biol Sci Med Sci. 2001;56(3):M146–56. https://doi.org/10.1093/gerona/56.3.m146.
2. Zhang Q, Ma Y, Lin F, Zhao J, Xiong J. Frailty and mortality among patients with chronic kidney disease and end-stage renal disease: a systematic review and meta-analysis. Int Urol Nephrol. 2020;52(2):363–70. https://doi.org/10.1007/s11255-019-02369-x.
3. Van Jacobs AC. Frailty assessment in patients with liver cir-rhosis. Clin Liver Dis (Hoboken). 2019;14(3):121–5. https://doi.org/10.1002/cld.825.
4. Heidelbaugh JJ, Bruderly M. Cirrhosis and chronic liver fail-ure: part I. Diagnosis and evaluation. Am Fam Physician. 2006;74(5):756–62.
5. Heidelbaugh JJ, Sherbondy M. Cirrhosis and chronic liver fail-ure: part II. Complications and treatment. Am Fam Physician. 2006;74(5):767–76.
6. Yadav A, Chang YH, Carpenter S, et al. Relationship between sarcopenia, six-minute walk distance and health-related quality of life in liver transplant candidates. Clin Transpl. 2015;29(2):134–41. https://doi.org/10.1111/ctr.12493.
7. Bauer JM, Sieber CC. Sarcopenia and frailty: a clinician's con-troversial point of view. Exp Gerontol. 2008;43(7):674–8. https://doi.org/10.1016/j.exger.2008.03.007.
8. Montano-Loza AJ, Meza-Junco J, Prado CM, et al. Muscle wasting is associated with mortality in patients with cirrhosis. Clin Gastroenterol Hepatol. 2012;10(2):166–173.e1. https://doi.org/10.1016/j.cgh.2011.08.028.
9. Kahn J, Wagner D, Homfeld N, Müller H, Kniepeiss D, Schemmer P. Both sarcopenia and frailty determine suitability of patients

for liver transplantation-a systematic review and meta-analysis of the literature. Clin Transpl. 2018;32(4):e13226. https://doi.org/10.1111/ctr.13226.

10. Kim WR, Biggins SW, Kremers WK, Wiesner RH, Kamath PS, Benson JT, Edwards E, Therneau TM. Hyponatremia and mortality among patients on the liver-transplant waiting list. N Engl J Med. 2008;359(10):1018–26. https://doi.org/10.1056/NEJMoa0801209.

11. Kardashian A, Ge J, McCulloch CE, et al. Identifying an optimal liver frailty index cutoff to predict waitlist mortality in liver transplant candidates. Hepatology. 2021;73(3):1132–9. https://doi.org/10.1002/hep.31406.

12. Montano-Loza AJ, Duarte-Rojo A, Meza-Junco J, et al. Inclusion of sarcopenia within MELD (MELD-Sarcopenia) and the prediction of mortality in patients with cirrhosis. Clin Transl Gastroenterol. 2015;6(7):e102. https://doi.org/10.1038/ctg.2015.31.

13. Bojko M. Causes of sarcopenia in liver cirrhosis. Clin Liver Dis (Hoboken). 2019;14(5):167–70. https://doi.org/10.1002/cld.851.

14. van Vugt JL, Levolger S, de Bruin RW, van Rosmalen J, Metselaar HJ, IJzermans JN. Systematic review and meta-analysis of the impact of computed tomography-assessed skeletal muscle mass on outcome in patients awaiting or undergoing liver transplantation. Am J Transplant. 2016;16(8):2277–92. https://doi.org/10.1111/ajt.13732.

15. McCabe P, Wong RJ. More severe deficits in functional status associated with higher mortality among adults awaiting liver transplantation. Clin Transpl. 2018;32(9):e13346. https://doi.org/10.1111/ctr.13346.

16. Tandon P, Reddy KR, O'Leary JG, et al. A Karnofsky performance status-based score predicts death after hospital discharge in patients with cirrhosis. Hepatology. 2017;65(1):217–24. https://doi.org/10.1002/hep.28900.

17. Thuluvath PJ, Thuluvath AJ, Savva Y. Karnofsky performance status before and after liver transplantation predicts graft and patient survival. J Hepatol. 2018;69(4):818–25. https://doi.org/10.1016/j.jhep.2018.05.025.

18. Wang CW, Lai JC. Reporting functional status in UNOS: the weakness of the Karnofsky performance status scale. Clin Transpl. 2017;31(7). https://doi.org/10.1111/ctr.13004.

19. Dunn MA, Josbeno DA, Schmotzer AR, et al. The gap between clinically assessed physical performance and objective physi-

cal activity in liver transplant candidates. Liver Transpl. 2016;22(10):1324–32. https://doi.org/10.1002/lt.24506.

20. Kasiske BL, Salkowski N, Wey A, Zaun D, Israni AK, Snyder JJ. Response to Bui et al, "patient functional status at transplant and its impact on Posttransplant survival of adult deceased-donor kidney recipients". Transplantation. 2020;104(2):e59. https://doi.org/10.1097/TP.0000000000002926.

21. Sinclair M, Poltavskiy E, Dodge JL, Lai JC. Frailty is independently associated with increased hospitalisation days in patients on the liver transplant waitlist. World J Gastroenterol. 2017;23(5):899–905. https://doi.org/10.3748/wjg.v23.i5.899.

22. Lai JC, Feng S, Terrault NA, Lizaola B, Hayssen H, Covinsky K. Frailty predicts waitlist mortality in liver transplant candidates. Am J Transplant. 2014;14(8):1870–9. https://doi.org/10.1111/ajt.12762.

23. Lai JC, Covinsky KE, Dodge JL, et al. Development of a novel frailty index to predict mortality in patients with end-stage liver disease. Hepatology. 2017;66(2):564–74. https://doi.org/10.1002/hep.29219.

24. Haugen CE, McAdams-DeMarco M, Holscher CM, et al. Multicenter study of age, frailty, and waitlist mortality among liver transplant candidates. Ann Surg. 2020;271(6):1132–6. https://doi.org/10.1097/SLA.0000000000003207.

25. Wang CW, Lebsack A, Chau S, Lai JC. The range and reproducibility of the liver frailty index. Liver Transpl. 2019;25(6):841–7. https://doi.org/10.1002/lt.25449.

26. Wang CW, Feng S, Covinsky KE, et al. A comparison of muscle function, mass, and quality in liver transplant candidates: results from the functional assessment in liver transplantation study. Transplantation. 2016;100(8):1692–8. https://doi.org/10.1097/TP.0000000000001232.

27. Williams FR, Berzigotti A, Lord JM, Lai JC, Armstrong MJ. Review article: impact of exercise on physical frailty in patients with chronic liver disease. Aliment Pharmacol Ther. 2019;50(9):988–1000. https://doi.org/10.1111/apt.15491.

28. Chakravarthy MV, Neutel J, Confer S, et al. Safety, tolerability, and physiological effects of AXA1665, a novel composition of amino acids, in subjects with child–pugh A and B cirrhosis. Clin Transl Gastroenterol. 2020;11(8):e00222. https://doi.org/10.14309/ctg.0000000000000222.

29. Amer ME, El-Sayed SZ, El-Kheir WA, et al. Clinical and laboratory evaluation of patients with end-stage liver cell fail-

ure injected with bone marrow-derived hepatocyte-like cells. Eur J Gastroenterol Hepatol. 2011;23(10):936–41. https://doi.org/10.1097/MEG.0b013e3283488b00.

30. Sinclair M, Gow PJ, Grossmann M, Angus PW. Review article: sarcopenia in cirrhosis--aetiology, implications and potential therapeutic interventions. Aliment Pharmacol Ther. 2016;43(7):765–77. https://doi.org/10.1111/apt.13549.

31. Kalafateli M, Mantzoukis K, Choi Yau Y, Mohammad AO, Arora S, Rodrigues S, de Vos M, Papadimitriou K, Thorburn D, O'Beirne J, Patch D, Pinzani M, Morgan MY, Agarwal B, Yu D, Burroughs AK, Tsochatzis EA. Malnutrition and sarcopenia predict post-liver transplantation outcomes independently of the Model for End-stage Liver Disease score. J Cachexia Sarcopenia Muscle. 2017;8(1):113–21. https://doi.org/10.1002/jcsm.12095; Epub 2016 Feb 1.

32. Lai JC, Sonnenday CJ, Tapper EB, et al. Frailty in liver transplantation: an expert opinion statement from the American Society of Transplantation liver and intestinal Community of Practice. Am J Transplant. 2019;19(7):1896–906. https://doi.org/10.1111/ajt.15392.

Chapter 7
Non-alcoholic Fatty Liver Disease

David Koeckerling, Thomas Marjot, and Jeremy Cobbold

Key Learning Points
- NAFLD represents a major global health burden and is closely associated with features of the metabolic syndrome.
- The pathogenesis of NAFLD is complex and the disease progression highly variable between individuals.
- The severity of hepatic fibrosis is the key feature determining prognosis so consequently patients require risk stratification using non-invasive approaches.
- Optimal management includes a multidisciplinary approach with focus on addressing cardio-metabolic risk factors as well as liver specific investigation and management.

D. Koeckerling
Medical Sciences Division, University of Oxford, Oxford, UK

T. Marjot
Oxford Centre for Diabetes, Endocrinology and Metabolism, University of Oxford, Oxford, UK

J. Cobbold (✉)
Department of Gastroenterology and Hepatology,
Oxford University Hospitals NHS Foundation Trust,
Oxford, UK
e-mail: Jeremy.Cobbold@ouh.nhs.uk

© Springer Nature Switzerland AG 2022   127
T. Cross (ed.), *Liver Disease in Clinical Practice*, In Clinical Practice, https://doi.org/10.1007/978-3-031-10012-3_7

Case Presentation and Q&A

A 58-year-old man was seen by his general practitioner after a routine health check demonstrated elevated liver biochemistry, with an alanine aminotransferase (ALT) value of 45 IU/L. He had recently been diagnosed with hypertension with BP of 162/101 mmHg and type 2 diabetes mellitus (T2D) with a glycosylated haemoglobin (HbA1c) of 69 mmol/mol (20–42 mmol/mol) for which he was started on metformin. He had no other significant past medical history and took no other medications. He had smoked ten cigarettes a day for over 20 years but drank minimal alcohol only on special occasions. The patient was asymptomatic.

His clinical examination was normal, apart from an elevated body mass index (BMI) at 31.8 kg/m^2.

The remainder of his blood tests showed haemoglobin 14.8 g/dl (13–17), white cell count 5.18 × 10^9/L (4–11), platelet count of 145 × 10^9/L; aspartate aminotransferase (AST) 43 IU/L, bilirubin 16 umol/L (3–17), alkaline phosphatase (ALP) 100 IU/L (20–140) and albumin 39 g/L (35–50). He had an elevated total cholesterol of 6 mmol/L. An abdominal ultrasound scan showed an echogenic liver, but otherwise normal appearances.

His Fibrosis-4 (FIB-4) was calculated as 2.6, an indeterminate score for advanced fibrosis

1. How would you make a diagnosis of NAFLD?
2. What is the significance of an indeterminate FIB-4?
3. How would you proceed to investigate?
4. What would be your approach to management?

Introduction

Non-alcoholic fatty liver disease (NAFLD) is a chronic liver disease which is closely related to features of the metabolic syndrome. It involves the accumulation of liver fat in the absence of other hepatic insults such as viral hepatitis or excessive alcohol intake. NAFLD encompasses a histopathological spectrum of disease ranging from simple steatosis to inflammation with hepatocyte injury, and eventually to fibrosis and cirrhosis (Table 7.1). NAFLD represents the commonest cause of liver disease worldwide, with up to 30% of the developed world affected, 80% of patients with T2DM affected and an estimated global prevalence of one billion. This explosion in numbers likely reflects both the growing global epidemic of obesity and obesity-related disease and an increased understanding and awareness of the condition. As a result, NAFLD has become the fastest growing indication for liver transplantation in the developed world. The percentage of patients undergoing liver transplantation for NASH cirrhosis in Europe has increased from 1.2% in 2002 to 8.4% in 2016, with NAFLD now being the second leading aetiology in patients requiring liver transplantation, after alcohol-related liver disease [3, 4].

TABLE 7.1 A brief glossary of terminology used in non-alcoholic fatty liver disease

Terminology	Definition
Cryptogenic cirrhosis	Cirrhosis with no obvious aetiology. Metabolic risk factors are prevalent in these patients and many are likely to have had underlying NASH [1]
'Fatty liver disease' (hepatic steatosis)	Accumulation of triglyceride droplets within the hepatic parenchyma, affecting >5% of hepatocytes
Fibrosis 4 (FIB-4)	Non-invasive scoring system used to help stratify NAFLD patients into those with low, indeterminate or high risk of advanced fibrosis
"Metabolic-dysfunction associated fatty liver disease" (**MAFLD**)	A newer term which encompasses NAFLD that describes the pathophysiology and allows for co-existence of other factors (e.g. alcohol) [2]

(continued)

TABLE 7.1 (continued)

Terminology	Definition
'Non-alcoholic fatty liver' (**NAFL**) also called 'simple steatosis'	Subcategory of NAFLD Hepatic steatosis without steatohepatitis, particularly without evidence of hepatocellular injury (ballooning of hepatocytes) [1]
'Non-alcoholic fatty liver disease' (**NAFLD**)	(a) Hepatic steatosis on imaging or histology (b) Absence of secondary causes for hepatic steatosis, including Substantial alcohol consumption, steatogenic medications, hepatitis C infection [1]
'Non-alcoholic steatohepatitis' (**NASH**)	Subcategory of NAFLD Hepatic steatosis + inflammation with evidence for hepatocyte injury (ballooning) +/− lobular or portal inflammation+/− hepatic fibrosis [1]
NASH with advanced fibrosis	Subcategory of NAFLD NASH with bridging fibrosis or cirrhosis, i.e. stage 3 or 4 out of 4, according to Kleiner and Brunt
NASH cirrhosis	Subcategory of NAFLD Advanced liver fibrosis with nodule formation in the context of current or previous NAFL/NASH [1]

Pathophysiology

Obesity and insulin resistance lead to hepatic steatosis through mechanisms including: (1) increased free fatty acid delivery from peripheral adipose tissue to the liver; (2) decreased fatty acid clearance through beta-oxidation; (3) increased hepatic de novo lipogenesis (DNL); and (4) decreased fat export from the liver in the form of very-low density lipoprotein (VLDL). The reason why some patients who develop steatosis also develop inflammation (NASH) and/or fibrosis is not entirely understood, but likely occurs through the complex interplay of genetic, environmental and gut microbial factors as 'multiple parallel hits.' Genetic factors such as polymorphisms in PNPLA3 and TM6SF2 have been shown to be determinant of inter-individual differences in hepatic fat content as well as a determinant of NASH and progressive hepatic injury. Ongoing insulin resistance derived from a sedentary lifestyle coupled with a Westernized diet rich in refined carbohydrates and soft drinks as well as a high daily total energy intake have been implicated in disease progression. Particularly the consumption of fructose, the main component of the widely used sweeteners sucrose and corn syrup, and its metabolism to uric acid have been linked to increased hepatic fat accumulation and higher fibrosis stages. The precise mechanism underlying the connection between obesity and NAFLD remains unknown, but adipose tissue dysfunction leads to reduced production of adiponectin, an adipokine with extensive hepatoprotective effects. Increasing evidence also suggests that the chronic low-grade systemic inflammatory state conferred by obesity is strongly associated with worsening insulin resistance and progressive NAFLD. The influence of the gut, particularly the gut microbiota on features of the metabolic syndrome and hepatic inflammation is also well recognized. Decreased microbiome quality and diversity as well as reductions in the quantity of *Bacteroidetes* have been implicated in gut–liver axis dysfunction with increased nutrient energy absorption, intestinal permeability and translocation of bacteria into the portal circulation [5, 6].

Natural History

Progression of NAFLD is variable and does not necessarily follow a linear pathway from NAFL through to NASH and fibrosis. NAFL in isolation tends to run a benign clinical course and despite its very high prevalence only a minority will go on to develop progressive disease [7]. Furthermore, those who do develop NASH may over time resort back to a non-inflammatory state. It is the evolution of fibrosis which is most clinically significant and represents the only histological feature to predict overall mortality, liver transplantation and liver-related events (Fig. 7.1) [8, 9]. As with other causes of chronic liver disease, inflammation is considered necessary for fibrogenesis, but histological NASH, although closely associated with fibrosis, does not seem to be a prerequisite. As a result, longitudinal studies have shown that NASH alone is not a reliable lesion to determine prognosis but may be associated with more rapid fibrosis progression [10]. In terms of clinical outcome, patients with a diagnosis of NAFLD have an increased overall mortality compared with the general

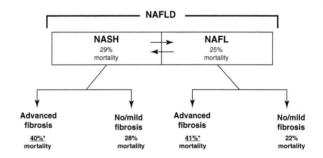

% Mortality/liver transplantation over 12.6 yrs
Angulo et al 2015

*p < 0.05 in multivariate analysis

Figure 7.1 The natural history of non-alcoholic fatty liver disease (NAFLD). *NAFL* non-alcoholic fatty liver, *NASH* non-alcoholic steatohepatitis, *HCC* hepatocellular carcinoma [8]

population, but this is accounted for by those who have developed fibrosis. The co-existence of NAFLD and type 2 diabetes mellitus (T2DM) is common, and the presence of T2DM is believed to drive fibrogenesis in patients with NAFLD. The degree of glycaemic control has been linked directly to the severity of fibrosis on liver biopsy in patients with NAFLD and T2DM, with every 1% rise in HbA1c transferring 15% increased odds of higher fibrosis stage [11].

By far the most common cause of death is from cardiovascular disease (CVD) followed by non-liver cancers, complications of cirrhosis and hepatocellular carcinoma (HCC) [8]. Importantly, the development of HCC can occur in the absence of cirrhosis.

Making the Diagnosis of NAFLD

In practice, NAFLD is most commonly identified in those with a combination of elevated aminotransferase values and/or hepatic steatosis on imaging, in the presence of one or more metabolic risk factors. However, NAFLD can exist in the absence of these features. Unfortunately, given the non-specific presentation of NAFLD, the absence of a single reliable diagnostic test and limited awareness of NAFLD's capability to progress, some patients will only be diagnosed once they develop features of cirrhosis and decompensated chronic liver disease.

Clinical History and Examination

By definition, a diagnosis of NAFLD requires the absence of excessive alcohol consumption, which is typically defined as 21 units per week on average in men and < 14 units on average per week in women (1 unit equals 10 ml or 8 g ethanol), although criteria vary. Other secondary aetiologies for steatosis should be excluded, including medications(e.g. corticosteroids, tamoxifen, amiodarone, highly active anti-retroviral therapy), hepatitis C infection, parenteral nutrition and Wilson's disease. A history of T2D, hypertension, dyslipidemia and obesity all increase the likelihood of a diagnosis of NAFLD and are risk factors for more aggressive disease. Most patients with NAFLD will be asymptomatic or have nonspecific symptoms such as disturbed sleep and fatigue. Occasionally some patients may present with right upper quadrant pain. As a result, for many patients NAFLD will be found incidentally on imaging as part of investigation for another condition. There are no specific physical examination findings for NAFLD, but abdominal obesity and hepatomegaly are common. Once cirrhosis has developed, patients may develop stigmata of chronic liver disease and features of portal hypertension.

Blood Tests

Liver enzymes are not a sensitive marker of NAFLD and up to 84% of patients diagnosed with NAFLD will have an alanine aminotransferase (ALT) within normal range. Furthermore, elevated aminotransferase values (ALT and AST) do not correlate with histology or predict disease progression. The current 'normal values' for aminotransferases are likely to be too high given that they were developed historically from populations which included an undiagnosed burden of Hepatitis C virus and NAFLD. As a result, lower cut-off values have been suggested in order to reflect true normal ranges, but these have yet to be adopted in mainstream practice. Whilst liver biochemistry is insensitive for diagnosis of NAFLD, for those who do have elevated aminotransferase levels, NAFLD is a common underlying condition. In over 350 patients referred for liver biopsy with elevated aminotransferase values and a negative chronic liver disease screen, 66% had NAFLD on histology [12].

Imaging

Several imaging techniques are available to help diagnose and quantify the degree of hepatic steatosis. Abdominal ultrasound has a good sensitivity when hepatic steatosis is greater than 33% but falls significantly when fat content drops below 30% and in obese individuals. The controlled attenuation parameter (CAP), acquired at the time of transient elastography (described below), has emerged as a promising tool for hepatic steatosis, which measures the attenuation of the amplitude of ultrasound waves passing through the liver and this technique is subject to ongoing validation. Magnetic resonance imaging and spectroscopy can not only detect a liver fat content of over 5% with near 100% accuracy but, with appropriate analysis, are also able to quantify steatosis. The role of such techniques in clinical practice has yet to be established.

Non-invasive Markers of Fibrosis in NAFLD

Scoring Systems

As the presence of advanced hepatic fibrosis predicts adverse clinical outcomes, non-invasive tools are needed to find such patients. Several non-invasive scoring systems have been developed to help predict those likely to have developed advanced stages of disease. Many scores incorporate liver biochemistry, particularly the AST/ALT ratio, which tends to rise above 0.8 in significant disease, with other blood and demographic parameters. The FIB-4 takes into account AST, ALT, platelet count and age, whilst an alternative scoring system is the NAFLD fibrosis score (NFS) which combines the AST/ALT ratio with age, BMI, T2DM or impaired glucose tolerance, platelets and albumin. It is worth noting the emphasis this score places on metabolic features (BMI and insulin resistance) as predictors of fibrosis. Both scores can easily be calculated from readily accessible online calculators. Both the FIB-4 and NFS help stratify patients into those at low, indeterminate or high risk of liver fibrosis. Those with low-risk scores can be reassured as the negative predictive value (NPV) for advanced fibrosis exceeds 93% (Table 7.2), the positive predictive values (PPV) however are poorer (<62%) meaning that those with indeterminate or high-risk scores warrant further investigation.

The Enhanced Liver Fibrosis (ELF™) test is an example of a panel of direct fibrosis markers validated in a number of chronic liver diseases, incorporating assessment of factors involved in fibrogenesis (Table 7.2). When used in NAFLD, it has been found to have a high sensitivity and specificity for the identification of advanced fibrosis.

Transient Elastography

Scarred or fibrotic liver tends to be stiff, which can be measured using a bedside or portable device to perform a liver stiffness measurement (LSM) using ultrasound-based elastography. A number of techniques are used, but vibration-controlled transient elastography, marketed as FibroScan® is widely used. This relatively quick and accessible technique quantifies stiffness using ultrasound to plot the progression of a pulsed shear wave and generates a LSM as a correlate of fibrosis. A low stiffness (<8 kPa) carries a reassuring negative predictive value of >97%, while the low positive predictive value of scores >8 kPa should prompt further investigation. Interpretations of elastography are also limited in obese patients. For obese patients, use of a larger FibroScan XL probe that acquires the reading from a deeper region of interest is associated with fewer measurement failures (1.1% vs. 16%) than the conventional probe, but even still, a significant discrepancy in degree of fibrosis exists between LSM and liver biopsy in 10%. Prospective series using magnetic reso-

TABLE 7.2 Non-invasive scores for advanced fibrosis. NPV; negative predictive value, PPV; positive predictive value. ELF, European Liver Fibrosis; HA, hyaluronic acid; TIMP1, tissue inhibitor of matrix metalloproteinase 1; PIIINP, amino terminal of procollagenase III

Non-invasive staging tool	Components	Scoring cut offs for advanced hepatic fibrosis
NAFLD fibrosis score	AST/ALT ratio, age, BMI, insulin resistance, platelet count, albumin	Low-risk score < −1.455 (NPV 93%) Indeterminate score 1.455–0.675 (43.6%) High-risk score > 0.675 (PPV 61.1%)
FIB-4	AST, ALT, platelet count, age	Low-risk score < 1.30 (NPV 95%) Indeterminate score 1.30–2.67 (PPV 50.6%) High-risk score > 2.67 (59.1)
BARD score	BMI, AST:ALT ratio, T2DM	Low-risk score < 2 (NPV 81.3%) High-risk score ≥ 2 (PPV 45.2%)
Transient elastography using FibroScan	Liver stiffness measurement (LSM) using handheld pulsed ultrasound	Low-risk score < 8.0 kPa (NPV 97%) Score ≥ 8 kPa (PPV 52%)
ELF panel	HA, TIMP1, PIIINP	<0.3576 NPV 94% >0.3576 PPV 71%

nance elastography (MRE) have also shown good accuracy in distinguishing between early and advanced fibrosis (86% sensitivity, 91% specificity) but the technique remains expensive and is not widely available. Newer multiparametric MRI techniques have shown promise in quantifying steatosis, fibrosis/inflammation and iron deposition all of which are associated with more aggressive disease.

The majority of patients with NAFLD are looked after in primary care, but those with more advanced disease are likely to benefit from more intensive management in a secondary care setting. In order to identify patients with advanced disease earlier and simultaneously reduce unnecessary referrals of low-risk patients to secondary care, non-invasive scoring systems were combined to form 'two-tiered' risk assessment pathways. Initially, advanced fibrosis is detected or excluded using either the NFS or FIB-4 as an inexpensive first screen. Patients who achieve indeterminate scores undergo retesting with more accurate and costly tests, such as ELF testing or transient elastography. One such model which has been successfully validated and implemented into clinical practice is the 'Camden and Islington NAFLD Pathway' which combines FIB-4 and ELF testing as first and second tiers, respectively (Fig. 7.2). FIB-4 and ELF testing have advantages over transient elastography in that they require no specialist equipment or training and have a lower diagnostic failure

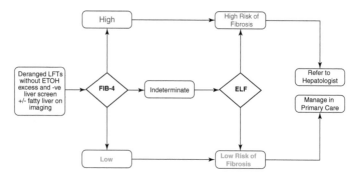

FIGURE 7.2 An example of a two-tiered risk stratification algorithm [13]

rate. In this pathway, patients deemed as low risk remain in primary care for management of their cardiometabolic risk factors and repeated risk assessment of advanced fibrosis in 3–5 years. High-risk patients are referred for further assessment by a specialist. Introduction of this pathway into clinical practice led to an 80% reduction in unnecessary referrals, while the detection of advanced fibrosis and cirrhosis increased fivefold and threefold, respectively [13].

The 'Nottingham liver disease stratification pathway' delivered an alternative algorithm to identify patients at risk of progressive liver disease in primary care. In this pathway, patients with-risk factors for NAFLD undergo BARD scoring, and those patients with a high score ($\geq$2) go on to have transient elastography at their community practices. Patients with a high-risk score on FibroScan (>8.0 kPa) are referred to specialist care. Implementation of this diagnostic pathway into GP practices in Nottingham resulted in a 140% increase of diagnosed cases of cirrhosis [14].

The Role of Liver Biopsy

Liver biopsy, despite being invasive and limited by sampling error, remains the reference standard for the evaluation of NAFLD and has a role in:

1. Confirming diagnosis of NAFLD and diagnosing hepatic co-morbidity.

    Often the diagnosis of NAFLD can be made on clinical grounds alone using liver biochemistry, imaging and history of metabolic risk factors. Liver biopsy, however, may be helpful diagnostically in patients who present atypically or who may have dual liver pathology, for example in those taking multiple medications, who have low-titres of auto-antibodies or with elevated iron indices.

2. Identification and staging of fibrosis.

    Although risk stratification tools described above allow for fibrosis to be screened for non-invasively, liver biopsy can be helpful to determine the fibrosis stage where non-invasive tests do not provide a clear answer, for example, where there are indeterminate measurements or where discrepancies between non-invasive tests or the clinical presentation exist.

3. Interventional clinical trials.

Histological examination of liver tissue obtained by liver biopsy to determine change in liver fibrosis and features of NASH remains the reference tool for primary outcome measurement in most pharmacological therapeutic clinical trials in NAFLD/NASH and is often obtained at baseline and intervals thereafter to determine efficacy of new treatments.

Management

The management of NAFLD should focus on reducing the cardiovascular risk seen in these patients and improving liver-related morbidity and mortality. The number and severity of metabolic syndrome components, and the severity of the liver disease serve to identify those patients in whom limited resources should be concentrated. Given the range of risk factors, interventions and complications, the management of NAFLD should be multidisciplinary, holistic and patient-centred (Fig. 7.3). This approach has been shown to improve

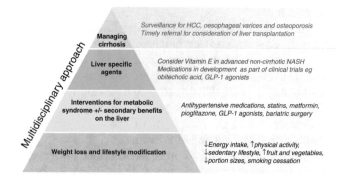

FIGURE 7.3 Management of non-alcoholic fatty liver disease (NAFLD)

surrogate markers of liver injury and cardiovascular risk including LFTs, dyslipidaemia, systolic blood pressure and BMI.

Weight Loss and Lifestyle Modification

There is consistent evidence that lifestyle interventions designed to promote healthy eating, reduce energy intake and/or increase physical activity reduce liver steatosis and improve insulin sensitivity in patients with NAFLD [15]. There is more limited data that lifestyle intervention leads to a reduction hepatic fibrosis. The optimal diet in NAFLD is not known and until further evidence is available patients should be advised to reduce consumption of saturated fat and refined carbohydrates and to calorie-restrict in an attempt to lose 0.5–1 kg/week. Evidence suggests that greater degrees of weight loss correspond to greater improvements in NAFLD histology including regression of inflammation and fibrosis, especially in those patients who achieve >10% body weight reduction [16]. Hence patients should ideally aim to lose >10% of their baseline body weight, but even in a clinical trial setting the proportion of patients managing to achieve this is less than 50% [17]. Bariatric surgery represents a more definitive way of achieving sufficient and sustained weight loss. Despite there being no formal recommendations for bariatric surgery in the context of NAFLD, recent meta-analysis of studies reporting pre- and postoperative liver histology has demonstrated a significant reduction in the incidence of steatosis (−50.2%), lobular inflammation (−50.7%) and fibrosis (−11.9%) after >12 months follow-up [18].

Smoking is significantly associated with death or liver transplantation in NAFLD (HR 2.62) [8] and cessation advice should form part of routine clinical practice. The poorer outcomes seen in smokers are predominantly due to increased number of cardiovascular events, but also through increased risk of hepatic fibrosis with a 10 pack-year history of smoking conferring an odds ratio of 2.48 for advanced fibrosis. Advising patients regarding alcohol consumption is more complex. The combination of metabolic syndrome with excessive alcohol intake is synergistic for liver fibrosis progression and the clinician should be alert to the co-existence of dual aetiologies.

Interventions for Metabolic Syndrome +/– Secondary Benefits on the Liver

Given the high cardiovascular morbidity and mortality associated with NAFLD optimization of cardiometabolic risk factors is central to management of NAFLD. In patients with diabetes, good glycaemic control should be achieved with agents that also promote weight loss and improved cardiovascular outcomes.

Metformin is currently the first line therapeutic agent in the management of patients with T2DM, improving insulin sensitivity without weight gain. Rodent models have shown that metformin reduces hepatic steatosis and inflammation, but these observations have not translated into humans. Metformin may, however, confer an overall survival benefit in patients with NAFLD and cirrhosis and reduce the risk of developing HCC.

Glucagon-like peptide-1 receptor agonists (GLP-1 RAs) promote the incretin effect, inducing satiety and weight loss, and have shown benefit in NASH, with a 48-week treatment course clearing histological NASH in 39% versus 9% in placebo group [19]. Semaglutide is another GLP-1 agonist with a similar mechanism of action to that of liraglutide, but with more potent metabolic effects. In a phase II trial, semaglutide was superior to placebo in resolving NASH, but did not lead to significant improvements in fibrosis stage [20]. It is still unclear how much of this histological benefit is mediated through improved weight loss and glycaemic control, or whether GLP-1 RAs have direct action specifically on the liver. Larger phase III trials are now underway to evaluate efficacy.

The sodium-glucose co-transporter 2 (SGLT-2) is predominantly expressed in the kidneys and reabsorbs the vast majority of glucose that is filtered by the glomerulus. SGLT-2 inhibitors are anti-hyperglycaemic agents which induce glycosuria and strengthen tubuloglomerular feedback. Independent of their glucose-lowering properties, SGLT-2 inhibitors have been shown to promote weight loss and improve cardiorenal endpoints, giving them attractive therapeutic potential beyond their original indication of improving glycaemic control in T2DM. The excretion of 60–80 g of glucose per day through glycosuria results in significant caloric loss and subsequent weight loss. In multiple landmark cardiovascular outcome trials, SGLT-2 inhibitors were able to reduce the rate of major cardiovascular events and hospitalizations for heart failure, as well as slow the progression of renal disease and albuminuria. The cardiorenal benefits of SGLT-2 inhibitors occurred, at least in part, independent of their anti-hyperglycaemic properties, yet the mechanism underlying these pleiotropic effects remains to be understood. Emerging clinical data also suggests that SGLT-2 inhibition may modulate NAFLD. In small randomized and open-label trials SGLT-2 inhibition led to improvements in liver biochemistry and reductions in liver fat content on MRI. Although there is potential for significant clinical benefits of SGLT-2 inhibition in patients with NAFLD, evidence from large, randomized trials with hard clinical or histological endpoints is currently lacking [21].

The thiazolidinedione class of antidiabetic medications such as pioglitazone, have indicated improvements in steatosis, inflammation and, possibly, fibrosis. However ongoing concern regarding fluid retention, weight gain, increased limb fracture risk and possible increase in prevalence of bladder cancer with these medications has limited their widespread use to date.

Statin use, including high intensity statin regimens, are safe in NAFLD and should be used even in those with cirrhosis or elevations in ALT or AST: often an elevated ALT or AST is found in primary care during blood monitoring after introduction of a statin, but this is more likely to reflect underlying NAFLD than statin induced liver injury. Furthermore, in patients referred for liver biopsy for suspected NASH, statin use was associated with protection from steatosis (OR 0.09), NASH (OR 0.25) and fibrosis (OR 0.42).

Liver-Specific Agents

Vitamin E has antioxidant and anti-inflammatory properties and demonstrated a significant improvement in the histological features of NASH in the PIVENS study [22]. Widespread use however has been limited by concerns regarding increased all-cause mortality with antioxidant supplementation and lack of standardized preparations.

The bile acid derivative, obeticholic acid, a potent farnesoid X receptor (FXR) agonist, has also been shown to improve histological indices of NASH and fibrosis in a phase 2 study. In the FLINT trial the proportion of participants achieving histological improvement, without worsening of fibrosis was 45% in the obeticholic acid group versus 21% in the placebo group. Fibrosis also improved in 35% of participants in the obeticholic acid group versus 19% in placebo group. The long term risks and benefits of this medication are being evaluated in a phase III clinical trial prior to widespread use in clinical practice [23]. In a planned interim analysis of this large phase III trial, one of its primary endpoints—fibrosis improvement without worsening of NASH—was achieved, with 18–23% of patients in the intervention arm experiencing fibrosis improvement compared to 12% of placebo recipients [24]. A further phase III trial of obeticholic acid in compensated NASH cirrhosis has completed enrolment of participants and follow-up of patients is ongoing, but full evaluation by the Food and Drug Administration is awaited.

Monitoring Cirrhosis, Liver Transplantation and the Multidisciplinary Approach

Patients who have developed cirrhosis as a result of NASH should be entered into standard surveillance programmes for hepatocellular carcinoma, oesophageal varices and osteoporosis. Consideration of transplantation should be along conventional guidelines.

Future Directions

The greatest effect on NAFLD will come from reducing international levels of obesity. Legislation and health policy must try to facilitate this aim, through a combination of education and behavioural change, which may include approaches such as taxation on sugar-rich soft drinks, unified food labelling, urban planning to promote physical activity, nutritional standards in schools and restricting television advertising of unhealthy food products.

At present there is insufficient data to recommend screening for NAFLD of at-risk groups such those with T2DM. This may change with emerging evidence that non-invasive techniques such as FibroScan and ELF testing may have a role in screening. Any screening strategy, however, must first undergo a robust health economic assessment before moving into clinical practice. Novel therapeutic avenues will continue to be explored including bile acid analogues, modification of the microbiome, antioxidants and further repurposing of existing medications.

Answers
1. **How would you make a diagnosis of NAFLD**
   This patient has already been found to have a raised ALT, an echogenic liver suggesting fatty infiltration and several co-existing metabolic risk factors including hyper-

tension, obesity and T2DM. A full liver screen should be performed to exclude alternative diagnoses and if negative, a diagnosis of NAFLD can confidently be diagnosed clinically.

2. **What is the significance of a high FIB-4 or NFS?**

The FIB-4 and NFS are non-invasive scoring system which help to identify patients with NAFLD at risk of advanced hepatic fibrosis. They combine age, liver biochemistry and platelet count; thrombocytopenia is often seen in cirrhosis due to increased sequestration of platelets in the spleen secondary to portal hypertension. The NFS also includes albumin and other components of the metabolic syndrome (insulin resistance and obesity) which are associated with progressive disease. Low FIB-4 and NFS scores have a high negative predictive value and advanced fibrosis can be reliably excluded, whereas indeterminate or high scores have a low positive predictive value and should prompt further investigation. Increasingly, FIB-4 and NFS are being incorporated into two-tiered risk stratification systems, in which patients with indeterminate scores undergo more accurate and costly non-invasive tests such as ELF testing or transient elastography. Patients deemed at low risk of significant fibrosis remain in primary care for management of their cardiometabolic risk factors, whereas high-risk patients should be referred for further assessment by a specialist.

3. **How would you proceed to investigate?**

The aims of further investigation should be to help confirm the presence of significant or advanced hepatic fibrosis. Fibrosis is of particular significance given that it is the histological feature which predicts long-term outcome. Either transient elastography to measure liver stiffness as a correlate of hepatic fibrosis or ELF test would be reasonable, non-invasive next investigations, depending on local resources and expertise. If there is discordance between clinical findings and non-invasive tests, or diagnostic uncertainty, then a liver biopsy may be considered.

4. **What would be your approach to management?**

The approach to management should be to assess and optimize cardiovascular risk factors as cardiovascular disease is the commonest cause of death among such patients, and to address fibrotic liver disease and its complications. The mainstay of treatment involves lifestyle interventions including weight loss through dietary measures, exercise and smoking cessation. Several medications used to treat other components of the metabolic syndrome may also have secondary benefits on the liver including metformin, statins, GLP-1 RAs and thiazolidinediones.

Obeticholic acid has shown promise in phase II and III studies, and subject to ongoing evaluation. If cirrhosis is confirmed, the patient should undergo surveillance for oesophageal varices and HCC.

References

1. Chalasani N, Younossi Z, Lavine JE, et al. The diagnosis and management of non-alcoholic fatty liver disease: practice guideline by the American Association for the Study of Liver Diseases, American College of Gastroenterology, and the American Gastroenterological Association. Hepatology. 2012;55:2005–23. https://doi.org/10.1002/hep.25762.
2. Eslam M, Sanyal AJ, George J, et al. MAFLD: a consensus-driven proposed nomenclature for metabolic associated fatty liver disease. Gastroenterology. 2020;158:1999–2014.e1. https://doi.org/10.1053/j.gastro.2019.11.312.
3. Haldar D, Kern B, Hodson J, et al. Outcomes of liver transplantation for non-alcoholic steatohepatitis: a European liver transplant registry study. J Hepatol. 2019;71:313–22. https://doi.org/10.1016/j.jhep.2019.04.011.
4. Younossi ZM, Stepanova M, Ong J, et al. Nonalcoholic steatohepatitis is the Most rapidly increasing indication for liver transplantation in the United States. Clin Gastroenterol Hepatol. 2021;19:580–589.e5. https://doi.org/10.1016/j.cgh.2020.05.064.

5. Marjot T, Moolla A, Cobbold JF, et al. Nonalcoholic fatty liver disease in adults: current concepts in etiology, outcomes, and management. Endocr Rev. 2020;41:bnz009. https://doi.org/10.1210/endrev/bnz009.

6. Koeckerling D, Tomlinson JW, Cobbold JF. Fighting liver fat. Endocr Connect. 2020;9:R173–86. https://doi.org/10.1530/EC-20-0174.

7. McPherson S, Hardy T, Henderson E, et al. Evidence of NAFLD progression from steatosis to fibrosing-steatohepatitis using paired biopsies: implications for prognosis and clinical management. J Hepatol. 2015;62:1148–55. https://doi.org/10.1016/j.jhep.2014.11.034.

8. Angulo P, Kleiner DE, Dam-Larsen S, et al. Liver fibrosis, but no other histologic features, is associated with long-term outcomes of patients with nonalcoholic fatty liver disease. Gastroenterology. 2015;149:389–397.e10. https://doi.org/10.1053/j.gastro.2015.04.043.

9. Ekstedt M, Hagström H, Nasr P, et al. Fibrosis stage is the strongest predictor for disease-specific mortality in NAFLD after up to 33 years of follow-up. Hepatology. 2015;61:1547–54. https://doi.org/10.1002/hep.27368.

10. Singh S, Allen AM, Wang Z, et al. Fibrosis progression in nonalcoholic fatty liver vs nonalcoholic steatohepatitis: a systematic review and meta-analysis of paired-biopsy studies. Clin Gastroenterol Hepatol. 2015;13:643–654.e9. https://doi.org/10.1016/j.cgh.2014.04.014.

11. Alexopoulos A, Crowley MJ, Wang Y, et al. Glycemic Control Predicts Severity of Hepatocyte Ballooning and Hepatic Fibrosis in Nonalcoholic Fatty Liver Disease. Hepatology. 2021;74(3):1220–33. https://doi.org/10.1002/hep.31806.

12. Skelly MM, James PD, Ryder SD. Findings on liver biopsy to investigate abnormal liver function tests in the absence of diagnostic serology. J Hepatol. 2001;35:195–9. https://doi.org/10.1016/S0168-8278(01)00094-0.

13. Srivastava A, Gailer R, Tanwar S, et al. Prospective evaluation of a primary care referral pathway for patients with non-alcoholic fatty liver disease. J Hepatol. 2019;71:371–8. https://doi.org/10.1016/j.jhep.2019.03.033.

14. Chalmers J, Wilkes E, Harris R, et al. Development and implementation of a commissioned pathway for the identification and stratification of liver disease in the community. Frontline Gastroenterol. 2019;11:86–92. https://doi.org/10.1136/flgastro-2019-101177.

15. Thoma C, Day CP, Trenell MI. Lifestyle interventions for the treatment of non-alcoholic fatty liver disease in adults: a systematic review. J Hepatol. 2012;56:255–66. https://doi.org/10.1016/j.jhep.2011.06.010.
16. Vilar-Gomez E, Martinez-Perez Y, Calzadilla-Bertot L, et al. Weight loss through lifestyle modification significantly reduces features of nonalcoholic steatohepatitis. Gastroenterology. 2015;149:367–378.e5. https://doi.org/10.1053/j.gastro.2015.04.005.
17. Musso G, Cassader M, Rosina F, et al. Impact of current treatments on liver disease, glucose metabolism and cardiovascular risk in non-alcoholic fatty liver disease (NAFLD): a systematic review and meta-analysis of randomised trials. Diabetologia. 2012;55:885–904. https://doi.org/10.1007/s00125-011-2446-4.
18. Bower G, Toma T, Harling L, et al. Bariatric surgery and non-alcoholic fatty liver disease: a systematic review of liver biochemistry and histology. Obes Surg. 2015;25:2280–9. https://doi.org/10.1007/s11695-015-1691-x.
19. Armstrong MJ, Gaunt P, Aithal GP, et al. Liraglutide safety and efficacy in patients with non-alcoholic steatohepatitis (LEAN): a multicentre, double-blind, randomised, placebo-controlled phase 2 study. Lancet. 2016;387:679–90. https://doi.org/10.1016/S0140-6736(15)00803-X.
20. Newsome PN, Buchholtz K, Cusi K, et al. A placebo-controlled trial of subcutaneous Semaglutide in nonalcoholic steatohepatitis. N Engl J Med. 2021;384(12):1113–24. https://doi.org/10.1056/nejmoa2028395.
21. Bonora BM, Avogaro A, Fadini GP. Extraglycemic effects of SGLT2 inhibitors: a review of the evidence. Diabetes Metab Syndr Obes. 2020;13:161–74. https://doi.org/10.2147/DMSO.S233538.
22. Sanyal AJ, Chalasani N, Kowdley KV, et al. Pioglitazone, vitamin E, or placebo for nonalcoholic steatohepatitis. N Engl J Med. 2010;362:1675–85. https://doi.org/10.1056/nejmoa0907929.
23. Neuschwander-Tetri BA, Loomba R, Sanyal AJ, et al. Farnesoid X nuclear receptor ligand obeticholic acid for non-cirrhotic, non-alcoholic steatohepatitis (FLINT): a multicentre, randomised, placebo-controlled trial. Lancet. 2015;385:956–65. https://doi.org/10.1016/S0140-6736(14)61933-4.
24. Younossi ZM, Ratziu V, Loomba R, et al. Obeticholic acid for the treatment of non-alcoholic steatohepatitis: interim analysis from a multicentre, randomised, placebo-controlled phase 3 trial. Lancet. 2019;394:2184–96. https://doi.org/10.1016/S0140-6736(19)33041-7.

Chapter 8
Chronic Hepatitis B

Navjyot Hansi, Loey Lung-Yi Mak, Upkar Gill, and Patrick Kennedy

Key Learning Points
- To recognise that universal vaccination of newborns against HBV is effective to prevent CHB infections in the infants and bring down CHB prevalence in the post-vaccination era.
- To appreciate the viral structure and viral cycle of HBV.
- To understand and interpret different serological markers and viral markers in diagnosis and workup of CHB with regard to the phase of disease.

N. Hansi
Addenbrooke's Hospital, Cambridge, UK

L. L.-Y. Mak
Division of Gastroenterology & Hepatology, Blizard Institute, London, UK

Barts and The London SMD, QMUL, London, UK
e-mail: lungyi@hku.hk

U. Gill
Hepatologist, Immunobiology Centre QMUL, Blizard Institute, Barts and The London SMD, QMUL, London, UK
e-mail: u.gill@qmul.ac.uk

P. Kennedy (✉)
Translational Hepatology, Blizard Institute, Barts and The London SMD, QMUL, London, UK
e-mail: p.kennedy@qmul.ac.uk

© Springer Nature Switzerland AG 2022
T. Cross (ed.), *Liver Disease in Clinical Practice*, In Clinical Practice, https://doi.org/10.1007/978-3-031-10012-3_8

- To learn the types of approved antiviral therapy, and the fact that newer drugs are being developed.
- To appreciate the indications of treatment and adjunct management in CHB patients and special populations.

Chapter Review Questions

1. What is the recommended immunisation protocol for infants born to HBsAg+ve mother?

   (a) HBV vaccine at 0, 1, 6 months.
   (b) HBV vaccine at 0, 1, 6 months + HBIg within 12–24 h.
   (c) HBV vaccine at 0, 1, 6 months + HBIg within 12–24 h + antiviral therapy for the mother if maternal serum HBV DNA level > 200,000.
   (d) HBV vaccine at 0, 1, 6 months + HBIg within 12–24 h + antiviral therapy for the mother if maternal HBeAg is positive.

2. Which of the following statement about HBV is true?

   (a) HBV is an RNA virus.
   (b) HBV enters the hepatocyte by sodium taurocholate cotransporting polypeptide.
   (c) HBV does not enter the nucleus of hepatocytes.
   (d) HBV is cytopathic and leads to robust inflammatory response within the liver.

3. HBsAg +ve, HBeAg −ve, ALT high, DNA high. Which of the following correctly describes the disease phase?

   (a) HBeAg-positive chronic hepatitis.
   (b) HBeAg-positive chronic infection.
   (c) HBeAg-negative chronic hepatitis.
   (d) HBeAg-negative chronic infection.

4. Which of the following is NOT an approved therapy for CHB?

   (a) Therapeutic vaccine.
   (b) Pegylated interferon.
   (c) Entecavir.
   (d) Tenofovir.

5. Which of the following patient does not require prophylactic antiviral therapy?

   (a) HBsAg−/anti-HBc + patient about to undergo haematopoietic stem cell transplantation.
   (b) HBsAg−/anti-HBc + patient about to receive rituximab.
   (c) HBsAg+/anti-HBc + patient about to receive high dose corticosteroid for newly diagnosed systemic lupus erythematosus.
   (d) HBsAg+/anti-HBc + patient about to receive a one-week course of prednisolone 20 mg daily for Bell's palsy.

Introduction

In 1965 Blumberg discovered the "Australia antigen" later to be known as hepatitis B surface antigen (HBsAg), the hallmark of chronic infection [1]. Several decades later chronic hepatitis B (CHB) remains a major public health challenge despite the availability of a vaccine since the early 1990s. Furthermore, despite access to established antiviral therapies, the currently available treatment strategies in CHB are non-curative, thus even treated patients require lifelong supervision in the majority of cases. This chapter summarises the diagnosis, natural history, virology, treatment, and management options in CHB for todays' physician.

Epidemiology

An estimated 292 million people are chronically infected globally [2]. In recognition of this in May 2016 the World Health Assembly released a target aim to significantly reduce the considerable morbidity and mortality found in individuals with chronic hepatitis B infections by the year 2030 [3]. Chronic infection remains highly prevalent in resource poor countries where it remains concentrated due to economical and logistical limitations. Transmission of hepatitis B virus (HBV) is through exposure to infected blood or body fluids containing virus. In areas of endemic disease; Asia, Africa, and the Middle East, the principal mode of transmission is perinatal. In the western world prevalence is considered to be low, but as a consequence of global migration patterns prevalence in the UK has increased over recent years to reflect this.

Preventative Measures

Screening

CHB is the leading cause of primary liver cancer worldwide; the complications of chronic infection, cirrhosis, and HCC account for an estimated 890,000 deaths per year [4]. Efforts to reduce the morbidity and mortality of CHB start with case finding, screening of at-risk subjects and those from endemic areas. In addition to case finding, screening of family members, vaccination of household contacts, and referral to specialist care where appropriate are the mainstay of public health policy. However, it is estimated that only 9% HBV-infected subjects have been diagnosed and 8% of those who are eligible for treatment received appropriate therapy [4].

Immunisation

At the heart of hepatitis B prevention is vaccination, which has been available since the mid-1980s. In 1992 the World Health Organisation (WHO) recommended global vaccination against hepatitis B, and a significant number of member states have integrated hepatitis B vaccination in to their infant vaccination schedules. Newborns to all HBsAg-positive women should receive a course of three doses of HBV vaccine (at birth, 1 and 6 months). Postvaccination testing occurs between 9 and 15 months. In addition, infants born to CHB mothers are recommended to receive hepatitis B immunoglobulin (HBIg) in addition to the HBV vaccination course within 12–24 h [5]. Mothers with high viral load titres (defined as HBV DNA >200,000 IU/mL) will also be prescribed antiviral therapy at the beginning of their third trimester to further reduce the risk of vertical transmission of virus. Although vaccination uptake remains low in some countries, successful implementation of immunoprophylaxis has had a marked impact in reducing the rate of perinatal transmission in recognised endemic areas. In Taiwan and Hong Kong prevalence has fallen from 10% to 15% to less than 1% amongst children and young adults.

Diagnosis and Disease Work-Up

Persistence of hepatitis B surface antigen (HbsAg) in the blood for more than 6 months is the basis on which a diagnosis of CHB is made (Table 8.1). Following acute exposure, HbsAg can be detected within 6 weeks in the majority of cases. The resolution of acute infection, with the subsequent disappearance of HbsAg is accompanied by the emergence of antibodies to HBs (anti-HBs), but there may be a period during which neither HbsAg nor anti-HBs is detected; loss of HbsAg and the detection of anti-HBs signify resolution of acute HBV.

Anti-HBc IgM titres are elevated in acute HBV and are used to confirm acute infection in the clinic, but anti-HBc IgM can also be elevated during reactivation of CHB. Titres of anti-HBc IgG usually persist if there is chronic infection but are also present along with anti-HBs in individuals who have recovered from acute HBV and thus can experience reactivation during immunosuppression/chemotherapy.

Quantitative HBV DNA is a direct measure of replication activity of the virus. Although genotype testing is not widely implemented there is strong evidence it can influence the natural history of CHB and response of antiviral therapy. There are ten major genotypes (A to J) with distinct geographic distributions.

TABLE 8.1 Definition and interpretation of serological tests in hepatitis B virus

Marker	Clinical interpretation
HBsAg	Hallmark of infection Positive in early phase of acute infection Persistently positive in chronic infection
Anti-HBs	Recovery from acute infection (or chronic) Immunity following vaccination
HBeAg	"e" (envelope) antigen positivity Positive in HBeAg-positive chronic infection (formerly referred to as immune tolerant disease) and HBeAg-positive chronic hepatitis (formerly referred to as immune clearance phase) Initially positive in acute infection Associated with high viral load
Anti-HBe	Loss of "e" antigen—seroconversion to develop antibody against HBe Present in HBeAg-negative chronic infection (formerly referred to as inactive carrier or low replicative phase)—low viral load Present in HBeAg-negative chronic hepatitis (formerly referred to as immune escape)—higher viral load
Anti-HBc (IgM)	Positive in acute infection Positive during some exacerbations of chronic infection
Anti-HBc (IgG)	Exposure to infection Present in association with HBsAg in chronic infection Present in association with anti-HBs after recovery of infection Isolated presence may indicate seropositive occult HBV

TABLE 8.1 (continued)

Marker	Clinical interpretation
Tests	
HBsAg (−) Total anti-HBc (+) Anti-HBs (+)	Immune due to natural infection
HBsAg (−) Total anti-HBc (−) Anti-HBs (+)	Immune due to Hepatitis B vaccination
HBsAg (+) Total anti-HBc (+) Anti-HBc IgM (+) Anti-HBs (−)	Acute infection (or exacerbation of chronic infection)
HBsAg (+) Total anti-HBc (+) Anti-HBc IgM (−) Anti-HBs (−)	Chronic infection
HBsAg (−) Total anti-HBc (+) Anti-HBs (−)	Interpretation unclear; number of possibilities (a) Resolved infection (common) (b) False-positive anti-HBc (c) "Low level" chronic infection/ occult HBV (d) Resolving acute infection (e) Chronic infection with surface antigen mutation

Further laboratory investigations including serum alanine aminotransferase (ALT) and aspartate transaminase (AST) are used as surrogates for disease activity. Additional parameters such as platelet count, prothrombin time, serum bilirubin, and albumin are evaluated to assess synthetic liver function and the severity of liver disease.

Additional viral serology is indicated to exclude hepatitis type C and delta (HDV) in addition to HIV co-infection. HDV is a satellite virus that only exists in the presence of HBV. The latter can accelerate liver fibrosis and consideration for early antiviral therapy is mandated.

Basic imaging such as liver ultrasound is indicated as part of initial disease work-up and assessment, while more detailed cross-sectional imaging has a role in confirming chronicity, the severity of chronic liver disease and the presence of portal hypertension. Non-invasive modalities to assess liver fibrosis such as serum markers and transient elastography (TE) have largely replaced liver biopsy. APRI and FIB-4 scores have been most extensively studied and validated with evidence base substantiated in large meta-analyses. Acoustic radiation force impulse (ARFI) imaging and MR elastography have respective advantages and limitations. However, liver biopsy remains the only means and gold standard for the assessment of necro-inflammation and fibrosis stage, although procedural risks such as bleeding, pain, and perforation remain.

Establishing disease phase involves serial assessments of liver function in addition to viral parameters and due to the dynamic nature of HBV, newly diagnosed patients are seen three-monthly in the specialist clinic for the first year to confirm clinical phenotype. Quantitative HbsAg level has an emerging role when combined with HBV DNA and serum ALT levels for disease stratification. Serum HbsAg levels are perceived as a surrogate of intrahepatic transcriptionally active covalently closed circular (ccc) DNA and can provide complementary information to enhance disease assessment and evaluation of treatment response [6].

Virology

Structure

The HBV virion particle, also known as the Dane particle (Fig. 8.1), is approximately 42 nm in size and composed of an outer envelope (Hbsag), which surrounds a nucleocapsid containing a small DNA genome of 3.2Kb. The genome is circular, partially double stranded encoding four overlapping open reading frames (ORF). The activities of the major viral proteins (polymerase, core, envelope, X, and e antigen) are shown in Fig. 8.1.

Viral Replication

HBV belongs to the family of hepadnaviruses, where stealth infection of host hepatocytes, the major cell type in the liver, with HBV virions allows the HBV genome to be converted to covalently closed circular (ccc) DNA providing a template

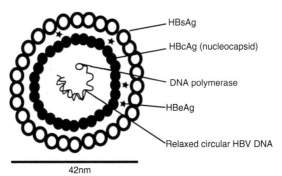

There are four protein-coding regions in the genome:
(i) The first reading frame codes for the proteins making up Hepatitis B surface antigen (HBsAg)
(ii) The second for pre-core/core encoding the core protein (HBcAg), a structural unit of the nucleocapsid, and the non-structural pre-core protein, the secreted e-Antigen (HBeAg)
(iii) The third for the DNA viral polymerase 'pol' required for RNA encapsidation and DNA synthesis, and (iv) Fourthly the 'X ORF' encoding the small viral regulatory X protein (HBx), which is essential for viral replication. The function of the latter is not fully understood but appears to be associated with HCC.

FIGURE 8.1 Diagram of the Dane particle

for transcription of messenger RNA/ pre-genomic RNA and translation of all the viral proteins. The functional importance of persistence of cccDNA in the nucleus of infected hepatocytes is the basis of HBV chronicity.

A turning point in understanding the mechanisms of viral replication and the potential development of novel therapeutic interventions has been the recent identification of a liver bile acid transporter, the sodium taurocholate cotransporting polypeptide (NTCP), as a functional receptor for HBV [7].

Natural History and Immunology

Acute HBV Infection

Age of viral acquisition and immune status of the host are critical to the successful clearance of infection. The majority of healthy adults (>90%) will recover from acute infection and develop long lasting immunity. Previous animal studies have demonstrated that resolution of HBV infection is largely mediated by the adaptive immune response but there is growing recognition of the role of the innate immune response in viral control [8].

Phases of Chronic HBV Infection

The disease course of established HBV infection remains unpredictable, although our understanding of hepatitis B immunopathogenesis and virology has improved in recent years.

Traditionally CHB is thought to progress through four distinct disease phases (Fig. 8.2) and this terminology has been updated within guidelines to be based on the description of the two main characteristics of chronicity; infection versus hepatitis [9, 10]. Better disease stratification is central to improve disease outcomes [11].

Perinatal or early infection in childhood is typically associated with high levels of virus, normal ALT, minimal inflam-

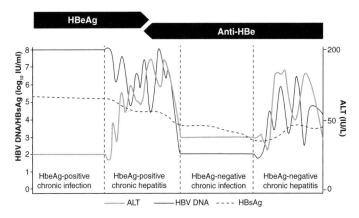

FIGURE 8.2 Clinical parameters during disease phases of Chronic Hepatitis B

mation, and mild or no fibrosis on liver biopsy. Historically defined as the "immune tolerant" (IT) disease phase, there was emerging data challenging this clinical phenotype with features of a signature immune profile of these patients to be more compromised than traditionally viewed [12] and this is now defined as "HbeAg-positive chronic infection". This is an important development in the field, as the classical disease phases have been the premise on which treatment decisions are made.

The immune active (previous nomenclature of "immune clearance") phase is now defined as "HbeAg-positive chronic hepatitis" thought to represent an awakening of the immune response with more marked immune activity reflected in perturbation of the serum ALT. Persistence of this disease phase is thought to result in progressive liver damage and thus treatment is indicated to avert the development of fibrosis and cirrhosis. HbeAg seroconversion marks the end of this phase and combined with low HBV DNA and normal serum ALT represents immune control. Classically this immune control phase, often referred to as the inactive or asymptomatic carrier phase, now renamed as "HbeAg-negative chronic infection" marks the end of immune mediated liver damage and therefore in the majority is associated with minimal or no fibrosis. This phase is characterised by the presence of anti-Hbe, HBV DNA is <2000 IU/mL, and normal serum ALT. HbeAg seroconversion and progression to this phase of disease before the age of 30 is associated with reduced risk for the development of HCC [13, 14].

A proportion of these patients will develop disease reactivation with the emergence of viral escape mutants, reflected in elevated HBV DNA levels and changes in serum ALT. HbeAg is not expressed owing to mutations in the pre-core or core promoter areas of the virus, thus this clinical picture is referred to as "HbeAg-negative chronic hepatitis". This phase is associated with low rates of spontaneous remission and prognostically is associated with a poor outcome.

Management of Hepatitis B

In line with national and international guidelines, CHB patients should be under long-term specialist follow-up to monitor disease progression. Spontaneous HbsAg seroclearance in untreated CHB patients occurs in <1% per year. Persistence of HbsAg—a risk factor for disease progression and the development of HCC—mandates lifelong specialist supervision [15].

The major challenge in CHB is the lack of curative therapies to achieve eradication of cccDNA representing a complete cure, let alone eradication of integrated HBV DNA which represents sterilising cure. Previously, the therapeutic goal in CHB was viral suppression and normalisation of serum ALT but today the "gold standard" treatment endpoint is HbsAg loss defined as "functional cure", which is associated with favourable clinical outcomes including lower risks of liver decompensation, liver transplantation, HCC, and death [16–18]. Current treatment strategies in CHB are aimed at avoiding the complications of disease and reducing liver-related morbidity and mortality. Approved antiviral agents broadly fall into two categories; nucleos(t)ide analogs (NUCs) or pegylated-interferon (Peg-IFN).

Nucleos(t)ide Analogs (NUCs)

NUCs achieve viral suppression by inhibiting reverse transcription of the pre-genomic RNA into HBV DNA. Rates of HbsAg seroclearance in e-antigen negative patients on oral antiviral treatment are equivalent to spontaneous seroclearance and thus treatment in the majority is lifelong. Despite this, NUCs are perceived as advantageous owing to their good tolerability profile and high genetic barrier to resistance. Furthermore, they are considered first-line therapy in specific patient subgroups, such as those who have decompensated disease, or patients who are intolerant to Peg-IFN or have poor predictors of response and/or co-morbidities that preclude the use of Peg-IFN. There have been some reports of renal toxicity, hypophosphatemia, Fanconi-like syndrome, and reduced bone mineral density have been reported with use of adefovir (now no longer recommended) and tenofovir disoproxil fumarate (TDF), but this appears largely restricted to those with pre-existing renal risk factors [19]. Moreover, tenofovir alafenamide (TAF), another prodrug of tenofovir, has been approved by the U.S. Food and Drug Administration (FDA) for use since year 2015 which demonstrated improved renal and bone safety with same efficacy as TDF [20, 21]. Recent studies have demonstrated histological reversal of fibrosis with long-term NUC therapy [22, 23]. Emerging data suggest the potent first-line NUCs (i.e. entecavir or tenofovir) are associated with reduction in HCC risk [24, 25].

Pegylated-Interferon (Peg-IFN)

Peg-IFN has an immune modulatory effect such that off-treatment immune control can be achieved; however, its use in clinical practice is limited due to systemic effects and the fact that patients with decompensated cirrhosis are contraindicated for PEG-IFN. Although it can be used in both e-Antigen positive and negative phases with compensated disease, appropriate patient selection is central to achieving

TABLE 8.2 Stopping rules for HBeAg negative and positive patients treated with Peg-IFN

	HBeAg negative	**HBeAg positive**
Week 12	Genotype D: No decline in qHBsAg and < $2\log_{10}$ IU/mL decline in HBV DNA	Genotypes A and D: No decline in qHBsAg Genotypes B and C: qHBsAg levels >20,000 IU/mL
Week 24	Not applicable	Genotypes A-D: qHBsAg >20,000 IU/mL

sustained immune control. Peg-IFN represents a finite treatment option and the utility of early stopping rules (Table 8.2) has optimised treatment in Peg-IFN treated patients leading to an early switch strategy to NUC therapy in those with an unfavourable response.

Patient Selection/Who to Treat

Due to the dynamic nature of CHB, the timing of antiviral therapy is critical and treatment decisions should be made on an individual basis.

Although International guidelines lack uniformity in their recommendations for first line-therapies, this allows flexibility and physician discretion. Various treatment algorithms have been proposed, and therapy is currently recommended for those with evidence of chronic active disease. Treatment criteria focus specifically on age; as the development of fibrosis, cirrhosis, and HCC increases significantly with advancing age; the level of HBV DNA and perturbation in serum ALT. Antiviral therapy is recommended in adults aged >30 years with HBV DNA >2000 IU/mL and abnormal ALT, on two consecutive tests 3 months apart; or if aged <30 years with HBV DNA >2000 IU/mL, abnormal ALT and evidence of necro-inflammation or fibrosis on liver biopsy or a TE score of >6 kPa (fibrosis F2 or higher). HBV DNA level of >20,000 IU/mL is a clear indication for treatment, irrespective of age and this recommendation is consistent across all international guidelines (AASLD, EASL, and APASL) [9, 10, 26]. There has been some debate as to what constitutes a normal ALT level and historical data have revised these thresholds on a number of occasions, initially favouring Prati criteria (an abnormal ALT is defined as >30 U/L in an adult male and > 19 U/L in an adult female) with more recent updated guidelines adjusting these limits again (AASLD; >25 U/L women and >35 U/L in men).

e-Antigen Positive

In hepatitis B e-Antigen (HbeAg) positive disease, patients completing 48 weeks of Peg-IFN demonstrated a favourable response with 25–30% achieving HbeAg seroconversion (tested 24 weeks post-treatment), and a proportion of these patients went on to achieve HbsAg loss [27]. Predictors of response are similar in both groups; younger age, female gender, higher serum ALT, and lower HBV DNA levels are considered more favourable factors for response to Peg-IFN. Genotype A and B patients have historically been reported to be more responsive to Peg-IFN therapy.

The aim of treating HbeAg positive disease is to achieve HbeAg seroconversion as delayed HbeAg clearance increases the risk of progression to fibrosis, cirrhosis, and HCC. Achieving HbeAg loss or seroconversion with NUC monotherapy can be achieved in 30–40% of patients but this can take up to 3–5 years in some patients.

At present, there are no data to suggest a clinical benefit in treating patients in the HbeAg-positive chronic infection phase, formerly referred to as the IT phase, however, there is growing evidence that not all patients designated IT are truly tolerant [12]. Therefore a proportion of these patients may benefit from earlier intervention or at the very least closer supervision and monitoring [28].

e-Antigen Negative

In this cohort the response rate to Peg-IFN (<25%) is lower than in HbeAg positive disease, however, this still remains higher than HbsAg seroclearance with NUC therapy alone. A decision to start a young patient on NUC therapy will require a discussion of the pros and cons of the prospect of lifelong therapy. Guidelines recommend that at lower thresholds of HBV DNA (>2000 or >20,000 IU/mL) additional factors should be taken into account such as patient age, family history of HCC, and family planning. The subgroup of patients who have a normal ALT, but persistent fluctuations in HBV DNA (between 2000 and 20,000 IU/mL) may have evidence of significant fibrosis and treatment may be warranted in these patients [28].

Special Populations

Cirrhotic

AASLD and EASL recommend treatment with NUC in cirrhotic patients with any detectable HBV DNA and ALT in addition to six-monthly ultrasound surveillance for HCC. Furthermore, NUC therapy in the cirrhotic patient should be lifelong to prevent the risk of reactivation, decompensation, and the development of HCC.

Immunosuppressed

In HbsAg positive (HBsAg+) patients or HBsAg negative (HbsAg-) but anti-HBc positive (anti-HBc+) patients on immunosuppressive agents, chemotherapy or undergoing haematopoietic stem cell transplantation, the risk of HBV reactivation is variable and therefore NUCs maybe mandated during treatment for a period of 6 months, and in some instances, to up to 2 years after completing chemotherapy or discontinuing immunosuppression. If the anticipated risk of reactivation is high (i.e., >10%), such as patients receiving B cell depleting therapy or HbsAg+ patients receiving anthracycline derivatives, prophylactic NUCs are required. Where the anticipated risk of viral reactivation is moderate (i.e., 1–10%), such as patients receiving anti-tumour necrosis factor or tyrosine kinase inhibitors, these patients may either be started on prophylactic antiviral or be carefully monitored with frequent serum ALT and DNA levels. Patients who receive traditional immunomodulators (e.g., azathioprine, 6-mercaptopurine, methotrexate) or low dose (<10 mg prednisolone or equivalent) corticosteroids for any duration do not need routine antiviral prophylaxis due to a low risk of HBV reactivation (i.e., <1%) [29]. Therefore, patients with any history of HBV exposure should be risk-stratified during immunosuppression to decide on the management strategy.

Pregnancy

Based on safety data from Tenofovir treated HIV-infected mothers and the low risk of teratogenicity, Tenofovir is recommended as the NUC of choice in CHB mothers with high levels of HBV DNA in the last trimester of pregnancy. HBIg is administered to newborns of CHB mothers (in addition to vaccination) regardless of whether NUC was taken to prevent vertical transmission.

Biomarkers

Loss of HbsAg or functional cure is the desired treatment endpoint in studies of novel HBV therapies. Thus, a reduction in qHBsAg levels is a measure of efficacy of new therapies, be that through an antiviral effect or as a result of immune-mediated clearance of infected hepatocytes. Levels have been shown to correlate with HBV DNA and cccDNA in HbeAg positive patients [30]. In addition, studies have demonstrated a role for qHBsAg levels to identify patients who may be suitable for treatment discontinuation (qHBsAg levels <100 IU/mL) and higher HbsAg levels correlate with HCC risk [31].

Another marker Hepatitis B core related antigen (HbcrAg) has been found to correlate well with cccDNA. Whilst on antiviral therapy, HbcrAg declines at a slower rate than HBV DNA, and as such, it can be regarded as a marker of persistence of HBV and correlates with intrahepatic cccDNA in liver biopsy studies [32]. Independently levels have been found to predict hepatocarcinogenesis in untreated and treated patients, however, currently there are no published risk models that incorporate this as there is not yet a consensus on a cut-off level to help inform the decision.

HBV RNA has emerged as a novel biomarker, which is detectable in the serum as encapsidated virion-containing pre-genomic RNA [33]. HBV RNA has been shown to mirror levels of HBV DNA (1–2 logs higher than RNA) in untreated subjects and demonstrated a distinct profile depending on the phase of infection [34, 35]. In treated subjects, HBV RNA has been shown to predict off-NUC virological relapse [36] and HCC development [37]. HBV RNA is also commonly measured in drug trials to prove target engagement. Standardisation of assays for HBV RNA are needed prior to its acceptance more broadly as a biomarker in clinical practice.

HCC Surveillance

International guidelines are fairly consistent in their approach to initiate oral antivirals in cirrhotic patients and 6-monthly HCC surveillance with ultrasound with or without serum alfa-feto protein measurement. In non-cirrhotics, HCC surveillance is recommended if there is a family history of HCC and using risk calculators such as REACH-B (validated in Asian CHB cohort) and PAGE-B score (good predictability for HCC in Caucasian CHB cohort) which incorporate non-modifiable risk factors such as age and ethnicity, as well as widely available parameters such as platelets. However, metabolic syndrome is emerging as an important co-aetiology with CHB and current early risk stratification scores do not yet incorporate this when evaluating HCC risk. In particular, diabetes mellitus is being increasingly recognised as a risk factor for HCC, and thus the CAMD scoring system (incorporating cirrhosis, age, male gender, diabetes mellitus) has been derived [38] and early validation studies have been published [39].

Future Therapies

Eradicating HBV and achieving a sterilising cure is the ultimate treatment goal but remains an elusive outcome. Novel strategies to maximise the efficacy of currently available treatments (NUCs & Peg-IFN), including the combination of these agents or their use in sequence has also been investigated, but without demonstrating superior treatment outcomes [40]. The discovery of the HBV entry receptor, NTCP, has been an important development in the field such that cell culture systems can provide an accessible platform to study new therapeutic targets. Novel agents in clinical phase of development are designed to inhibit viral replication by alternative mechanisms (other than inhibition of DNA polymerase) or antigen reduction, which include viral entry inhibitors, core protein allosteric modulators, RNA interference-based therapy, and nucleic acid polymers that prevent surface antigen export. Another approach is to boost or restore the host immune response against HBV using toll like receptor agonists, immune checkpoint inhibitors, soluble bispecific fusion molecules, therapeutic vaccination, and engineered monoclonal antibodies are also under investigation [41, 42]. The majority of these strategies have had proven efficacy in suppression of viral protein and/or nucleic acids, but the durability of therapeutic effects is unknown. Despite these advances in HBV therapy, the question arises whether such agents will be affordable in areas where HBV is endemic. Moreover, long-term safety data is awaited, and together with this, it is also likely these strategies will be combined with NUCs and/or Peg-IFN in the short term, therefore, the therapies used in today's clinic are likely to constitute a central component of treatment strategies for the foreseeable future [43].

Conclusion

There is renewed focus on treatment and management of CHB in light of the recent advances in the hepatitis B field. A better understanding of the complex HBV life cycle, clinical phenotypes as well as the host–virus interplay will lead to the development of curative treatment strategies in the future and hopefully, novel therapeutic approaches that are able to achieve sustained off-treatment responses in the majority of cases.

Chapter Review Questions

1. What is the recommended immunisation protocol for infants born to HBsAg+ve mother?

    (a) HBV vaccine at 0, 1, 6 months.
    (b) HBV vaccine at 0, 1, 6 months + HBIg within 12–24 h.
    (c) HBV vaccine at 0, 1, 6 months + HBIg within 12–24 h + antiviral therapy for the mother if maternal serum HBV DNA level > 200,000.
    (d) HBV vaccine at 0, 1, 6 months + HBIg within 12–24 h + antiviral therapy for the mother if maternal HBeAg is positive.

2. Which of the following statement about HBV is true?

    (a) HBV is an RNA virus.
    (b) HBV enters the hepatocyte by sodium tarocholate cotransporting polypeptide.
    (c) HBV does not enter the nucleus of hepatocytes.
    (d) HBV is cytopathic and leads to robust inflammatory response within the liver.

3. HBsAg +ve, HBeAg −ve, ALT high, DNA high. Which of the following correctly describes the disease phase?

    (a) HBeAg-positive chronic hepatitis.
    (b) HBeAg-positive chronic infection.
    (c) HBeAg-negative chronic hepatitis.
    (d) HBeAg-negative chronic infection.

4. Which of the following is NOT an approved therapy for CHB?

   (a) Therapeutic vaccine.
   (b) Pegylated interferon.
   (c) Entecavir.
   (d) Tenofovir.

5. Which of the following patient does not require prophylactic antiviral therapy?

   (a) HBsAg−/anti-HBc + patient about to undergo haematopoietic stem cell transplantation.
   (b) HBsAg−/anti-HBc + patient about to receive rituximab.
   (c) HBsAg+/anti-HBc + patient about to receive high dose corticosteroid for newly diagnosed systemic lupus erythematosus.
   (d) HBsAg+/anti-HBc + patient about to receive a one-week course of prednisolone 20 mg daily for Bell's palsy.

Answers

1. (c)
2. (b)
3. (c)
4. (a)
5. (d)

References

1. Blumberg BS, Alter HJ, Visnich S. A "New" antigen in leukemia sera. JAMA. 1965;191:541–6.
2. Polaris Observatory Collaborators. Global prevalence, treatment, and prevention of hepatitis B virus infection in 2016: a modelling study. Lancet Gastroenterol Hepatol. 2018;3(6):383–403.
3. Cox AL, El-Sayed MH, Kao JH, Lazarus JV, Lemoine M, Lok AS, et al. Progress towards elimination goals for viral hepatitis. Nat Rev Gastroenterol Hepatol. 2020;17(9):533–42.

4. World Health Organization. Global hepatitis report 2017. Geneva: World Health Organization; 2017. p. 2017.
5. [Centers for Disease Control (CDC) and Prevention webpage:]. https://www.cdc.gov/hepatitis/hbv/perinatalxmtn.htm.
6. Martinot-Peignoux M, Lapalus M, Asselah T, Marcellin P. HBsAg quantification: useful for monitoring natural history and treatment outcome. Liver Int. 2014;34(Suppl 1):97–107.
7. Yan H, Zhong G, Xu G, He W, Jing Z, Gao Z, et al. Sodium taurocholate cotransporting polypeptide is a functional receptor for human hepatitis B and D virus. elife. 2012;1:e00049.
8. Rehermann B. Natural killer cells in viral hepatitis. Cell Mol Gastroenterol Hepatol. 2015;1(6):578–88.
9. European Association for the Study of the Liver. Electronic address: easloffice@easloffice.eu, European Association for the Study of the Liver. EASL 2017 clinical practice guidelines on the management of hepatitis B virus infection. J Hepatol. 2017;67(2):370–98.
10. Terrault NA, Lok ASF, McMahon BJ, Chang KM, Hwang JP, Jonas MM, et al. Update on prevention, diagnosis, and treatment of chronic hepatitis B: AASLD 2018 hepatitis B guidance. Hepatology. 2018;67(4):1560–99.
11. Liaw YF, Chu CM. Hepatitis B virus infection. Lancet. 2009;373(9663):582–92.
12. Bertoletti A, Kennedy PT. The immune tolerant phase of chronic HBV infection: new perspectives on an old concept. Cell Mol Immunol. 2015;12(3):258–63.
13. Chen CJ, Yang HI, Su J, Jen CL, You SL, Lu SN, et al. Risk of hepatocellular carcinoma across a biological gradient of serum hepatitis B virus DNA level. JAMA. 2006;295(1):65–73.
14. Yang HI, Lu SN, Liaw YF, You SL, Sun CA, Wang LY, et al. Hepatitis B e antigen and the risk of hepatocellular carcinoma. N Engl J Med. 2002;347(3):168–74.
15. Liu J, Yang HI, Lee MH, Lu SN, Jen CL, Batrla-Utermann R, et al. Spontaneous seroclearance of hepatitis B seromarkers and subsequent risk of hepatocellular carcinoma. Gut. 2014;63(10):1648–57.
16. Yuen MF, Wong DK, Fung J, Ip P, But D, Hung I, et al. HBsAg Seroclearance in chronic hepatitis B in Asian patients: replicative level and risk of hepatocellular carcinoma. Gastroenterology. 2008;135(4):1192–9.
17. Yip TC, Chan HL, Wong VW, Tse YK, Lam KL, Wong GL. Impact of age and gender on risk of hepatocellular carci-

noma after hepatitis B surface antigen seroclearance. J Hepatol. 2017;67(5):902–8.

18. Anderson RT, Choi HSJ, Lenz O, Peters MG, Janssen HLA, Mishra P, et al. Association between Seroclearance of hepatitis B surface antigen and long-term clinical outcomes of patients with chronic hepatitis B virus infection: systematic review and meta-analysis. Clin Gastroenterol Hepatol. 2021;19(3):463–72.

19. Gill US, Zissimopoulos A, Al-Shamma S, Burke K, McPhail MJ, Barr DA, et al. Assessment of bone mineral density in tenofovir-treated patients with chronic hepatitis B: can the fracture risk assessment tool identify those at greatest risk? J Infect Dis. 2015;211(3):374–82.

20. Lampertico P, Buti M, Fung S, Ahn SH, Chuang WL, Tak WY, et al. Switching from tenofovir disoproxil fumarate to tenofovir alafenamide in virologically suppressed patients with chronic hepatitis B: a randomised, double-blind, phase 3, multicentre non-inferiority study. Lancet Gastroenterol Hepatol. 2020;5(5):441–53.

21. Toyoda H, Leong J, Landis C, Atsukawa M, Watanabe T, Huang DQ, et al. Treatment and renal outcomes up to 96 weeks after tenofovir alafenamide switch from tenofovir disoproxil fumarate in routine practice. Hepatology. 2021;74(2):656–66.

22. Tsai NC, Marcellin P, Buti M, Washington MK, Lee SS, Chan S, et al. Viral suppression and cirrhosis regression with tenofovir disoproxil fumarate in Asians with chronic hepatitis B. Dig Dis Sci. 2015;60(1):260–8.

23. Marcellin P, Gane E, Buti M, Afdhal N, Sievert W, Jacobson IM, et al. Regression of cirrhosis during treatment with tenofovir disoproxil fumarate for chronic hepatitis B: a 5-year open-label follow-up study. Lancet. 2013;381(9865):468–75.

24. Hosaka T, Suzuki F, Kobayashi M, Seko Y, Kawamura Y, Sezaki H, et al. Long-term entecavir treatment reduces hepatocellular carcinoma incidence in patients with hepatitis B virus infection. Hepatology. 2013;58(1):98–107.

25. Papatheodoridis GV, Idilman R, Dalekos GN, Buti M, Chi H, van Boemmel F, et al. The risk of hepatocellular carcinoma decreases after the first 5 years of entecavir or tenofovir in Caucasians with chronic hepatitis B. Hepatology. 2017;66(5):1444–53.

26. Sarin SK, Kumar M, Lau GK, Abbas Z, Chan HL, Chen CJ, et al. Asian-Pacific clinical practice guidelines on the management of hepatitis B: a 2015 update. Hepatol Int. 2016;10(1):1–98.

27. Sonneveld MJ, Rijckborst V, Boucher CA, Hansen BE, Janssen HL. Prediction of sustained response to peginterferon alfa-2b for hepatitis B e antigen-positive chronic hepatitis B using on-treatment hepatitis B surface antigen decline. Hepatology. 2010;52(4):1251–7.

28. Zoulim F, Mason WS. Reasons to consider earlier treatment of chronic HBV infections. Gut. 2012;61(3):333–6.

29. Reddy KR, Beavers KL, Hammond SP, Lim JK, Falck-Ytter YT. American Gastroenterological Association I. American Gastroenterological Association Institute guideline on the prevention and treatment of hepatitis B virus reactivation during immunosuppressive drug therapy. Gastroenterology. 2015;148(1):215–9; quiz e16–7.

30. Sonneveld MJ, Hansen BE, Brouwer WP, Chan HL, Piratvisuth T, Jia JD, et al. hbsag levels can be used to rule out cirrhosis in hbeag positive chronic hepatitis b: results from the sonic-b study. J Infect Dis. 2020;225(11):1967–73.

31. Tseng TC, Liu CJ, Yang HC, Su TH, Wang CC, Chen CL, et al. High levels of hepatitis B surface antigen increase risk of hepatocellular carcinoma in patients with low HBV load. Gastroenterology. 2012;142(5):1140–1149.e3; quiz e13–4.

32. Wong DK, Seto WK, Cheung KS, Chong CK, Huang FY, Fung J, et al. Hepatitis B virus core-related antigen as a surrogate marker for covalently closed circular DNA. Liver Int. 2017;37(7):995–1001.

33. Wang J, Shen T, Huang X, Kumar GR, Chen X, Zeng Z, et al. Serum hepatitis B virus RNA is encapsidated pregenome RNA that may be associated with persistence of viral infection and rebound. J Hepatol. 2016;65(4):700–10.

34. Butler EK, Gersch J, McNamara A, Luk KC, Holzmayer V, de Medina M, et al. Hepatitis B virus serum DNA andRNA levels in Nucleos(t)ide analog-treated or untreated patients during chronic and acute infection. Hepatology. 2018;68(6):2106–17.

35. Mak LY, Cloherty G, Wong DK, Gersch J, Seto WK, Fung J, et al. HBV RNA profiles in patients with chronic hepatitis B under different disease phases and antiviral therapy. Hepatology. 2021;73(6):2167–79.

36. Seto WK, Liu KS, Mak LY, Cloherty G, Wong DK, Gersch J, et al. Role of serum HBV RNA and hepatitis B surface antigen levels in identifying Asian patients with chronic hepatitis B suitable for entecavir cessation. Gut. 2021;70(4):775–83.

37. Mak LY, Huang Q, Wong DK, Stamm L, Cheung KS, Ko KL, et al. Residual HBV DNA and pgRNA viraemia is associated with hepatocellular carcinoma in chronic hepatitis B patients on antiviral therapy. J Gastroenterol. 2021;56(5):479–88.

38. Hsu YC, Yip TC, Ho HJ, Wong VW, Huang YT, El-Serag HB, et al. Development of a scoring system to predict hepatocellular carcinoma in Asians on antivirals for chronic hepatitis B. J Hepatol. 2018;69(2):278–85.

39. Kim SU, Seo YS, Lee HA, Kim MN, Kim EH, Kim HY, et al. Validation of the CAMD score in patients with chronic hepatitis B virus infection receiving antiviral therapy. Clin Gastroenterol Hepatol. 2020;18(3):693–9. e1

40. Thimme R, Dandri M. Dissecting the divergent effects of interferon-alpha on immune cells: time to rethink combination therapy in chronic hepatitis B? J Hepatol. 2013;58(2):205–9.

41. Yang N, Bertoletti A. Advances in therapeutics for chronic hepatitis B. Hepatol Int. 2016;10(2):277–85.

42. Yuen MF, Chen DS, Dusheiko GM, Janssen HLA, Lau DTY, Locarnini SA, et al. Hepatitis B virus infection. Nat Rev Dis Primers. 2018;4:18035.

43. Ye J, Chen J. Interferon and hepatitis B: current and future perspectives. Front Immunol. 2021;12:733364.

Chapter 9
Chronic Hepatitis C

Ruth Tunney, Martin Prince, and Varinder Athwal

Key Learning Points
- Chronic Hepatitis C (CHC) is a global disease estimated to affect 170 million people worldwide and to cause 350,000 deaths per annum.
- Hepatitis C is a bloodborne virus, and the most common modes of transmission are injecting drug use and unsafe health care practices, including incompletely sterilised medical equipment.
- Most patients exposed will go on to develop chronic infection and have a risk of progression to cirrhosis and primary liver cancer over time.
- Current antiviral medication is very efficacious and very well tolerated. Diagnosis and access to therapy remain the main barriers to cure.

R. Tunney
North-West Deanery, Manchester, UK

M. Prince · V. Athwal (✉)
Manchester University NHS Foundation Trust, Manchester, UK
e-mail: varinder.athwal@mft.nhs.uk

© Springer Nature Switzerland AG 2022   177
T. Cross (ed.), *Liver Disease in Clinical Practice*, In Clinical Practice, https://doi.org/10.1007/978-3-031-10012-3_9

Case Study

Jane is a 56-year-old lady referred to liver clinic with a positive hepatitis C antibody after presenting to her GP with tiredness. She has no active medical history, takes no regular medication and denies any intravenous drug use in the past. She informs you on further questioning that she had a road traffic accident in 1980 and underwent surgery on a left femoral fracture. At this time, she was given blood products. She drinks between 2 and 3 bottles of wine per week and works as a teaching assistant. Clinical examination is remarkable for the presence of palmar erythema only. Blood testing reveals positive for HCV antibody.

RNA viral load is log 8.3 IU/ml.
Genotype 1, subtype A.
ALT 81.
AST 59.
Albumin 36.
Bilirubin 12.
INR 1.1.
Platelets 99.
Creatinine 71 (eGFR >90).

Questions

1. Which of the below is not a method to non-invasively assess liver fibrosis:

   (a) Liver biopsy.
   (b) Ultrasound scan liver with acoustic radiation force impulse (ARFI) imaging.
   (c) Shear wave transient elastography (e.g. FibroScan™).
   (d) AST to Platelets ratio index (APRI).
   (e) FIB-4 index.

2. Non-invasive assessment reveals the likelihood of cirrhosis. Which of the below would be the most suitable first-line treatment option:

   (a) Advise to wait for newer therapies.
   (b) Treat with Pegylated interferon-α and Ribavirin for 24 weeks.

   (c) Treat with Sofosbuvir, Ledipasvir and Ribavirin for 12 weeks.

   (d) List for liver transplant.

   (e) Treat with Sofosbuvir, Velpatasvir, Voxilaprevir for 12 weeks.

3. Treatment is successful at clearing the virus and Jane achieves SVR at 12 weeks. How would you follow-up this patient?

   (a) Discharge from liver service.

   (b) Annual repeat HCV RNA PCR to ensure clearance of virus.

   (c) 6-monthly ultrasound scan of liver with assessment of synthetic liver function and alpha-fetoprotein (AFP).

   (d) 3-monthly alpha-fetoprotein (AFP) assessment.

   (e) 6-monthly LFTs and liver biopsy to assess fibrosis between 1–5 years after SVR.

Background

Chronic Hepatitis C (CHC) is a global disease estimated to affect 170 million people worldwide and to cause 350,000 deaths per annum. Despite recent advancements in therapy, it is still a leading indication for liver transplantation. The estimated prevalence in the UK population is 0.25%, having dropped since the introduction of [1]. The majority of infected people are unaware of their status.

The hepatitis C virus (HCV) was first categorised in the mid-1970s but was not identified and formally named until 1989, after the development of diagnostic testing. The hepatitis C virus is a small, enveloped RNA virus of the Flavivirus family. It has a viral genome of 9.6 kb, encoding a single polyprotein. This is further processed to three structural proteins (one core and two envelope proteins) and seven non-structural (NS) regulatory proteins. The non-structural proteins are essential for viral replication and hence are key targets for directly acting antiviral drugs (DAAs).

Cellular entry occurs via a variety of cell surface receptors and the virion. Viral replication occurs predominantly within hepatocytes, though replication may occur in peripheral lymphocytes, giving rise to some of the non-hepatic manifestations seen in chronic infection. Viral infection of hepatocytes induces metabolic stress, direct and indirect cytopathic effects and hepatic steatosis, inducing inflammation, apoptosis and necrosis. The resultant activation of hepatic stellate cells leads to liver fibrosis, cirrhosis and hepatocellular cancer.

Fibrosis progresses in a non-linear process and appears to increase in rate as fibrosis advances.

Approximately 20% of infected individuals will develop advanced liver fibrosis or cirrhosis after 20 years of chronic infection. Risk factors for the development of cirrhosis are older age at infection, male sex, central obesity/metabolic syndrome, coexistent infections (for example, hepatitis B or HIV) and alcohol intake. Coffee consumption appears to be protective against fibrosis [2].

The mode of viral transmission is predominantly blood to blood. In developed countries intravenous drug use leads to up to 90% of new infections. In the developing world the majority of infections are iatrogenic through reuse of incompletely sterilised equipment or inadequate testing of blood products.

Large outbreaks of infection have been linked to use of clotting factors in patients with haemophilia prior to universal testing in the early 90s and to the schistosomiasis eradication programme in Egypt in the 1960s [3].

Sexual and vertical transmission are rare with risks of 2% and 3%, respectively. The latter is more likely if the mother is co-infected with HIV. The risk of sexual transmission appears to be higher in HIV infected men who have sex with men. The risk falls upon commencement of anti-retroviral therapy. Transmission may also occur through sharing of products in contact with mucus membranes (e.g. drug snorting paraphernalia and toothbrushes) and tattoos.

5–10% of cases occur in people where no risk factors can be identified. Immunity post-infection is ineffective and repeated infections have been reported after successful treatment.

HCV is an exceptionally variable virus and up to eight genotypes have been defined by genome analysis and homology. Each genotype is numerically designated and has greater than 30% nucleotide variation. Six major genotypes are recognised for choosing therapy. Genotypes are further divided into subtype with more than 80 subtypes identified. Subtypes are categorised alphabetically.

Genotype 1 is the most common worldwide (approximately 50% of infections) but there is wide geographic variation [2]. Genotype 1 predominates in northern Europe, northern America and Japan. Egypt has predominantly genotype 4 infection and genotype 3 is endemic in south Asia and the Indian subcontinent. Figure 9.1 shows the distribution of genotypes worldwide.

Viral genotype remains an important factor to consider, as some therapies are less effective against some genotypes. Moreover, genotype may have an effect on rate of fibrosis progression.

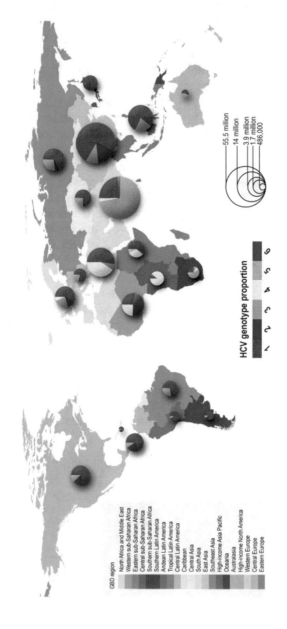

FIGURE 9.1 Prevalence of Hepatitis C and genotype by region (reproduced with permission from Messina et al. [9])

Presentation

The incubation for HCV infection is between 2 and 10 weeks. 80% of patients are asymptomatic during acute infection. Symptomatic patients present with an insidious onset of acute hepatitis with anorexia, nausea, fatigue and fevers. Jaundice is seen in 25% of patients. Fulminant hepatitis is extremely rare (<1%).

After infection, 25% of patient will clear the virus spontaneously over a period of 2–6 months. The remaining 75% of patients develop chronic infection, defined by persistent HCV RNA more than 6 months after index infection.

The majority of chronically infected patients are asymptomatic and have a normal clinical examination or have non-specific symptoms like tiredness and poor concentration ("brain fog").

Chronic infection is most often picked up through screening of at-risk individuals (for example, at needle exchange programmes or through the incidental finding of abnormal liver function tests). If not picked up incidentally, chronic infection does not normally present until patients develop complications of cirrhosis such as ascites, variceal bleeding, encephalopathy or impaired synthetic function. Up to 19% of untreated patients with cirrhosis will eventually develop hepatocellular carcinoma. The progression from exposure to decompensated cirrhosis or HCC is between 20 and 30 years. Concomitant alcohol use and co-infection with hepatitis B or HIV worsens prognosis and increases rate of disease progression. Effective anti-retroviral therapy improves outcomes in HIV co-infection.

Extrahepatic manifestations in CHC are relatively common and occur in up to 74% of patients, although they may not be identified as related to CHC by the patient or their care team. The most common presenting symptoms include arthralgia, paraesthesia and myalgia. Circulating immune complexes, autoimmune processes and mononuclear cell dysfunction are key in the pathogenesis of these non-liver phenomena. Chronic infection is linked to an increase in insulin resistance and type-2 diabetes mellitus. Consequently, infection increases cardiovascular risk, in particular cerebrovascular disease.

Circulating immune complexes may lead to a mixed (type 2a) cryoglobulinaemia that can present in variety of ways, ranging from asymptomatic detection of circulating mixed cryoglobulin complexes (seen in 40–50% of CHC patients) to cryoglobulinaemic vasculitis. Serum cryoglobulin and complement levels do not correlate with disease severity. Clinical manifestations include purpuric skin lesions, arthralgia, polyneuropathy and membranoproliferative glomerulonephritis.

CHC infection is associated with auto-antibody production and many autoimmune diseases have been described. Immune Thrombocytopenic Purpura (ITP) is an autoimmune condition with antibodies against platelet membrane proteins. CHC is frequently seen in conjunction with ITP, in a significantly higher incidence than the general population.

Links between HCV infection and lung disease have been reported, in particular pulmonary fibrosis. The mechanism of disease, at present, is not fully defined. Lichen planus is a pruritic dermatological condition from a cell-mediated immune response and is seen with increased incidence in patients with CHC infection, and vice versa. Other conditions associated with CHC include porphyria cutanea tarda, Sjogren's syndrome and lymphoproliferative disorders, in particular non-Hodgkin B-cell lymphoma.

Investigations

Hepatitis C is usually identified on blood testing. A finding of a positive hepatitis C antibody indicates previous exposure to the virus. Polymerase chain reaction (PCR) testing to identify the presence of circulating viral RNA distinguishes chronic infection from spontaneous clearance or successfully treated past infection. PCR is also used to identify viral genotype, which may be of benefit in planning therapy (unless pangenotypic therapy is preferred). Negative anti-HCV with RNA positivity suggests acute infection, with the time from infection to RNA positivity being approximately 2 weeks. Antibody seroconversion may take 3 months or more and may be significantly delayed in HIV positive people with a low CD4 count, who require RNA testing to confirm diagnosis. HCV core antigen may be used as a substitute marker for HCV RNA in diagnosis and treatment monitoring.

Screening for HCV should be offered to all intravenous drug users, HIV-positive people, pre-1990 blood product recipients and men who have sex with men (MSM) who engage in high-risk sexual activities. Testing should also be offered to sex workers, tattoo recipients, migrants from high prevalence regions, alcohol dependent people and former prisoners [4].

Assessment of liver fibrosis remains important, especially with regard to follow-up care and planning. As all patients with CHC should be offered prompt therapy, it should not be used to prioritise care in developed health systems. All patients should receive a liver ultrasound. Traditionally liver biopsy with semi-quantitative staging of fibrosis was thought to be the gold standard investigation. However, this is invasive and carries the risk of serious complications and is not appropriate for repeated use or in patient with coagulopathy (either due to severe liver disease or primary clotting disorders). Biopsy still has a role in the event of diagnostic uncertainty, such as suspected mixed aetiology liver disease where biopsy results will influence clinical decision-making. Non-invasive methods for estimating liver fibrosis are therefore the primary choice for fibrosis assessment and may be based on either blood tests or imaging technology.

Blood panels to assess liver fibrosis may consist of composite indices of readily available clinical parameters (for example, the APRI index or the FIB-4 score which are based on serum ALT, AST, platelet values and the patient's age) or may be based on patented algorithms where samples are analysed by a commercial company to give a measure of liver fibrosis (for example, the Enhanced Liver Fibrosis, or ELF™ test).

Imaging based techniques typically use shear wave propagation technology through the liver to assess liver stiffness as a surrogate for hepatic fibrosis (for example, transient elastography or FibroScan™). Liver stiffness values are correlated to estimate fibrosis. In most resource rich countries FibroScan™ has become the standard method for fibrosis assessment. Alternative liver stiffness measurements, such as using acoustic radiation force imaging (ARFI), can also provide a reliable method to detect advanced fibrotic disease.

Management

The management of CHC goes beyond just antiviral therapy. Patients should be fully informed about the condition and advised about behaviour modification to reduce transmission risk, including protected sexual intercourse and avoiding sharing toothbrushes, razors or drug injecting equipment. Hepatitis A and B testing should be undertaken and vaccination offered to susceptible individuals. The treatability and tolerability of hepatitis C with newer agents should be communicated clearly to enhance adherence to treatment as there remains misconceptions from earlier therapy modalities.

Prior to 2014, the treatment of hepatitis C was comprised of PEGylated (the addition of a polyethylene glycol polymer) alpha interferon-based regimens, commonly combined with ribavirin. Interferon is associated with multiple problems including the need for it to be administered by injection, a significant side effect profile, long treatment duration and only modest efficacy in hepatitis C. Treatment courses ranged from 24 to 48 weeks with variable cure rates (45% for genotype 1 and 4, approximately 80% for genotype 2 and 3). Long treatment courses and side effects affected adherence and thus efficacy. Moreover, risks of serious complication are markedly increased in patients with advanced liver fibrosis/cirrhosis who also had a much higher rate of treatment failure. The limitations of interferon-based regimens meant that treatment was traditionally offered most frequently to patients with more advanced fibrosis, after liver transplantation (where the rate of fibrosis progression is highest) and to people injecting drugs to prevent onward infection.

The treatment of hepatitis C has been revolutionised in recent years by the advent of directly acting antiviral agents (DAAs), with treatment initiation rates accelerating following the improved access to DAAs since 2014/15. DAAs target viral replication, and as hepatitis C is an RNA virus with no reservoirs of infection, profound direct inhibition of viral replication will allow host clearance of infection and cure.

The intention of treatment is cure, in order to reduce progression of liver fibrosis, cirrhosis, hepatocellular carcinoma and thereby reduce mortality. Cure is defined as a sustained viral response with undetectable HCV RNA or HCV core antigen 12 or 24 weeks after treatment completion (SVR 12 or SVR 24). SVR rates in the treatment of CHC with DAAs usually exceed 90%. Successful treatment of CHC leads to an 80% reduction in the risk of decompensation in patients with compensated cirrhosis and higher levels of protection in patients with early-stage fibrosis.

DAAs have been developed by direct analysis of viral genome and proteins. At present three classes of DAA are licenced. These are protease (or NS3/4A serine) inhibitors—for example, grazoprevir and glecaprevir, polymerase (or NS5B) inhibitors—for example, sofosbuvir and dasabuvir and NS5A inhibitors—for example, ledipasvir [5]. Their modes of action are summarised in Fig. 9.2. The high levels of

Current Antiviral Targets and Drug Classes

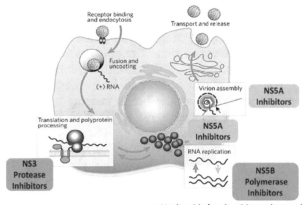

FIGURE 9.2 Current Antiviral Targets and Drug Classes. In house prepared slide (Courtesy Prof A M Geretti)

viral heterogeneity and development of resistance mutations with single agent antiviral therapy mean that combination therapy is required. Combination therapy can be with multiple classes of DAAs or with DAAs and ribavirin. These are frequently co-formulated to reduce pill burden and enhance adherence. Combination therapy with alpha-interferon has now become unnecessary. Several pangenotypic regimens exist. Choice of regimen should be tailored to the individual patient and is dependent on availability, cost, previous treatments, virology and presence of cirrhosis or decompensated liver disease.

People with acute hepatitis C should have their HCV RNA checked four-weekly and considered for treatment if their HCV RNA shows a less than 2 $\log_{10}$ decline by week 4 or remains detectable at week 12. In practice, most centres with ready access to DAA therapy will treat acute hepatitis C to reduce risk of onward transmission and public health benefit.

All adults with chronic hepatitis C should be considered for treatment with DAAs. Treatment should be commenced rapidly in the presence of significant fibrosis (METAVIR F2-F3) or cirrhosis (F4), significant extrahepatic manifestations, HCV recurrence post-transplant and in high-risk individuals (e.g. current intravenous drug users). In most nations with access to DAA therapy, all patients infected with hepatitis C are triaged rapidly to therapy and minimising delay has become part eradication plan. Treatment may not be indicated if life expectancy is significantly truncated due to comorbidities unrelated to liver disease, such as advanced cancer. The issues to consider before starting treatment are outlined in Table 9.1 and a list of baseline investigations required are given in Table 9.2.

Regimen lengths are typically 8–16 weeks and are associated with SVR rates above 95% typically reported. SVRs rates may be slightly lower in patients with more advanced liver disease (especially decompensated cirrhosis) and in patients with resistance associated substitutions (RAS). Patients without evidence of clinically significant liver disease or fibrosis can be discharged from services once SVR is

TABLE 9.1 Medical history in the work-up of CHC patient

History to Elicit	Importance
Risk factors for re-infection (e.g. continued drug use, high-risk occupation)	Long-term management may require education and risk modification
Likely duration of infection	Advanced fibrosis/cirrhosis more likely in patients infected for longer
Previous failed treatments for CHC	May alter treatment regimen and length. Also increases likelihood of resistance associated substations
Previous discontinuation/ adverse events with CHC treatments	May exclude some treatment options
Complete drug history	Drug-drug interactions with antiviral medications
Previous hepatic decompensation and cirrhosis	Will alter choice of treatment, addition of ribavirin, and potentially lengthen duration.
Comorbidities (e.g. diabetes mellitus, ITP, etc.)	Treatments can affect glycaemic control and induce to thrombocytopaenia
Pregnancy, risk of pregnancy or breastfeeding	Ribavirin has a teratogenic risk
Alcohol history	Chronic alcohol dependence increases rate of fibrosis progression

achieved. The remainder may need to remain under hepatology services for ongoing management of cirrhosis surveillance for hepatocellular carcinoma. Well controlled HIV, previous unsuccessful treatment with interferon, a history of liver transplantation and host genetic status, especially IFNL3 (previously IL28B) status, do not appear to affect the success rates of combination DAA treatment.

Special consideration may be required for certain population groups. For example, in hepatitis B co-infected individu-

TABLE 9.2 Important investigations in work-up of CHC patients

Investigation	Importance
Genotype (+/− subtype)	Will influence drug choice and duration
RNA viral load	Assess success of treatment and likelihood of success.
Non-invasive assessment of fibrosis (e.g. transient elastography, magnetic resonance elastography, serum biomarkers and biomarker panels)	Define presence/absence of advanced fibrosis and cirrhosis. Method to ration treatments, especially the newer costlier therapies, to those with the greatest need.
Assessment of transplant suitability in patients with cirrhotic	Patients with advanced disease may require liver transplant, irrespective of viral eradication
Check for concomitant infections.	Those co-infected with chronic hepatitis B or HIV may need alteration to treatment regim
Assess for co-existing liver diseases	Other chronic liver disease may need management after viral clearance
Liver biopsy	May be needed to assess level of fibrosis, if non-invasive markers display discordancy. Will also give information about presence of co-existing liver disease

als there is a rare risk of HBV reactivation following DAA treatment [6]. Treatment of HBV may be necessary before commencing HCV treatment, where eligible. Sofosbuvir-based regimens are not recommended in severe renal impairment (eGFR <30 ml/min/1.73 m^2) [5]. Protease inhibitors should be avoided in those with a history of decompensated cirrhosis due to increase toxicity risk and further episodes of decompensation. In the event of hepatic decompensation successful treatment with a protease inhibitor free regimen may lead to improvement in liver function and avoid the need for liver transplantation. Treatment timing will depend on waiting lists and the urgency of transplantation, with pre-transplantation treatment of hepatitis C being favoured except in the most advanced cases of liver disease [7]. Hepatitis C recurrence is universal post-transplant if the individual has not had treatment. In liver transplant recipients with either new infection or recurrence treatment should be initiated early to minimise graft dysfunction and disease.

The World Health Organisation has set a target to eliminate viral hepatitis as a public health threat by 2030, with the intention of increasing rates of diagnosis, reducing the incidence of new infections, treating at least 80% of those eligible and reducing liver disease-related mortality [8]. An estimated 13 million new infections and 1.1 million deaths could be prevented by 2030 through elimination, with a significant public health cost. Despite the high SVR rates of DAAs, barriers to treatment still exist. Widely available access to testing and treatment is still lacking in many countries worldwide, with specific focus needed for at-risk populations such as users of injectable drugs, MSM and individuals from high prevalence areas. Public health initiatives should also be targeted at destigmatising viral hepatitis and encouraging take-up of screening by informing the public of the high cure rates of hepatitis C.

Although DAAs have radically changed the success rates and tolerability of HCV treatment they have not been without problems. One problem is the development of viral resistance. Resistance associated substitution (RAS) testing is not routine practice but should be offered to every patient who fails to achieve an SVR with DAA therapy. The potential for resistance development is the most worrying issue for DAA usage. Resistance to one DAA confers significant cross resistance to other drugs in the same class. Avoidance of resistance requires that patients have excellent compliance for the duration of treatment. In patients who fail therapy, careful and individualised assessment of the resistance patterns is needed to choose the optimal second-line regimen. This may include extended courses of standard therapies or reserved regimens (e.g., triple combination salvage regimens). At present it is not clear how future treatment should be directed for patients who fail treatment with combination DAA therapy and the optimal time for repeat treatment. Resistance may persist for many years (currently unknown) after unsuccessful therapy.

Summary

Chronic hepatitis C is a world health problem with significant associated morbidity and mortality. We now have the tools to potentially eradicate hepatitis C, but success will be dependent on improving diagnosis, especially in harder to reach populations where CHC is more prevalent. Moreover, access and affordability of DAA therapies is critical for success.

Answers to Questions

1. (a)

Liver biopsy is considered the gold standard for the assessment of fibrosis but is an invasive test with limitations and associated morbidity. As such non-invasive methods have been developed. These broadly divide into serological marker panels (e.g. APRI, ELF™, Fibrotest™ and FIB-4) and physical methods that predominantly assess stiffness or elasticity of the liver using a waveform (e.g. FibroScan™, ARFI and MR elastography). Ultrasound scanning is important to assess for portal hypertension as a consequence of cirrhosis, assess for the presence of liver lesions and will give some information regarding the physical properties of the liver but does not directly assess the level of fibrosis.

2. (c)

From these options C is the best response. Waiting in a patient with well compensated cirrhosis is not advised as the window for treatment may be missed. Current regimens are highly efficacious and well tolerated in patients with genotype 1 CHC with cirrhosis. Similarly, her cirrhosis is compensated (Childs-Pugh-Turcotte A, MELD 7) and there is not have clear liver transplant indications. Treatment can be undertaken with DAAs at this point and prevent the future necessity of transplant. Alternative interferon-free regimes have similar efficacy and tolerability to Sofosbuvir, Ledipasvir and Ribavirin for 12 weeks (for example, 16 week therapy with Elbasvir, Grazoprevir and Ribavirin). Treatment with Sofosbuvir, Velpatasvir and Voxilaprevir is usually reserved for first-line treatment failures.

3. (c)

Jane has a high likelihood of liver cirrhosis and should not be discharged. Current guidelines recommend 6-monthly imaging of the liver as surveillance for hepatocellular carcinoma in patients with cirrhosis who could have treatment in the event of a detectable lesion. There is no need to repeat her HCV RNA viral load regularly. AFP may be considered as an adjunct to US surveillance but should not be used on its own. Assessing her synthetic function is sensible to ensure that there is not a deterioration that may require further management. Biopsy would not routinely be applied for this purpose.

References

1. Hughes G. Hepatitis C in the UK 2020: working to eliminate hepatitis C as a major public health threat. Publ Health Engl. 2020.
2. Spearman CW, Dusheiko GM, Hellard M, Sonderup M. Hepatitis C. Lancet. 2019;394(10207):1451–66.
3. Frank C, Mohamed MK, Strickland GT, Lavanchy D, Arthur RR, Magder LS, et al. The role of parenteral antischistosomal therapy in the spread of hepatitis C virus in Egypt. Lancet. 2000;355(9207):887–91.
4. World Health Organisation. Guidelines for the care and treatment of persons diagnosed with chronic hepatitis C virus infection. Geneva: WHO Guidelines Approved by the Guidelines Review Committee; 2018.

5. European Association for the Study of the Liver. EASL recommendations on treatment of hepatitis C: final update of the series. J Hepatol. 2020;73:1170–218.

6. Serper M, Forde KA, Kaplan DE. Rare clinically significant hepatic events and hepatitis B reactivation occur more frequently following rather than during direct-acting antiviral therapy for chronic hepatitis C: data from a national US cohort. J Viral Hepat. 2018;25(2):187–97.

7. World Health Organization. Winning the race to eliminate hepatitis C: accelerating efforts together to reach the World Health Organization's 2030 elimination targets. Geneva: World Health Organization; 2020.

8. World Health Organisation. Global Health Sector Strategy on Viral Hepatitis, 2016–2021.

9. Messina JP, Humphreys I, Flaxman A, Brown A, Cooke GS, Pybus OG, Barnes E. Global distribution and prevalence of hepatitis C virus genotypes. Hepatology. 2015 Jan;61(1):77–87.

Chapter 10
Autoimmune Hepatitis and Overlap Syndromes

Kristel K. Leung and Gideon M. Hirschfield

Key Learning Points

This chapter aims to leave readers with the ability to:

- Describe the epidemiology of autoimmune hepatitis (AIH), including associated genetic and environmental factors;
- Apply clinical, biochemical, immunological, and histopathological criteria to diagnose AIH;
- Describe the management of patients with AIH, including treatment options and goals of treatment;
- Appreciate the challenges when considering diagnosing autoimmune overlap syndromes.

K. K. Leung
Division of Gastroenterology and Hepatology, Department of Medicine, Toronto Centre for Liver Disease, University Health Network, University of Toronto, Toronto, ON, Canada
e-mail: kristel.leung@uhn.ca

G. M. Hirschfield (✉)
Division of Gastroenterology and Hepatology, Department of Medicine, Toronto Centre for Liver Disease, Toronto General Hospital, University Health Network, University of Toronto, Toronto, ON, Canada
e-mail: gideon.hirschfield@uhn.ca

© Springer Nature Switzerland AG 2022   195
T. Cross (ed.), *Liver Disease in Clinical Practice*, In Clinical Practice, https://doi.org/10.1007/978-3-031-10012-3_10

Chapter Review Questions

A 41-year-old woman presents with a 6-month history of lethargy and vague abdominal pain and has been referred to your clinic with elevated liver enzymes. Her past medical history includes Graves' disease for which she now takes thyroxine. There is no given history of prescribed or non-prescribed medications otherwise. Physical examination is unremarkable. Notable blood test results include ALT 190 U/L, AST 180 U/L, ALP 100 U/L, bilirubin 10 μmol/L, albumin 40 g/L, INR 1.1, and immunoglobulin G (IgG) 22.4 g/L. An ultrasound abdomen was normal.

1. What key investigations would you be looking to do next?

    (a) Hemochromatosis genotyping
    (b) Alpha-1-antitrypsin levels
    (c) Hepatitis B, C, and autoimmune serology
    (d) Liver biopsy

2. The blood tests reveal positive results: Anti-SMA titre is 1:80 and ANA 1:160. The rest of the liver screen and TSH is unremarkable. You suspect a diagnosis of AIH. What is the next appropriate management step?

    (a) Start the patient on prednisolone and azathioprine and explain treatment is for life
    (b) Repeat the bloodwork in 2 weeks to see if the anti-SMA titre and IgG values change to higher titres
    (c) Request a liver biopsy to aid confirmation of diagnosis, severity, and further exclude alternate cause of liver injury
    (d) Send blood for further serology (anti-SLA)

3. A liver biopsy demonstrated features of chronic hepatitis with a plasma cell-rich interface hepatitis without alternative aetiologies suggested. Some fibrosis was reported. The

patient was started on a combination of prednisolone and subsequently azathioprine. Her liver biochemistry and IgG values normalized by 6 months of therapy. How long should treatment be continued?

(a) Treatment can be stopped now that her liver biochemistry has normalized
(b) Treatment should be continued indefinitely as risk of relapse is high
(c) Treatment should be continued for 2–5 years with maintenance of normal biochemistry values; a trial off therapy can be considered with monitoring
(d) Her treatment should be continued for 1 year with maintenance of normal biochemistry values, then stopped

Introduction

Autoimmune hepatitis (AIH) is an uncommon immune-mediated liver disease with a fluctuating and generally progressive course. The disease has a varied presentation that spans sub-clinical disease to fulminant liver failure. For the majority of patients, effective treatment is available to prevent complications of chronic liver disease. The aetiology of AIH is unknown but is thought to be due to a complex interaction between genetic and environmental factors. Also, AIH patients frequently have co-existing autoimmune diseases. The pathogenesis of AIH is characterized by cell and antibody-mediated destruction of hepatocytes. Although there is a female predilection, it also affects males as well as all age groups.

The diagnosis of AIH can be challenging. One should first exclude alternate causes of liver injury; practically speaking, common viral and drug injuries predominate in the differential. Subsequently, identifying supportive hepatitis biochemistry, autoimmune serology and consistent histology is needed to reach a diagnosis of AIH. In the context of increased serum aminotransferase activity, characteristically there is elevation of immunoglobulin G (IgG) concentrations and presence of circulating autoantibodies frequently associated with AIH. A liver biopsy is generally required to confidently establish a diagnosis, grade disease severity, exclude alternate competing causes, and justify long-term immunosuppression which underpins treatment. Initial disease is treated to the point of remission, with maintenance therapy thereafter to prevent relapse. Definitions of remission are varied. Recently, inducing both biochemical and histologic remission has been the goal, albeit the true impact of such a strict definition remains to be confirmed, particularly given the range of disease presentation by severity and the breadth of age at diagnosis [1]. Notably, historic data clearly demonstrates that untreated severe disease is associated with a very poor survival and is a course that corticosteroids and azathioprine can strikingly change.

Epidemiology

AIH is a disease that affects all age groups, both sexes, and is seen across all ethnicities and geographic areas. The pooled worldwide annual incidence and prevalence of AIH is 1.37 and 17.44 per 100,000 persons, respectively, with similar incidence worldwide and a higher prevalence in Europe and America compared to the Asian population [2]. Early series highlighted a bimodal age distribution for disease: the first peak between the ages of 10 and 30 years and second between 40 and 50 years. However, more contemporary descriptions highlight diagnosis across all ages, particularly elderly patients, with recent studies demonstrating peak rates in patients aged over 60 years [2], as well as a peak incidence in men at age 65 and women at age 70 [3]. Overall, pooled incidence and prevalence estimates in women are fourfold to fivefold more than in men [2]. Men tend to present younger, have more disease flares, but better survival than women [4].

The clinical presentation and disease course of AIH varies according to region and ethnicity. Clinicians should be mindful of varying patterns of presentation and severity that have been described, e.g., in African Americans, Somalian males, and North American Aboriginals. One should seek to exclude locally relevant environmental toxins such as khat.

Aetiology and Pathogenesis

The aetiology of AIH is unknown, and it is highly unlikely that there is a single aetiologic agent. Disease aetiology is likely multifactorial with genetic and environmental factors playing a role in disease pathogenesis. As with other autoimmune conditions, AIH is strongly associated with genetic variation within the human leukocyte antigen (HLA) region. The HLA system is involved in immune regulation and HLA class II DRB1 alleles have a particularly strong association with AIH risk, with possession of HLA DR3 (*DRB1*0301*) and DR4 (*DRB1*0401*) increasing overall susceptibility risk. The carriage of HLA DR3 is predictive of more aggressive disease whilst HLA DR4 predicts later onset. Recently a genome-wide association study (GWAS) identified a gene locus previously associated with other autoimmune disease, *SH2B3*, is also associated with the development of AIH [5]. Other common non-HLA associated genetic risk associations were not confirmed in this GWAS study, whilst very rare single gene associations with AIH (AIRE, GATA-2) have predominantly proved of relevance for highlighting pathways to liver injury (most notably regulatory T cell dysfunction).

Environmental triggers include reports of AIH developing following viral liver disease such as Hepatitis A and even severe acute respiratory syndrome coronavirus 2. In addition, there are well recognized forms of drug-induced AIH with medications including nitrofurantoin, minocycline, and halothane that can sometimes be self-limiting following drug cessation. The rise in AIH in the elderly may also reflect pan-exposure to more drugs but this remains speculative. Mechanistically, environmental triggers may be presented immunologically in a manner that triggers molecular mimicry, particularly if the individual has a genetic predisposition to altered immune regulation, albeit subtle. Breakdown of self-tolerance mechanisms to liver autoantigens is presumed to result in T cell-mediated destruction of hepatocytes. Disturbance in the regulatory mechanism of regulatory T cells has been proposed to result in an immune attack against liver autoantigens. Lymphocytes, plasma cells, and macrophages are activated and release cytokines, which results in further hepatocyte damage. Underpinning changes in B cell regulation of T cell responses are also relevant.

Clinical Features

The clinical presentation of AIH ranges from asymptomatic disease through to acute fulminant liver failure. Around 25% of patients are asymptomatic at diagnosis, including some with cirrhosis, with these cases only being picked up due to slightly elevated liver enzymes on routine bloodwork. Some non-specific symptoms commonly seen in patients include fatigue, weight loss, abdominal pain, nausea, amenorrhea, rash, and flitting joint pains. Clinicians must be wary that a common unfortunate misconception is that AIH cannot be fluctuating in its presentation.

AIH presents acutely in approximately 25% of cases. This is either due to acute exacerbation of chronic hepatitis or true acute AIH without any chronic features on histology. Patients may complain of similar symptoms reported in acute viral or drug-induced hepatitis. Acute AIH can lead to fulminant liver failure; these patients are jaundiced and have features of liver failure.

Approximately 30% of patients are cirrhotic at presentation, amongst whom some may present with features of decompensation such as jaundice, ascites, encephalopathy, and/or variceal bleeding.

Patients may also have co-existing autoimmune diseases, including thyroiditis (most common), type I diabetes, inflammatory bowel disease, rheumatoid arthritis, primary Sjogren's syndrome or coeliac disease. There may be a family history of autoimmune conditions and having relatives with AIH increases individual risk.

There are no specific signs on physical examination. Patients with acute hepatitis may have fever, jaundice, hepatomegaly, and upper abdominal tenderness. Young women may manifest marked acne with acute severe presentations. There may be signs of chronic liver disease and/or decompensation.

Diagnosis

A diagnosis of AIH requires a combination of compatible biochemical, immunological, and histological findings associated with AIH, with exclusion of alternate liver disease [6]. A thorough history assessing for risk factors of liver disease including a detailed drug/herbal remedy history of new and long-established drugs is essential.

Biochemical

Serum alanine aminotransferase (ALT) and aspartate aminotransferase (AST) activities are usually raised and are indicative of hepatic inflammatory activity. In comparison, alkaline phosphatase (ALP) values are either normal or mildly raised.

Elevated gammaglobulins, specifically serum IgG concentrations, are found in 85% of patients. Conversely, immunoglobulin A and M concentrations are predominantly normal, although there may be minor increments. Occasionally at the time of presentation, 5–10% of patients may have IgG concentrations within the limits defined by the laboratory.

Immunological

If a diagnosis of AIH is suspected, serum autoantibodies should be sought and interpreted in the context of the clinical presentation [7]. Circulating non-organ specific autoantibodies add weight and are key to the diagnosis of AIH. Serology, just as histology, needs to be considered in the clinical context of the individual patient, and serology alone is insufficient to make a diagnosis and treatment plan for any patient with autoimmune liver disease.

Serology is also used to sub-classify AIH serologically into type 1 and type 2 diseases (Table 10.1). Positive anti-smooth muscle antibody (ASMA) and/or anti-nuclear antibody (ANA) characterize type 1 AIH, whilst positive anti-liver kidney microsomal antibody 1 (LKM-1) and/or anti-liver cytosolic 1 (LC-1) define type 2 AIH. The female to male ratio in type 1 is 3:1 and type 2 is 9:1, with type 1 seen more in adults and type 2 seen more in children.

Anti-soluble liver antigen/liver-pancreas (SLA/LP) antibodies are positive in 10–30% of patients. These antibodies are the only specific antibodies associated with AIH (specificity 99%) and may aid in the diagnosis when conventional autoantibodies are negative. Positive SLA/LP antibody status is associated with worse prognosis, with higher risk of severe disease and risk of relapse. Anti-SLA/LP antibody assays may not be readily available outside of the setting of a specialist centre; of interest the presence of anti-Ro antibodies is often a good surrogate for SLA reactivity.

Other antibodies that may be positive include anti-mitochondrial antibodies (AMA; most commonly diagnostic of primary biliary cholangitis/cirrhosis), with 8–12% of patients with AIH being AMA positive throughout their disease with no features of biliary disease. Antibodies to actin and atypical peripheral anti-neutrophilic cytoplasm

TABLE 10.1 Type 1 and Type 2 autoimmune hepatitis

	Type 1	Type 2
Percentage of cases	80%	20%
Geography	Worldwide	More common in Northern Europe
Female:male ratio	3:1	9:1
Age of presentation	All ages	Usually childhood and young adults
Presentation	Variable	Severe. Mostly acute presentation; lower IgG values than type 1
Autoantibodies	ANA, anti-SMA, anti-SLA	Anti-LKM1, anti-LC-1
HLA	HLA DR3/DR4	HLA DR3/DR7
Prognosis	Good	More aggressive and difficult to treat, high relapse risk and inevitable need for long-term maintenance immunosuppression

(p-ANCA) may also be seen in type 1 AIH but are not specific, therefore have limited diagnostic benefit. SMA in AIH is mainly directed against F-actin, and reports suggest that most patients with type 1 AIH have antibodies to F-actin as well as being seropositive for SMA; hence testing for F-actin antibodies may be helpful in certain settings. However, reliance only on anti F-actin specificity of SMA may miss a diagnosis of AIH, as F-actin is not the only target of SMA, therefore lack of detection of anti F-actin does not exclude AIH [6].

At initial presentation, 20% of patients may have undetectable or very low titres of autoantibody levels. If clinical suspicion remains high, autoantibody tests should be repeated; on occasion it is appropriate to liaise with the immunology laboratories to ensure technical issues are not interfering with assay interpretation, e.g., failure to adequately dilute sera.

Pathology

Liver biopsy continues to have an important role in the diagnosis and management of AIH, albeit definitive features histologically do not exist, and clinicopathologic correlation is always required. It is generally recommended that all patients have liver histology evaluation at baseline, unless there are strong clinical contraindications e.g., severe coagulopathy. Its role complements exclusion of alternate aetiologies (in particular, fatty infiltration and viral infection), evaluating severity of liver inflammation, identification of overlapping biliary injury, and staging liver fibrosis. Histology is characterized by interface hepatitis, a lymphoplasmacytic infiltrate predominantly in the portal area (Fig. 10.1) but may breach the junction between portal tract and liver parenchyma [8]. Although plasma cells are typically abundant, this is not always the case, and their paucity does not exclude AIH. The abundance of plasma cells may help in differentiating it from viral hepatitis. Interface hepatitis is often associated with ballooning and rosetting of peri-portal hepatocytes (regenerating hepatocytes) as well as emperipolesis (i.e., penetration of lymphocytes into peri-portal hepatocytes); this latter feature is sensitive for a diagnosis of AIH and should be actively sought. Disease severity is characterized by presence and degree of necro-inflammatory activity and fibrosis; upwards of one-third of patients will be cirrhotic at presentation. Interface hepatitis causes peri-portal fibrosis. In more severe cases, this can progress to bridging necrosis and nodule formation. This is predicative of later development of cirrhosis and associated with poor outcomes. Occasionally, there is

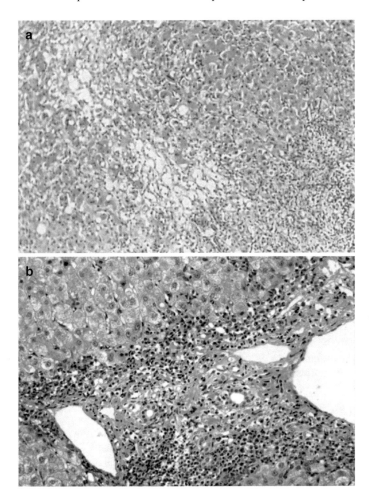

FIGURE 10.1 Histology of active autoimmune hepatitis. (**a**) Evidence of portal inflammation consisting mainly of lymphocytes (H&E). (**b**) Evidence of severe portal inflammation with interface hepatitis close to visible portal tracts, with necroinflammatory foci present (H&E)

mild bile duct inflammation without destruction. With a severe inflammatory insult, there may be bile duct damage or loss. This does not tend to be extensive and is not usually observed following remission, which may help distinguish AIH from cholestatic liver disease.

Differential Diagnosis

The differential diagnosis of AIH is broad but of most importance to consider are viral infections, drugs (e.g., checkpoint inhibitors, nitrofurantoin, minocycline, herbal remedies, new biologic medications), metabolic liver disease, and infiltrative aetiologies (further outlined in Table 10.2).

TABLE 10.2 Differential diagnosis for autoimmune hepatitis

Condition	Notes
Drug-induced liver injury	
• Checkpoint inhibitors • Nitrofurantoin, minocycline • Herbal therapies	It may be difficult to differentiate from autoimmune hepatitis. Thorough drug history both old and new (prescribed and non-prescribed) is vital
Viral hepatitis	
• Hepatitis A • Hepatitis B (± Hepatitis D) • Hepatitis C • Hepatitis E • Epstein–Barr virus • Cytomegalovirus • Severe acute respiratory syndrome coronavirus 2	Autoantibodies including low titres of ANA, SMA, and LKM can be detectable in viral hepatitis. This is particularly the case with hepatitis C

Table 10.2 (continued)

Condition	Notes
Metabolic disease	
• Non-alcoholic steatohepatitis	Low titres of autoantibodies including ANA and SMA may be positive in non-alcoholic steatohepatitis
• Wilson's disease	
• Alpha 1 antitrypsin deficiency	
• Haemochromatosis	
Alcohol related liver disease	Low titres of autoantibodies including ANA and SMA may be positive in alcohol related liver disease
Other autoimmune liver diseases	
• Primary biliary cholangitis	The presence of anti-mitochondrial antibodies is suggestive of primary biliary cholangitis
• Primary sclerosing cholangitis	Biliary tree pathology may suggest primary sclerosing cholangitis Failure to respond to immunosuppression as well as cholestatic liver biochemistry should lead to consideration of cholestatic liver disease

Scoring Systems Used in Diagnosis

The International Autoimmune Hepatitis Group (IAIHG) has produced revised simplified criteria for the diagnosis of AIH (Table 10.3). It constitutes a scoring system that is simple, useful, and easily applied [9]. These criteria serve as an

TABLE 10.3 Simplified diagnostic criteria for autoimmune hepatitis (International Autoimmune Hepatitis Group) [11]

Variable	Cut-off	Points
ANA or SMA	Titre ≥1:40	1[a]
One or more of:		
ANA or SMA	≥1:80	
LKM	≥1:40	2[a]
SLA	Positive	
Serum immunoglobulin G	>Upper limit of normal	1
	≥1.1 × upper limit of normal	2
Liver histology	Compatible	1
	Typical	2
Absence of viral hepatitis	No	0
	Yes	2

A total score of ≥6 indicates probable autoimmune hepatitis while a score of ≥7 indicates definite autoimmune hepatitis
[a]Addition of points achieved for all autoantibodies (maximum of 2 points)

aid to diagnosis with 95% sensitivity and 90% specificity, albeit require clinical judgement to use appropriately. This is especially important in acute onset AIH or fulminant AIH, as using the criteria may fail to diagnose patients, as immunoglobulin levels may be normal and circulating antibodies undetectable. Equally, where there is a clear alternate diagnosis, its application is inappropriate, and likely to confuse.

Other Investigations

A liver screen including viral serology, blood tests to exclude alpha 1 antitrypsin deficiency and Wilson's disease should be performed to exclude other differential diagnoses. A liver ultrasound should be performed early in initial investigations to exclude overt biliary pathology and assess for splenomegaly, which may indicate portal hypertension. It is recommended that children/young adults who have a diagnosis of AIH should have magnetic resonance cholangiopancreatography (MRCP) to exclude biliary pathology, which if present, is suggestive of autoimmune sclerosing cholangitis/primary sclerosing cholangitis.

Management

The treatment of AIH is based on case series and relatively few controlled trials, and although effective in improving survival benefit and preventing worsening outcomes, the exact mechanisms behind therapy effectiveness are unclear. Guidelines on treatment exist from American Association for the Study of Liver Disease [10], European Association for the Study of the Liver [11], and British Society of Gastroenterology [12], with wide variation in the management of patients with AIH even amongst experts [13]. Figure 10.2 describes a treatment algorithm that may be used. Predniso(lo)ne with or without azathioprine is a mainstay of therapy for treatment induction [14]. IgG values are also useful to monitor response to therapy and as a sign of relapse. However, one must remember that pan-hypergammaglobulinaemia can be seen in cirrhosis, and care should be taken to assess IgG values on treatment even when within normal range.

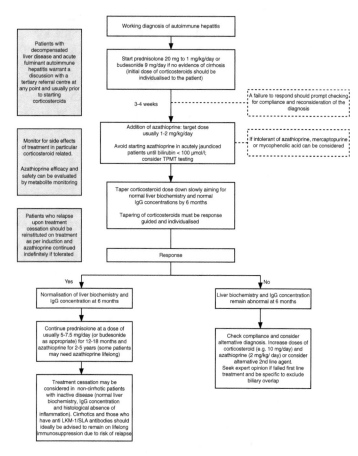

FIGURE 10.2 Summary treatment algorithm for autoimmune hepatitis. This figure is a representation of our treatment approach. It is important to note that at any point patients can be considered for transplant assessment or an opinion from a tertiary referral centre sought

Who Should Be Treated?

Most patients with AIH require treatment. The British Society of Gastroenterology guidelines suggest that treatment should be offered to all patients with AIH and evidence of moderate or severe inflammation, those who have cirrhosis and active disease, younger patients in the hope of preventing cirrhosis in the future, and symptomatic patients [12].

Patients who may not need treatment are elderly patients with mild disease activity and/or significant co-morbidity where the risk of immunosuppression outweighs the benefit. In this cohort of patients, uncontrolled trials have showed that survival is similar to those on treatment. Studies have also demonstrated that patients with inactive cirrhosis (histologically absent or minimal inflammation) but with serological evidence of disease do not benefit from treatment.

If a decision has been made to withhold treatment, patients should be followed up (e.g., every 3–6 months), monitored for deteriorating liver enzyme values and liver function, and re-evaluated as appropriate. AIH is a lifelong disease, therefore all patients with this diagnosis should be regularly followed up, regardless of whether they are on treatment. Patients on treatment should be monitored at both the primary and secondary care level.

Pharmacological Treatment

Prednisolone is usually the drug of choice initially to induce remission. Similarly, prednisone is also used, although it requires hepatic metabolism to convert the medication to its active form. The starting dose varies from 20 mg daily to 1 mg/kg/day. Of note, despite the wide variation in starting dose, no significant differences in rates of normalization of transaminases have been found between high-dose versus low-dose groups [15]. Fundamentally, whilst there are guide-lines for managing AIH, an individualized approach is key to successful care. The prednisolone dose is slowly weaned to the minimum dose required to maintain normal liver bio-chemistry and immunoglobulin levels over 3 months. It is kept on for a period of 12–18 months usually at a dose of around 5–7.5 mg for remission, with uptitration of dosage as needed with elevation in liver enzymes. Dose titrations should be guided by response and individualized. A slow and prolonged course of treatment is particularly essential to induce and maintain remission.

Budesonide, a synthetic corticosteroid, may be used as an alternative to prednisolone in patients with no evidence of cirrhosis for induction in those with early disease and mild fibrosis. Budesonide undergoes first pass metabolism via the liver, therefore should not be used if portal hypertension or a portal vein clot exists. It has fewer side effects and been shown to be as effective as prednisolone in non-cirrhotic patients. The starting dose is 9 mg/day followed by gradual down titration. Budesonide has yet to be approved for maintenance therapy.

Azathioprine is a key agent used in managing AIH and is commonly used to maintain remission as a corticosteroid sparing agent. This is a purine metabolite that is started concurrently or 3–4 weeks after initiation of corticosteroid. Azathioprine in conjunction with predniso(lo)ne is also used as a combination therapy for induction with a dose of azathioprine of 50 mg daily or 1–2 mg/kg/day and prednisolone 30 mg daily. Mercaptopurine can also be used in AIH, most frequently if azathioprine use is associated with side effects such as nausea.

A delay in starting azathioprine allows the clinician time to assess for corticosteroid responsiveness, which is an important confirmatory diagnostic intervention. Commencement of azathioprine is also to be delayed in patients who are jaundiced. The initial target azathioprine dose for maintaining remission is 1 mg/kg/day, with higher doses reserved for those with more difficult disease to control. It is usually continued for 2–5 years but may be indefinite in certain cases. The combination of corticosteroids and azathioprine seems to be more beneficial in achieving histological remission and has fewer side effects than corticosteroids alone (given the ability to use lower doses of corticosteroids). Failure to start azathioprine (or equivalent) is thought to be one of the factors associated with poor long-term outcomes.

Managing Medication Side Effects and Treatment Considerations

Given the need for prolonged immunosuppression in patients with AIH, patients should be tested for immunity against hepatitis A and B infection and susceptible patients offered immunizations as soon as possible. Influenza and pneumococcal immunizations are also suggested for susceptible patients.

Ideally, side effect counselling should be carried out with patients who are being considered for treatment regarding the side effect profiles of medications used in AIH. Long-term use of corticosteroids is associated with significant side effects, which should be addressed and treated. These include diabetes, osteoporosis, hypertension, weight gain, cataracts, adrenal insufficiency, and increased risk of infections [10]. The treatment-associated side effects of corticosteroids are of great concern to patients, explains some of the non-compliance seen in clinical practice, and represent an unmet need for patients who seek equally effective therapy with a better side effect profile. All patients on corticosteroids should have a baseline and annual bone density scan and initiated on calcium and vitamin D supplements.

Side effects of azathioprine include development of photosensitive rash (thus, as a preventive measure, patients should be advised to use sunblock), pancreatitis, bone marrow toxicity, and increased long-term risk of cancer including haematological malignancies. Azathioprine metabolite monitoring can be of value in some patients with AIH, particularly those with difficult to control disease or compliance concerns. Thiopurine methyltransferase testing can be considered for patients prior to starting azathioprine treatment to identify those at increased risk of bone marrow toxicity. Patients on azathioprine should have regular interval monitoring of liver blood test and blood count.

The risk of hepatocellular carcinoma in AIH is elevated, and whilst individually rare, screening should be offered to cirrhotic patients as per standard guidelines.

Assessing Response to Treatment, Treatment Cessation, Outcomes, and Prognosis

Most patients respond to treatment. 80–90% of patients will have a reduction in transaminase activity following initiation of corticosteroids. This typically occurs within weeks of treatment, with gradual improvement of liver biochemistry and immunoglobulin values. Clinical remission is defined by complete normalization of transaminase and immunoglobulin levels. This may take 6–12 months. Histological remission, characterized by absence of interface hepatitis, typically lags behind biochemical remission by several months.

A small proportion of patients do not respond or are slow responders to corticosteroid and azathioprine therapy. Ensuring a patient is adherent is essential, as non-adherence to therapy is the most common reason for treatment failure. Alternative diagnoses including overlap syndromes should also be considered.

Occasionally, the disease may be severe enough to necessitate treatment alteration. An increase in the corticosteroid and azathioprine dose is suggested initially with variable success. Alternatively, second-line agents may be used such as mycophenolate mofetil (MMF), tacrolimus, ciclosporin, rituximab, and infliximab [14]. There is varied clinical opinion as to the choice of agent, and discussion/referral with a specialist is recommended.

The decision to stop immunosuppressants is always difficult. Transaminase and immunoglobulin levels should be normal for at least 18–24 months prior to considering stopping treatment. Furthermore, it is advisable to continue immunosuppressants long enough to allow histological remission, and this may take up to 2–5 years. A liver biopsy to determine histological remission may be considered prior to cessation, but relapse can occur even if the biopsy is normal; cirrhotic patients should rarely, if ever, consider treatment cessation. Patients with ongoing inflammation histologically should remain on treatment due to risk of relapse on cessation. Despite histological remission, 50–90% of patients relapse 12 months after stopping treatment. If a patient experiences a relapse, treatment as per induction should be reinstituted and azathioprine continued indefinitely if tolerated.

Poor prognosis is associated with patients who have cirrhosis, younger onset of disease and presence of SLA/LP, LKM-1, or LC-1 antibodies.

Liver Transplantation

Liver transplantation should be considered in decompensated liver disease or fulminant AIH. Patients with fulminant disease should be promptly transferred to a tertiary centre as they may require urgent liver transplantation. It may be reasonable to commence corticosteroids in those presenting with acute severe AIH; however, this should only be done following discussion with a tertiary centre. Lack of response after 1 week is a sign of poor prognosis.

Survival rates post-transplantation are good and exceed 75% at 5 and 10 years. Unfortunately, recurrence of disease is well described and is seen in 10–50% of patients in various studies, with re-transplantation required in 8–23% [16]. Interestingly, there are cases where an autoimmune type of hepatitis can occur in patients who have had a liver transplant for other causes. This is referred to as de novo AIH.

Special Circumstances

Pregnancy

AIH flares can occur at any stage of pregnancy; however, it is more common during the first 3 months postpartum (~20%). This can occur despite the disease being well-controlled during pregnancy, making it imperative that patients are regularly followed up and their disease controlled from conception to postpartum. Given the potential risk to the foetus of a flare, it is advisable to continue immunosuppression such as corticosteroids and azathioprine during pregnancy. Ideally, pregnancy care should be done conjointly with a high-risk obstetrical expert, with discussion of the risks and benefits of continuing immunosuppression during conception, pregnancy, and postpartum. With regard to MMF use, this medication is absolutely contraindicated in pregnancy and conception should be avoided until at least 6 weeks of cessation. Patients with severe liver disease and portal hypertension should be counselled carefully prior to conception, with discussion and appreciation of the risks of pregnancy, along with appropriate high-risk obstetric input as available.

Overlap Syndromes

AIH, primary biliary cholangitis (PBC), and primary sclerosing cholangitis (PSC) constitute the main spectrum of autoimmune liver disease. It is unsurprising that there is an overlap of biochemical, serological, radiological, and histological features in some patients. The term cross-over or overlap syndrome is used to describe the sequential or simultaneous co-existence of AIH with clear features of either PBC or PSC. There is absence of an exact clinical or pathological definition, therefore designation is arbitrary and imprecise. Given that there is no specific diagnostic test for autoimmune liver disease, clinically overlap syndrome should be considered when a patient's disease course deviates from that expected for the dominant underlying disease [17].

PBC-AIH Overlap

This designation describes patients who have PBC with additional overlapping features of AIH, such as significant elevations in serum aminotransferase activity and elevated IgG concentrations. When this arises, liver biopsy is important, with its interpretation requiring careful multi-disciplinary patient specific discussion. Non-response to treatment in

PBC should not be mistaken for AIH overlap. The presence of significant interface hepatitis on pathology may be suggestive of an overlap, but its presence depends on understanding the nature of the PBC presentation, e.g., treatment failure with ursodeoxycholic acid (UDCA) is much more common in those presenting before the age of 50. Diagnostic criteria proposed by Chazouilleres et al. is commonly used albeit no gold standard exists, fundamentally because defined aetiologic factors remain to be understood. Treatment is largely based on treating the predominant disease and is individualized. No randomized data exists to guide clinicians with treatment in these patients, although a combination of UDCA and corticosteroids is required in most patients to obtain a complete biochemical response [18].

PSC-AIH Overlap

The presence of radiological or histological evidence of typical PSC alongside strong histological features of AIH is suggestive of PSC-AIH overlap. Most commonly, the diagnosis of AIH precedes the development of PSC by years and tends to affect younger patients. PSC should always be considered in AIH patients who are treatment unresponsive. There is often marked elevation in serum ALP levels. Furthermore, patients may have co-existing inflammatory bowel disease. If PSC is suspected, MRCP is recommended to assess for beading and structuring of the biliary tree; many suggest routine MRCP in young patients who present with AIH, given the higher frequency of overlap associated with young age at diagnosis of AIH. Occasionally these radiological features may be delayed, therefore a liver biopsy may be helpful at looking for bile duct damage.

Both UDCA and immunosuppressants have been shown to improve liver biochemistry in PSC-AIH overlap patients, although UDCA is no longer recommended in PSC alone given the repeated lack of evidence for efficacy from randomized controlled studies. Treatment should be individualized, taking into consideration liver biochemistry, serology, radiology, and histology. If there is significant interface hepatitis, immunosuppression can be initiated, and addition of UDCA can be considered once inflammation has settled. Similarly, acute cholestasis can cause a rise in transaminase levels therefore it would be reasonable to trial UDCA prior to introduction of immunosuppressants and monitor for improvement in liver biochemistry.

Clinical Pearls
- Autoimmune hepatitis is an uncommon disease that has a varied clinical presentation ranging from asymptomatic disease to fulminant liver failure.
- Disease is often characterized by positive autoantibodies to ANA, ASMA, and LKM-1.
- Disease can be provoked by viral illnesses or drugs.
- Characteristic appearances of AIH on pathology include interface hepatitis and emperipolesis; histology supporting AIH is required as part of diagnosis.
- The disease responds well to immunosuppression, often with a combination of corticosteroids and azathioprine.
- Failure to respond to treatment should lead to an assessment of medication compliance, other diagnoses (including overlap syndromes), consideration of treatment change, as well as recognition of increased risk of decompensation and need for liver transplantation.

Chapter Review Answers
1. What key investigations would you be looking to do next?

   (a) Hemochromatosis genotyping
   (b) Alpha-1-antitrypsin levels
   (c) **Hepatitis B, C, and autoimmune serology**
   (d) Liver biopsy

   Answer: Correct answer (c). A thorough history is essential in order to elucidate clues for the possible causes of abnormal liver biochemistry. In particular, common illnesses like viral hepatitis types B and C should be evaluated with serology, along with clinical evaluation regarding risk factors for viral hepatitis (e.g., endemic country of origin, tattoos, previous intravenous drug use, remote blood transfusions). Blood tests investigating for a liver aetiology should also include liver autoantibodies (in particular, ANA and anti-SMA, followed by additional extended testing as appropriate especially in the context of a history of autoimmune thyroid disease (i.e. Graves' disease). Testing for hemochromatosis (a) or alpha-1-antitrypsin (b) can be considered if the above investigations were not helpful, and/or a family history comes to light. A liver biopsy (d) this early in the diagnostic work-up is not yet indicated, and hence is incorrect.

2. The blood tests reveal positive results: Anti-SMA titre is 1:80 and ANA 1:160. The rest of the liver screen and TSH is unremarkable. You suspect a diagnosis of AIH. What is the next appropriate management step?

(a) Start the patient on prednisolone and azathioprine and explain treatment is for life

(b) Repeat the bloodwork in 2 weeks to see if the anti-SMA titre and IgG values change to higher titres

(c) **Request a liver biopsy to aid confirmation of diagnosis, severity, and further exclude alternate cause of liver injury**

(d) Send blood for further serology (anti-SLA)

Answer: The elevation in serum aminotransferase activity, detection of anti-SMA and elevated IgG concentrations are all highly suggestive of a diagnosis of AIH. The next management step would be to recommend (c) a liver biopsy to aid confirmation of diagnosis, and further exclude alternate causes of liver injury. The patient is not currently in acute liver failure, and hence, starting therapy as in (a) at this stage in management is not yet indicated, and diagnosis should be confirmed first as well as exclude any alternate causes of liver injury. (B) is incorrect, as there is no role for repeating bloodwork to assess for changes in levels of anti-SMA and immunoglobulin G at this time while the patient has not received any treatment. Anti-soluble liver antigen (SLA) would not be helpful at this time with regard to furthering diagnostic clarification or management.

3. A liver biopsy demonstrated features of chronic hepatitis with a plasma cell-rich interface hepatitis without alternative aetiologies suggested. Some fibrosis was reported. The patient was started on a combination of prednisolone and subsequently azathioprine. Her liver biochemistry and IgG values normalized by 6 months of therapy. How long should treatment be continued?

(a) Treatment can be stopped now that her liver biochemistry has normalized

(b) Treatment should be continued indefinitely as risk of relapse is high

(c) **Treatment should be continued for 2–5 years with maintenance of normal biochemistry values; a trial off therapy can be considered with monitoring**

(d) Her treatment should be continued for 1 year with maintenance of normal biochemistry values, then stopped

Answer: Treatment paradigms in AIH need to be individualized but must account for the likelihood that in most patients, relapse rates are very high when all treatment is discontinued. Generally at the outset, corticosteroids are needed for at least 12–18 months and azathioprine for 2–5 years. For cirrhotic patients who are treated it is rare, if ever, sensible to stop immunosuppression. For new patients, particularly young ones, who are non-cirrhotic, and in whom after prolonged therapy (e.g. 2–5 years) have normal blood tests (including immunoglobulin G values) a single trial off therapy is reasonable with monitoring. Some advocate a liver biopsy before withdrawal of therapy, and whilst there can be some utility (e.g. for those with any activity treatment is continued and/or escalated) relapse can occur even in the presence of a normal biopsy. Our patient is non-cirrhotic, and as such, (c) is the most appropriate answer.

References

1. Trivedi PJ, Hubscher SG, Heneghan M, Gleeson D, Hirschfield GM. Grand round: autoimmune hepatitis. J Hepatol. 2019;70(4):773–84.
2. Lv T, Li M, Zeng N, Zhang J, Li S, Chen S, Zhang C, Shan S, Duan W, Wang Q, et al. Systematic review and meta-analysis on the incidence and prevalence of autoimmune hepatitis in Asian, European, and American population. J Gastroenterol Hepatol. 2019;34(10):1676–84.
3. Grønbæk L, Vilstrup H, Jepsen P. Autoimmune hepatitis in Denmark: incidence, prevalence, prognosis, and causes of death. A nationwide registry-based cohort study. J Hepatol. 2014;60(3):612–7.
4. Al-Chalabi T, Underhill JA, Portmann BC, McFarlane IG, Heneghan MA. Impact of gender on the long-term outcome and survival of patients with autoimmune hepatitis. J Hepatol. 2008;48(1):140–7.
5. de Boer YS, van Gerven NM, Zwiers A, Verwer BJ, van Hoek B, van Erpecum KJ, Beuers U, van Buuren HR, Drenth JP, den Ouden JW, et al. Genome-wide association study identifies variants associated with autoimmune hepatitis type 1. Gastroenterology. 2014;147(2):443–452.e445.
6. Liberal R, Grant CR, Longhi MS, Mieli-Vergani G, Vergani D. Diagnostic criteria of autoimmune hepatitis. Autoimmun Rev. 2014;13(4–5):435–40.
7. Terziroli Beretta-Piccoli B, Mieli-Vergani G, Vergani D. Serology in autoimmune hepatitis: a clinical-practice approach. Eur J Intern Med. 2018;48:35–43.
8. Hübscher SG. Role of liver biopsy in autoimmune liver disease. Diagn Histopathol. 2014;20(3):109–18.
9. Hennes EM, Zeniya M, Czaja AJ, Parés A, Dalekos GN, Krawitt EL, Bittencourt PL, Porta G, Boberg KM, Hofer H, et al. Simplified criteria for the diagnosis of autoimmune hepatitis. Hepatology. 2008;48(1):169–76.
10. Mack CL, Adams D, Assis DN, Kerkar N, Manns MP, Mayo MJ, Vierling JM, Alsawas M, Murad MH, Czaja AJ. Diagnosis and management of autoimmune hepatitis in adults and children: 2019 practice guidance and guidelines from the American Association for the Study of Liver Diseases. Hepatology. 2020;72(2):671–722.

11. European Association of the Study of the Liver (EASL). EASL clinical practice guidelines: autoimmune hepatitis. J Hepatol. 2015;63(4):971–1004.

12. Gleeson D, Heneghan MA. British Society of Gastroenterology (BSG) guidelines for management of autoimmune hepatitis. Gut. 2011;60(12):1611–29.

13. Liberal R, de Boer YS, Andrade RJ, Bouma G, Dalekos GN, Floreani A, Gleeson D, Hirschfield GM, Invernizzi P, Lenzi M, et al. Expert clinical management of autoimmune hepatitis in the real world. Aliment Pharmacol Ther. 2017;45(5):723–32.

14. Doycheva I, Watt KD, Gulamhusein AF. Autoimmune hepatitis: current and future therapeutic options. Liver Int. 2019;39(6):1002–13.

15. Pape S, Gevers TJG, Belias M, Mustafajev IF, Vrolijk JM, van Hoek B, Bouma G, van Nieuwkerk CMJ, Hartl J, Schramm C, et al. Predniso(lo)ne dosage and chance of remission in patients with autoimmune hepatitis. Clin Gastroenterol Hepatol. 2019;17(10):2068–2075.e2062.

16. Stirnimann G, Ebadi M, Czaja AJ, Montano-Loza AJ. Recurrent and de novo autoimmune hepatitis. Liver Transpl. 2019;25(1):152–66.

17. Trivedi PJ, Hirschfield GM. Review article: overlap syndromes and autoimmune liver disease. Aliment Pharmacol Ther. 2012;36(6):517–33.

18. Chazouillères O, Wendum D, Serfaty L, Rosmorduc O, Poupon R. Long term outcome and response to therapy of primary biliary cirrhosis-autoimmune hepatitis overlap syndrome. J Hepatol. 2006;44(2):400–6.

Chapter 11
IgG4-Related Hepato-Pancreato-Biliary Disease

Eoghan McNelis and Emma Culver

Key Learning Points
- IgG4-related disease (IgG4-RD) is a multiorgan condition presenting with 'inflammatory' mass lesions, strictures and/or 'fibrotic' encasement of body regions.
- All organs affected by IgG4-RD share similar histopathological features, specifically a lymphoplasmacytic infiltrate with abundant IgG4-positive plasma cells and a storiform pattern of fibrosis.
- Four broad disease subsets have been described, defined by the predominant pattern of organ involvement, with differences in age, gender, ethnicity, serum IgG4 concentrations and time to presentation.
- The new American College of Rheumatology/European League Against Rheumatism (ACR/EULAR) classification criteria for IgG4-RD (2019) focus on important exclusion criteria to help minimise misdiagnosis.

E. McNelis · E. Culver (✉)
Experimental Medicine Division, Level 5, University of Oxford,
John Radcliffe Hospital, Headington, UK
e-mail: emma.culver@nhs.net

© Springer Nature Switzerland AG 2022
T. Cross (ed.), *Liver Disease in Clinical Practice*, In Clinical Practice, https://doi.org/10.1007/978-3-031-10012-3_11

- IgG4-RD is typically corticosteroid-responsive. B cell depletion with rituximab is safe and efficacious in reducing disease relapse and corticosteroid-related adverse events.
- Disease progression with organ dysfunction, organ failure and an increased risk of malignancy can occur, warranting careful follow-up.

Introduction

IgG4-related disease (IgG4-RD) is a multisystem fibroinflammatory condition characterised by histopathological findings of a lymphoplasmacytic infiltrate with abundant IgG4-positive plasma cells and storiform pattern of fibrosis in affected organs. It usually presents insidiously with mass-like lesions and/or fibrotic plaques/strictures. Given its systemic manifestations, patients will present to a range of different generalists and sub-specialists. It is often mis-diagnosed as malignancy or other infective/inflammatory conditions and can be left untreated for a number of years after initial presentation.

Diagnosis is based upon a combination of clinical presentation, serological findings, radiological evidence, histopathology where available and excellent response to corticosteroid therapy. Both systemic and organ-specific criteria have been developed to improve diagnostic accuracy. Early intervention is important to reduce morbidity and mortality associated with progressive and fibrotic disease. Treatment aims to provide symptomatic benefit, reduce inflammatory burden and prevent disease progression. IgG4-RD should be managed with a holistic and multidisciplinary approach to ensure accurate diagnosis, patient support and education, optimal choice and timing of therapy and effective management of complications.

Disease Phenotypes

IgG4-RD has recently been sub-divided into four broad disease subsets defined by the predominant pattern of organ involvement. These groups incorporate the hepato-pancreato-biliary system, the retroperitoneum and aorta, limited head and neck involvement and systemic disease, although there are many overlapping features. These phenotypes differ in terms of age, gender, ethnicity, serum IgG4 concentrations and time to presentation (Fig. 11.1).

The most common hepato-pancreato-biliary presentations of IgG4-RD are IgG4-related sclerosing cholangitis, IgG4-related pancreatitis (autoimmune pancreatitis type-1), IgG4-related hepatopathy and IgG4-related cholecystitis (Table 11.1) [1].

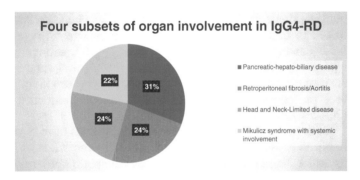

FIGURE 11.1 Disease phenotypes in IgG4-RD. Large crosssectional international patient cohort (765 cases) have identified four major patient groups including Pancreatic-Hepato-Biliary disease (31%), Retroperitoneal Fibrosis and/or Aortitis %) (24%), Head and Neck-Limited disease (24%) and classic Mikulicz syndrome with systemic involvement (22%)

TABLE 11.1 Definitions of IgG4-HBD

IgG4 related sclerosing cholangitis	IgG4-SC
IgG4 related pancreatitis (autoimmune pancreatitis type 1	AIP
IgG4 related hepatopathy	IgG4-H
IgG4 related cholecystitis	IgG4-C

Pathophysiology

We have witnessed a rapid expansion in our understanding of the pathophysiology of this condition. This has helped to better define its natural history and enabled more targeted therapies for those with active disease. Genetic studies have reported a human leucocyte antigen type II association, and multiple single-nucleotide polymorphisms have been defined linked to both the presence of AIP, extra-pancreatic organ involvement and risk of disease relapse. Autoantibodies against different antigens such as galectin-3, prohibin, annexin A11 and laminin 511-E8 have been reported. All are ubiquitous proteins and are expressed with variable frequencies (20–75%) in different involved organs.

Both the adaptive and innate immune systems have been implicated, with an emphasis on the role of memory B cells, T follicular helper (Tfh) and peripheral helper (Tph) cells, CD4+ cytotoxic lymphocytes (CTLs) and alternative macrophages. The expansion of clonally restricted CTLs SLAMF+ cells in the circulation and infiltrating tissue in patients with IgG4-RD may be central to its pathogenesis, producing a number of pro-fibrotic cytokines and interacting with B cells (antigen-driven). Depletion of B cells, e.g. rituximab therapy, leads to profound clinical and radiological improvement, as well as a decline in plasmablasts and CD4+ CTLs [2] (Fig. 11.2).

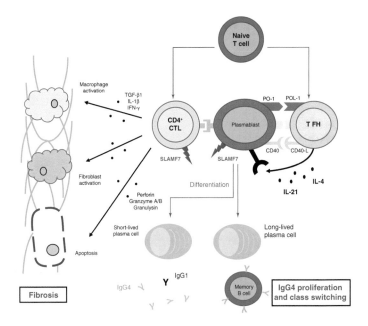

FIGURE 11.2 Diagram showing the presumed pathophysiology of IgG4-related disease

Epidemiology

The epidemiology of IgG4-HBD is poorly understood. The largest nationwide survey in Japan in 2009 defined an incidence of 1.4 per 100,000 and a prevalence of 4.6 per 100,000 cases of AIP, with an estimated 8000 patients in Japan with systemic IgG4-RD (62 per million inhabitants). IgG4-SC is the most common extra-pancreatic manifestation of AIP; isolated IgG4-SC accounts for only 8% of cases in Western cohorts [3]. Reported worldwide frequencies of AIP and IgG4-SC are shown in Table 11.2.

TABLE 11.2 Reported worldwide frequencies of IgG4-SC and AIP

Cohort	Country	Number of patients	Number of patients with IgG4-SC (%)	Number of patients with AIP (%)
AIP	Japan	918	311 (34)	918 (100)
IgG4-SC and AIP	UK	115	69 (60)	106 (92)
IgG4-SC and AIP	USA	53	53 (100)	49 (92)
IgG-RD	China	118	21 (18)	45 (38)
IgG4-RD	Japan	235	30 (13)	142 (60)
IgG4-RD	Spain	55	30 (4)	
IgG4-RD	Italy	41	4 (10)	17 (41)

Disease Associations

IgG4-SC has been linked to a history of chronic occupational exposure to chemicals and dusts, especially 'blue-collar work' in 60–88% of patients in UK and Dutch cohorts [4]. Clinical history of allergy and/or atopy has been described in 40–60% of AIP patients, in association with peripheral eosinophilia and elevated IgE levels [5]. Retroperitoneal fibrosis more specifically has been linked with smoking and asbestos exposure. A coexistent history of other autoimmune diseases (e.g. thyroid and coeliac disease) is found in up to 10% [3] (Table 11.3).

TABLE 11.3 Disease associations and risk factors

Occupational exposure e.g. chemicals, dusts, asbestos
Smoking
Atopy and/or allergy
Other autoimmune diseases

Demographics and Clinical Presentation

The disease has a male preponderance, mainly presenting in the sixth decade of life. Pancreatic involvement often presents with obstructive jaundice (70–80%), weight loss and abdominal pain. There may be symptomatic pancreatic exocrine and endocrine insufficiency, manifesting as anorexia, weight loss, steatorrhoea and new-onset diabetes mellitus. No specific symptoms allow reliable differentiation from other causes of a pancreatic mass or biliary obstruction.

Laboratory Parameters

Patients with IgG4-HPB disease can manifest with abnormal liver function tests, usually cholestasis. Liver screen demonstrates elevated serum IgG concentrations (can be normal despite an elevated IgG4 subclass) and positive antinuclear antibody titres in 50% of patients. Serum protein electrophoresis shows a polyclonal hypergammaglobulinaemia. Elevated inflammatory markers (C-reactive protein) are frequently seen and non-specific. Tumour markers, for example, carbohydrate antigen 19-9, can be raised irrespective of the cause of biliary obstruction.

Serum IgG4 concentrations are raised in most (65–80%) patients at diagnosis, but can also elevated in other malignant, inflammatory and autoimmune pathologies, and in 5% of healthy individuals. Serum IgE concentrations are raised in 35–60% of patients, and peripheral eosinophilia is found in one-third of cases, especially in those with known atopy.

Complement proteins (C3 and C4 levels) may be reduced, in particular in those with co-existing renal involvement.

Radiological Features

Although the classical imaging description of AIP is with a diffuse sausage-shaped pancreas and psuedocapsule on cross-sectional computerised tomography and/or magnetic resonance cholangio-pancreatogram, over half of patients have a discrete pancreatic head mass with distal common bile duct involvement because of a mass effect, which mimics pancreatic cancer (Fig. 11.3). Localised lymphadenopathy is common and does not distinguish it from malignancy. Evidence of

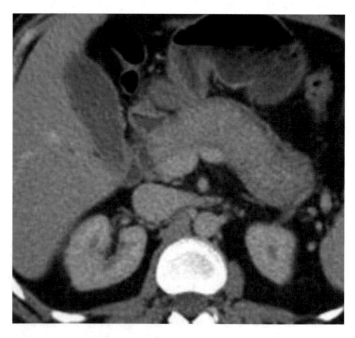

FIGURE 11.3 Portal-phase axial computed tomography of the pancreas, showing a classical sausage-shaped pancreas with a pseudocapsule in autoimmune pancreatitis

extra-pancreatic organ involvement supports the diagnosis. IgG4-SC can involve any part of the biliary tree and is best characterised by cholangiography (four classical patterns defined) (Fig. 11.4) [6]. Particular features include long (>1/3 length) and multifocal strictures, mild upstream dilatation, proximal biliary disease with pancreatic swelling and a thin, narrowed pancreatic duct. IgG4-H can present with a discrete liver mass/pseudotumour independent of pancreatic and biliary involvement. Renal and salivary gland manifestations are seen in up to 20% of patients with AIP/IgG4-SC and should be actively sought.

Type 1: low bile duct stricture, frequently associated with AIP, and corresponds with compression of the intrahepatic bile duct by fibroinflammation within the head of the pancreas.
Type 2: diffuse intrahepatic cholangiopathy with lower common bile duct stricture.
Type 3: hilar and lower common bile duct stricture.
Type 4: hilar stricturing alone.

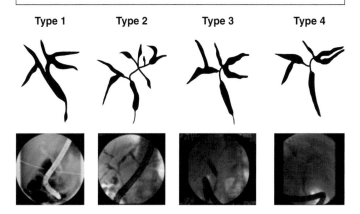

FIGURE 11.4 IgG4-SC with cholangiographic features. Type 1: low bile duct stricture, frequently associated with AIP, and corresponds with compression of the intrahepatic bile duct by fibroinflammation within the head of the pancreas. Type 2: diffuse intrahepatic cholangiopathy with lower common bile duct stricture. Type 3: hilar and lower common bile duct stricture. Type 4: hilar stricturing alone

Fluorodeoxyglucose positron emission tomography (FDG PET/CT) has shown diagnostic utility in IgG4-RD due to its ability to identify active inflammatory lesions and subclinical disease.

Histopathological Characteristics

Histological evaluation is important in supporting a diagnosis of IgG4-RD and excluding malignancy. Every effort should be made to obtain biopsy specimens before treatment is commenced. Whilst cytological samples from brushings of biliary strictures or fine-needle aspiration of a pancreas mass can detect malignant cells (sensitivity 20–50%) they do not provide sufficient material to diagnose IgG4-RD. Tissue biopsies from the ampulla, bile duct and/or pancreas obtained at cholangioscopy or endoscopic ultrasound are often small, yet have intact architecture necessary to detect plasma cell infiltration and fibrosis. Resection specimens are the most conclusive means of obtaining a histological diagnosis, which are made retrospectively.

Organs affected by IgG4-RD broadly share similar histopathological features. Classically these include storiform fibrosis (swirling pattern), obliterative phlebitis, a lymphoplasmacytic infiltrate with predominance of IgG4+ plasma cells and variable presence of eosinophils (Fig. 11.3). An IgG4+/IgG+ plasma cell ratio of >40% is required to support a histological diagnosis of IgG4-RD. The absolute numbers of IgG4+ plasma cells varies between affected organs and the size of the tissue specimen obtained (Fig. 11.5).

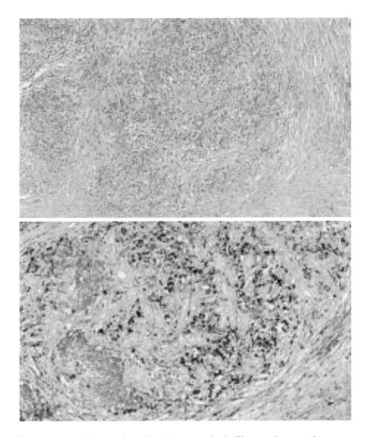

FIGURE 11.5 Dense lymphoplasmacytic infiltrate in autoimmune pancreatitis (H&E stain, 100× magnification). IgG4 immunostaining ×150 magnification demonstrated (>50 IgG4-positive plasma cells per high power field)

Diagnosis

The diagnosis of IgG4-RD is challenging, as it presents to multiple different specialists with often disconnected features and mimics a number of important malignant and inflammatory processes. Both general and organ-specific scoring systems have been developed to aid diagnosis. For HPB disease, the HISORt criteria (histology, imaging, serology, other organ involvement and response to therapy) and Japanese International Consensus Diagnostic Criteria (type I and II AIP) are most widely used. The Boston Consensus Histopathological Criteria are valuable where there are histological biopsy or resection specimens. The new American College of Rheumatology/European League Against Rheumatism (ACR/EULAR) Classification Criteria for IgG4-RD (2019) have defined exclusion criteria and a minimum point system to help minimise misdiagnosis (Tables 11.4 and 11.5) [7]. However, when applied to patients with pancreaticobiliary disease, whilst highly specific there was lower sensitivity in those with an atrophic pancreas or those with biliary-predominant disease. There is a broad differential diagnosis at presentation, and we advocate discussion of such complex patients in a specialist IgG4 multidisciplinary team.

TABLE 11.4 Exclusion criteria for a diagnosis of IgG4-RD

Clinical exclusions	Fever
	Unresponsive to steroids
	Leukopenia and thrombocytopaenia
	Peripheral eosinophilia (>3000/mm^3)
Serological exclusions	PR3 or MPO-ANCA positive
	Anti-Ro or Anti-La positive
	Extractable nuclear antibody positive
	Cryoglobulins
	Other disease specific antibody
Radiology exclusions	Rapid radiographic progression
	Large bone abnormality
	Splenomegaly
	High suspicion of infection or malignancy
Pathology exclusions	Primarily granulomatous inflammation
	Necrotising vasculitis
	Malignant infiltrate
	Prominent histiocytic infiltrate
	Prominent neutrophilic infiltrate
	Multicentric Castleman's pathology
	Prominent necrosis
	Inflammatory pseudotumour pathology

TABLE 11.5 Simplified ACR/EULAR 2019 classification criteria for IgG4-related disease. Must meet entry criteria and have no exclusion criteria. A score of >20 supports a diagnosis

Histopathology	
Uninformative biopsy	0
Dense lymphocytic infiltrate	+4
Dense lymphocytic infiltrate and obliterative phlebitis	+6
Dense lymphocytic infiltrate and storiform fibrosis with or without obliterative phlebitis	+13
Immunostaining	**0–16**, as follows: Assigned weight is **0** if the IgG4+:IgG+ ratio is 0–40% or indeterminate and the number of IgG4+ cells/high power field [hpf] is 0–9 Assigned weight is **+7** if (1) the IgG4+:IgG+ ratio is ≥41% and the number of IgG4+ cells/hpf is 0–9 or indeterminate; or (2) the IgG4+:IgG+ ratio is 0–40% or indeterminate and the number of IgG4+ cells/hpf is ≥10 or indeterminate Assigned weight is **+14** if (1) the IgG4+:IgG+ ratio is 41–70% and the number of IgG4+ cells/hpf is ≥10; or (2) the IgG4+:IgG+ ratio is ≥71% and the number of IgG4+ cells/hpf is 10–50 Assigned weight is **+16** if the IgG4+:IgG+ ratio is ≥71% and the number of IgG4+ cells/hpf is ≥51

TABLE 11.5 (continued)

Serum IgG4 concentration	
Normal or not checked	0
> Normal but >2× upper limit of normal	+4
2–5× upper limit of normal	+6
>5× upper limit of normal	+11
Bilateral lacrimal, parotid, sublingual and submandibular glands	
No set of glands involved	0
One set of glands involved	+6
Two or more sets of glands involved	+14
Chest	
Not checked or neither of the items listed is present	0
Peribronchovascular and septal thickening	+4
Paravertebral band-like soft tissue in the thorax	+10
Pancreas and biliary tree	
Not checked or none of the items listed is present	0
Diffuse pancreas enlargement (loss of lobulations)	+8
Diffuse pancreas enlargement and capsule-like rim with decreased enhancement	+11

TABLE 11.5 (continued)

Pancreas (either of above) and biliary tree involvement	+19
Kidney	
Not checked or none of the items listed is present	0
Hypocomplementemia	+6
Renal pelvis thickening/soft tissue	+8
Bilateral renal cortex low-density areas	+10
Retroperitoneum	
Not checked or neither of the items listed is present	0
Diffuse thickening of the abdominal aortic wall	+4
Circumferential or anterolateral soft tissue around the infrarenal aorta or iliac arteries	+8

Disease Monitoring

The IgG4-RD responder index was developed as a research tool but may be used in clinical practice to longitudinally track disease activity, organ progression and damage in individual patients. An elevated IgG4 at diagnosis can be tracked to suggest a response to treatment and disease flares and can also reflect the extent of disease. Elevated serum IgE concentrations and peripheral eosinophilia are often seen and can correlate with disease activity. Hypocomplementaemia (C3, C4) is most frequently seen in individuals with IgG4-related tubulo-interstitial nephritis and declines as disease activity worsens. Other potential biomarkers include circulating plasmablasts, Tfh-2 cells, CD4+ CTLs and chemokine CCL18, which have all been associated with disease activity and show declining concentrations with treatment.

Management

The main goals of treatment are to reduce and control inflammation, preserve organ function and prevent complications. All patients with active and symptomatic disease require treatment, some more urgently than others (e.g. biliary strictures causing obstructive jaundice and cholangitis). Even those who are asymptomatic can have vital organ involvement (e.g. peri-aortitis). Some individuals experience spontaneous improvement (e.g. IgG4-SC type 1, often related to reduced pancreatic and bile duct inflammation), however, recurrence in the same or other organs is frequent, and close follow-up is therefore warranted. Watchful waiting is appropriate in only a minority of patients.

Crucially, this condition should be managed via a multispecialty approach incorporating radiologists, histopathologists, gastroenterologists/hepatologists, rheumatologists, general physicians, alongside any other organ system specialties that need to be involved. The first inter-regional multidisciplinary team managing IgG4-RD was established between Oxford and University College London Hospitals, successfully guiding important diagnostic and management decisions [8].

Induction Treatment

Induction therapy aims to control inflammation rapidly. Corticosteroids are the first line agents used currently in IgG4-HPB disease [8]. B cell depletion with rituximab in a prospective open-label trial showed an excellent response, with complete remission in 40% of patients at 12 months from the induction dose alone. Methotrexate has been used for successfully, especially in those with more limited head and neck disease [9]. In certain situations, medical interventions such as temporary stent placement (biliary, ureteral) are complementary to medical therapies to prevent obstructive complications such as infection.

Glucocorticoids are the first-line treatment IgG4-RD, and those with 'inflammatory' subset disease typically respond well, within days to weeks. Steroid use has been shown to induce remission quicker, more consistently, and with a lower relapse rate than a conservative approach [10]. International consensus suggests an induction dose of 30–40 mg/day for 2–4 weeks, with higher doses considered if vital organs are involved, and lower doses in elderly individuals and those with co-morbidities. Tapering by 5 mg every 1–2 weeks is guided by clinical improvement, biochemistry and follow-up imaging. Remission is defined by substantial improvement and/or correction of biochemical and radiological abnormalities. Complete resolution of strictures and/or normalisation of liver biochemistry with steroids is reported in most (99%) patients with AIP and two-thirds of patients with IgG_4-SC [11]. An absence of response can represent a burnt-out fibrotic phenotype but should prompt a thorough search for an alternative diagnosis. The concept of a 'steroid trial to confirm diagnosis' in those with high suspicion of AIP/IgG4-SC should only be performed under close observation in experienced centres, after thorough exclusion of malignancy.

Maintenance Treatment

This is often individualised based on the perceived risk of relapse, to prevent disease progression and reduce corticosteroid-related adverse events. Patients with IgG4-SC are at high risk of relapse (50–60%), most within 6 months of discontinuing or tapering steroid treatment. Risk factors for relapse include male gender, IgG4-SC with proximal strictures, the number of organs involved at baseline, serum IgG4 and IgE concentrations at diagnosis and speed of tapering treatment.

Second-line immunosuppressive therapies, especially azathioprine, is commonly used in IgG4-HBD based on experience in autoimmune hepatitis and overlap conditions [12]. Whilst retrospective cohort data supports the use of azathioprine to reduce steroid adverse effects and maintain remission, there are no randomised or controlled studies of this agent in igG4-RD to date. Mycophenolate plus corticosteroids has been shown to reduce the risk of relapse compared to corticosteroids alone in those induced with steroids in a randomised controlled trial in IgG4-RD. Cyclophosphamide plus corticosteroids has been shown to reduce the risk of relapse compared to steroids alone in a non-randomised controlled trial of all comers with IgG4-RD, but middle-aged and elderly populations suffer from considerable adverse effects. Several studies have assessed rituximab therapy as a maintenance agent in IgG4-RD. One multicentre study assessing long-term efficacy and safety supported the use of maintenance rituximab to reduce relapse, although reported a high infection rate in one-third of patients. Other therapies such as inebilizumab (CD19 B cell depletion), abatacept (fusion protein of CTLA4 and FcIgG1), B cell inhibition with Xmab5871 (CD19 and FcgIIRB) and elotuzumab (anti-SLAM F7) are currently in clinical trials.

Outcome

If diagnosed and treated early, IgG4-HPB disease has a favourable prognosis. Delayed therapy and progressive disease can lead to complications including venous thrombosis, portal hypertension, liver cirrhosis and mortality [3]. An all-cause increased risk of malignancy (>two-fold) has been shown [3]. Adverse effects of immunosuppressive treatment, including diabetes, osteoporosis, opportunistic infections, can occur and patients require careful monitoring.

Questions

1. A 62-year-old man presents with painless jaundice and a 4-month history of weight loss. Abdominal CT scan showed a low-attenuating ring surrounding a sausage-shaped pancreas; there was no biliary disease evident on the CT scan. Once malignancy has been excluded and other necessary exclusion criteria were met, a diagnosis of IgG4-related disease was considered.

   Serum IgG4 level was 5.2 g/L (normal level <1.3 g/L). Biopsy of the pancreas revealed a dense lymphocytic infiltrate and obliterative phlebitis under the microscope; immunostaining showed the IgG4+:IgG+ cell ratio was 50%. Further imaging showed no extension of disease beyond the pancreas.

   According to the 2019 ACR/EULAR classification, this patient meets the classification criteria for IgG4-related disease.

   True or false?

2. A 65-year-old man with an existing diagnosis of IgG4-RD presents with a flare up of his IgG4-related sclerosing cholangitis. This is his second exacerbation in the last 18 months. Which management plan would be most appropriate for him?

   (a) Prednisolone induction and commence maintenance dose of immunosuppressive such as azathioprine.
   (b) Laparoscopic cholecystectomy.
   (c) Gemcitabine and cisplatin.
   (d) Therapeutic ERCP with stent insertion

3. Which departments should be involved in the multidisciplinary management of patients with IgG4-RD?

   (a) Radiology
   (b) Hepatology
   (c) Histopathology
   (d) Rheumatology

4. Which leucocytes have been implicated in the pathogenesis of IgG4-RD?

   (a) CD4+ cytotoxic lymphocytes
   (b) T follicular helper cells
   (c) Memory b cells
   (d) Peripheral helper cells
   (e) Alternative macrophages

5. Which of these is the most prominent risk factor implicated in the development of IgG4-RD?

   (a) Hepatitis B
   (b) Occupational exposure
   (c) Obesity
   (d) Female sex

Answers

1. **True.** As per ACR/EULAR criteria, once alternative diagnoses have been excluded, a diagnosis of IgG4-RD requires a score of >20. Histopathology: dense lymphocytic infiltrate and obliterative phlebitis (**+6**); immunostaining: IgG4+:IgG+ cell ratio 50% (**+14**); Serum IgG4 5.2 g/L (**+6**); low-attenuating ring surrounding a sausage-shaped pancreas on CT (**+11**). This score of 37 meets criteria for IgG4-RD diagnosis. It is important to remember that elevated serum IgG4 is not specific for IgG4-RD.

2. **Prednisolone induction and; commence maintenance dose of immunosuppressive such as azathioprine.** Corticosteroids have been shown to be very effective in the treatment of initial presentation of IgG4-RD or flare-ups. 30–40 mg prednisolone, weaned by 5 mg every 2 weeks might be a sensible dose. A maintenance therapy ought to be commenced due to the frequent flare ups; azathioprine and mycophenolate have been shown to be effective, particularly in HPB IgG4-RD.

3. **All of the above.** The best management of IgG4-RD is achieved via a cohesive multidisciplinary approach—this includes radiologists, rheumatologists, histopathologists,

hepatologists, general medics and any other specialty implicated by the patient's presentation (ENT, ophthalmology).
4. **All of the above**. All of the cells listed above have been implicated in the pathogenesis of IgG4-RD, through both the innate and adaptive immune responses.
5. Occupational exposures, especially blue collar workers, have been shown to be associated with IgG4-SC, along with smoking, atopy and other autoimmune conditions.

References

1. Smit WL, Culver EL, Chapman RW. New thoughts on immunoglobulin G4-related sclerosing cholangitis. Clin Liver Dis. 2016;20(1):47–65. https://doi.org/10.1016/j.cld.2015.08.004.
2. Maehara T, Moriyama M, Nakamura S. Pathogenesis of IgG4-related disease: a critical review. Odontology. 2019;107(2):127–32. https://doi.org/10.1007/s10266-018-0377-y.
3. Huggett MT, Culver EL, Kumar M, Hurst JM, Rodriguez-Justo M, Chapman MH, Johnson GJ, et al. Type 1 autoimmune pancreatitis and IgG4-related sclerosing cholangitis is associated with extrapancreatic organ failure, malignancy, and mortality in a prospective UK cohort. Am J Gastroenterol. 2014;109(10):1675–83. https://doi.org/10.1038/ajg.2014.223.
4. de Buy Wenniger LJM, Culver EL, Beuers U. Exposure to occupational antigens might predispose to IgG4-related disease. Hepatology. 2014;60(4):1453–4. https://doi.org/10.1002/hep.26999.
5. Culver EL, Sadler R, Bateman AC, Makuch M, Ferry B, Aalberse R, Barnes E, Rispens T. Immunoglobulin E, eosinophils and mast cells in atopic individuals provide novel insights in IgG4-related disease. J Hepatol. 2016;64:S646.
6. Culver EL, Barnes E. IgG4-related sclerosing cholangitis. Clin Liver Dis. 2017;10(1):9–16. https://doi.org/10.1002/cld.642.
7. Wallace ZS, Naden RP, Chari S, Choi H, Della-Torre E, Dicaire JF, Hart PA, et al. The 2019 American College of Rheumatology/European League Against Rheumatism classification criteria for IgG4-related disease. Arthritis Rheumatol. 2020;72(1):7–19. https://doi.org/10.1002/art.41120.

8. Goodchild G, Peters RJR, Cargill TN, Martin H, Fadipe A, Leandro M, Bailey A, et al. Experience from the first UK inter-regional specialist multidisciplinary meeting in the diagnosis and management of IgG4-related disease. Clin Med. 2020;20(3):e32–9. https://doi.org/10.7861/clinmed.2019-0457.

9. Della-torre E, Campochiaro C, Bozzolo EP, Dagna L, Scotti R, Nicoletti R, Stone JH, Sabbadini MG. Methotrexate for maintenance of remission in IgG4-related disease. Rheumatology. 2015;54(10):1934–6. https://doi.org/10.1093/rheumatology/kev244.

10. Hart PA, Kamisawa T, Brugge WR, Chung JB, Culver EL, Czakó L, Frulloni L, et al. Long-term outcomes of autoimmune pancreatitis: a multicentre, international analysis. Gut. 2013;62(12):1771–6. https://doi.org/10.1136/gutjnl-2012-303617.

11. Ghazale A, Chari ST, Zhang L, Smyrk TC, Takahashi N, Levy MJ, Topazian MD, et al. Immunoglobulin G4-associated cholangitis: clinical profile and response to therapy. Gastroenterology. 2008;134(3):706–15. https://doi.org/10.1053/j.gastro.2007.12.009.

12. Avşar AK, Gerçik Ö, Can G, Zengin B, Kocaer SB, Kılıç AO, Uslu S, et al. FRI0596 azathioprine and glucocorticoid combination might be a good treatment option to achieve remission in patients with IGG4-related disease. Ann Rheum Dis. 2019;78(Suppl 2):993–4. https://doi.org/10.1136/annrheumdis-2019-eular.4632.

Chapter 12
Hereditary Haemochromatosis

William J. H. Griffiths

Key Learning Points
- Understanding the pathophysiology of haemochromatosis
- Pathway for diagnosis
- Investigation and when/how to treat
- Non-HFE syndromes

Case

A 55-year-old moderately obese woman presents with a history of worsening arthralgia. Her serum ferritin level is raised at 650 µg/L with normal CRP, haemoglobin and liver function tests. What would you do next?

(a) Recommend venesection
(b) Arrange *HFE* genotyping
(c) Check the transferrin saturation
(d) Arrange a liver ultrasound

W. J. H. Griffiths (✉)
Cambridge Liver Unit, Cambridge University Teaching Hospitals NHS Foundation Trust, Addenbrooke's Hospital, Cambridge, UK
e-mail: bill.griffiths@addenbrookes.nhs.uk

© Springer Nature Switzerland AG 2022245
T. Cross (ed.), *Liver Disease in Clinical Practice*, In Clinical Practice, https://doi.org/10.1007/978-3-031-10012-3_12

The patient is diagnosed with HH (C282Y homozygous) following further investigation. Which of the following apply?

(a) The patient could be observed initially
(b) Therapeutic venesection should be commenced
(c) First degree relatives require only a ferritin check
(d) First degree relatives should have *HFE* genotyping

Background

Hereditary Haemochromatosis (HH) is an autosomal recessive disorder characterised by organ damage due to dietary iron accumulation; the condition may also be referred to as HFE-related or type 1 Haemochromatosis. The presentation occurs earlier, and with greater severity, in men due to the lack of specific iron losses that occur via menstruation in women. Typically, HH manifests above the age of 40 years. Iron is mainly deposited in the liver and in the synovial tissue of joints but eventually in the pancreas, skin, heart, the gonadotrophin-secreting cells of the anterior pituitary and rarely the adrenal and parathyroid glands. It is not clear why iron accumulates preferentially in certain extra-hepatic tissues. Disease manifestations thereby include hepatic fibrosis, arthropathy, diabetes mellitus due to lack of insulin, pigmentation, cardiomyopathy and impotence. Fatigue is a common early symptom and, together with arthralgia, affect quality of life in patients with HH. A serum ferritin >1000 µg/L at diagnosis equates to a five-fold relative mortality risk. Hepatic cirrhosis is associated with significantly reduced survival and a 100-fold increased risk of hepatocellular carcinoma (HCC), the commonest cause of death in HH [1]. The high rate of HCC is due to a combination of cirrhosis and the carcinogenic properties of iron, and the risk remains despite iron removal. The discovery of the *HFE* gene in 1996 provided a significant breakthrough for the diagnosis of HH [2]. Until then, genetic testing relied on HLA linkage following the identification of this association in the 1970s. Homozygosity for the C282Y mutation on chromosome 6p accounts for 90% of cases of HH; thus a specific tool was immediately available for non-invasive diagnosis, screening and prevalence estimation. The advent of HFE has enabled characterisation of the natural history and expression of HH, and a greater understanding of the hepatic siderosis associated with chronic liver disease.

Iron Pathophysiology

In normal individuals, gastrointestinal iron absorption is homeostatically regulated according to body iron status. An important concept is that there is no physiological mechanism in humans to excrete excess iron when overload occurs. In HH, the gene defect results in an inability to appropriately reduce iron absorption such that body iron accumulation ensues (Fig. 12.1). When following the natural history of the condition, the initial laboratory finding is that of a raised plasma transferrin saturation as iron absorbed from the intestine loads on to the transferrin carrier protein at an increased rate compared with normal individuals. Subsequently, as tissue iron loading occurs the serum ferritin starts to rise proportionately. Total body iron, which is 4 g in a normal adult, typically rises above 10 g in a patient with HH. In C282Y homozygotes serum ferritin concentrations >1000 μg/L are associated with the development of liver fibrosis.

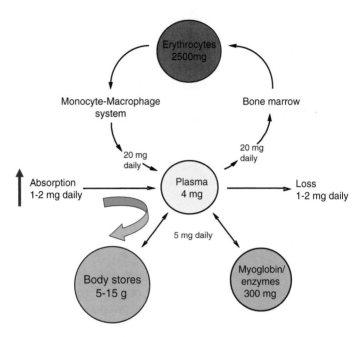

FIGURE 12.1 Iron pathophysiology in HH. Under normal circumstances iron absorption is regulated to match insensible losses with total adult body iron around 4 g. In haemochromatosis the iron storage compartment greatly increases due to unopposed intestinal uptake as normal feedback mechanisms are disrupted. Note the size of the transferrin iron pool, approximately 0.1% of total body iron, and that transferrin saturates early during the natural history of haemochromatosis

Disease Expression

After the discovery of HFE it was quickly recognised that around 0.5% of white people are homozygous for the C282Y mutation and thereby genetically predisposed to developed HH [3]. However, only a proportion of these individuals have evident symptoms or signs. Many will be presymptomatic with biochemical iron loading or have little or no evidence of iron loading, particularly pre-menopausal females (Fig. 12.2). When taking a history from a patient with HH it is prudent to

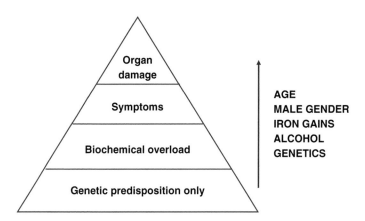

FIGURE 12.2 The iceberg of pathology in C282Y homozygotes ranging from genetic predisposition only to significant organ damage including cirrhosis, arthropathy and diabetes. Various factors determine progression as listed. Venesection prior to the onset of organ damage ensures normal survival and prior to the onset of symptoms prevents morbidity associated with the disorder

ask about previous iron gains (oral iron supplementation, amenorrhoea, early menopause) and iron losses (blood donation, gut pathology, menorrhagia). As a rule, symptoms tend not to occur until the serum ferritin level is elevated. Although significant hepatic fibrosis is unlikely with serum ferritin values <1000 µg/L, joint disease can certainly occur and may be irreversible. The 'penetrance' of C282Y homozygosity is generally described as 'low' but varies according to the definition and study population; for example, evidence of pathology may be seen in a third of males but biopsy-proven cirrhosis occurs in only 1% overall. A recent UK biobank study, which included nearly 3000 homozygotes, described significant a disease burden in HH [4]. Despite the evident disease burden and potential preventability, population screening is not currently recommended as effective pilot studies remain lacking. Environmental factors which modify iron loading and hence expression of the disease include excess alcohol, iron-rich diet and blood donation.

Other factors such as obesity may influence hepatic fibrosis per se. Genetic modifiers are important determinants of disease expression in C282Y homozygotes. Genome-wide association studies in HH have identified the transferrin gene and TMPRSS6 gene as direct modifiers of iron overload. In addition, variants which contribute to chronic liver disease progression have been associated with development of cirrhosis in homozygotes [5].

Diagnosis

HH can be diagnosed in most cases by non-invasive means. A compatible genotype combined with biochemical evidence of iron loading is sufficient. The combination of elevated serum ferritin and transferrin saturation (>50% in males and 45% in females) is highly suggestive of the condition—it is advisable to repeat these on a fasting sample in the first instance. Hyperferritinaemia with a normal transferrin saturation is typically due to excess alcohol and/or in the context of non-alcoholic fatty liver and the metabolic syndrome. As well as the common homozygous genotype C282Y/C282Y, which accounts for the majority of cases, the compound heterozygous form C282Y/H63D accounts for 5–10% of cases and is associated with mild iron burden. Of note, EASL guidelines recognise C282Y homozygosity as a diagnostic genotype for HH, whereas other genotypes such as C282Y/H63D and H63D/H63D require exclusion of additional causes of hyperferritinaemia [6]. Liver biopsy is reserved for those individuals without a recognisable genotype or in those where there is a risk of significant liver fibrosis. The latter is important to identify as surveillance for HCC is required in those with incipient or established cirrhosis. Histologically, iron is deposited initially in peri-portal hepatocytes with later spill over into bile duct epithelium and Kupffer cells (Fig. 12.3).

In terms of non-invasive exclusion of significant fibrosis, in homozygotes where serum aminotransferase values are normal, hepatomegaly is absent and the serum ferritin is below

1000 µg/L there is negligible risk [7]. In addition, a serum hyaluronic acid level >46.5 ng/mL is associated with 100% sensitivity and specificity for cirrhosis. Transient elastography has been shown to reduce the requirement for biopsy in at risk patients and can accurately classify severe fibrosis in around 60% of homozygotes with ferritin >1000 µg/L and raised transaminases [8]. Cirrhosis is less common at presentation over recent decades due to greater clinical awareness and access to *HFE* gene testing. Magnetic resonance imaging (MRI), specifically T2-weighted sequences, can be used to demonstrate hepatic iron deposition non-invasively and specific software may be used for quantification. This is not required in HH as serum ferritin and quantitative phlebot-

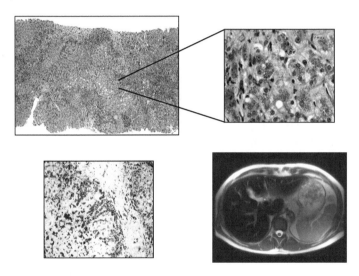

FIGURE 12.3 Biopsy and imaging findings in severe HH. The top left panel shows a low power haematoxylin and eosin stain demonstrating parenchymal nodules surrounded by fibrous tissue (cirrhosis). On high power (top right) brown pigment is noted within hepatocytes. With Perls' reagent (bottom left) the pigment stains blue and is confirmed as iron. Magnetic resonance imaging (MRI) demonstrates a low signal intensity liver compared with muscle on T2-weighted imaging (bottom right)

omy are reliable indicators of the degree of iron overload. However, the technique may be useful when HFE analysis is negative but iron overload is suspected biochemically. MRI can also be used to quantify levels of steatosis and fibrosis when characterising patients with unexplained significant hyperferritinaemia.

It is important to screen first degree relatives of C282Y homozygotes as there will be a significant pick up of pre-morbid disease and indeed those already with unrecognised symptoms due to HH—the so-called cascade screening approach. Children should not be tested until adulthood, as iron is required for growth, although spousal testing for C282Y heterozygosity (10–15% risk in Caucasian populations) may obviate this need.

Treatment

Regular removal of blood, typically approximately 500 mL every week, remains a proven and effective method to clear excess iron. As a rule this will drop the serum ferritin by around 50 µg/L per visit. It is advisable to venesect until the serum ferritin falls below 50 µg/L and, from a practical perspective, to then maintain a level between 20 and 100 µg/L long term. Some advocate maintaining the transferrin saturation below 50% at all times based on a recent French study which was retrospective in nature [9, 10]. Some patients do not tolerate venesection well and therefore may be restricted to a half unit or fortnightly removal instead. It is not necessary to check the serum ferritin at every visit when undergoing therapeutic venesection, particularly in the early stages when the ferritin level is high and can fluctuate. The haemoglobin level should be maintained above 12 g/dL for men and 11 g/dL for women—if the haemoglobin drops below these values a reduction in venesection frequency would be indicated. The frequency of maintenance phlebotomy depends on age, gender and the degree of initial iron accumulation although a typical interval is 3 months. Patients in the maintenance phase may be able to enrol as blood donors, certainly in the UK. Since October 2012, NHS Blood and Transplant have allowed stable patients with HH, who are otherwise eligible, to donate (up to every 6 weeks if necessary) and since 2018 they have been coded specifically to ensure regular phlebotomy whatever their blood group. This means for the majority of patients in the maintenance phase there is an option to give blood rather than have it discarded through a hospital or community venesection service. Younger homozygotes in the very early stages of iron accumulation should be encouraged to become donors from the start. HH blood donors will require separate measurement of serum ferritin which can be annual once established. Patients should be encouraged to join a patient society such as Haemochromatosis UK which also provides venesection booklets for recording of phlebotomies and laboratory values; the booklets are useful for the patient's clinician to see how they are progressing.

Venesection treatment prior to onset of cirrhosis or diabetes ensures normal survival, and has been associated with regression of hepatic fibrosis [11]. Interestingly, longitudinal studies have shown that rates of iron accumulation are variable and progressive iron loading does not always occur particularly in females [12]. This begs the question of whether all homozygotes require immediate treatment; asymptomatic pre-menopausal females with normal ferritin and well elderly patients could be observed. In addition, compound heterozygotes should have lifestyle advice offered and venesection only if there is convincing evidence of iron overload, e.g. via MRI or liver biopsy. Of note, HCC can occur in non-cirrhotic patients and despite iron depletion. HH is a relatively uncommon indication for liver transplantation, usually in the context of HCC, and outcomes are comparable with other forms of chronic liver disease.

Some patients do not tolerate venesection at all, although this is quite rare—typical reasons would be anaemia, poor veins or needle phobia. There is some evidence that proton pump inhibitors reduce iron absorption and the need for venesection during the maintenance phase. The once daily oral iron chelator deferasirox has shown reasonable efficacy for therapeutic iron depletion at a dose of 10 mg/kg in a phase 1/2 trial [13]. Novel therapies which interfere with iron homeostasis at a molecular level are in development.

Non-HFE Haemochromatosis

Since the discovery of the *HFE* gene, several other gene defects have been associated with primary iron overload (Table 12.1). Apart from the distinct phenotype associated with classical ferroportin disease, these other types resemble HFE-related disease though more severe. A number of private mutations in the *HFE* gene itself have also been identified which in some patients, often in conjunction with C282Y heterozygosity, explain the observed iron overload from a genetic perspective.

Juvenile haemochromatosis (JH) was first described in the late 1970s, is severe and seen typically under the age of 30 affecting both sexes equally. Inheritance is recessive and hypogonadism and cardiomyopathy are usually evident. Heart failure may indeed be life-threatening but salvageable

TABLE 12.1 Online Mendelian Inheritance in Man (OMIM) classification of inherited systemic iron overload. All are autosomal recessive apart from ferroportin iron overload (type 4) which is dominantly transmitted. Additional rare atypical disorders are listed beneath

Hereditary iron overload: OMIM classification			
Name	Type	Gene	Published
HFE	1	*HFE*	1996
Juvenile	2A	*HJV*	2004
	2B	*HAMP*	2003
TfR2	3	*TfR2*	2000
Ferroportin	4	*SLC40A1*	2001

Acaeruloplasminaemia, atransferrinaemia, H-ferritin, Neonatal

with aggressive iron-chelation therapy. Mutations in the *HJV* gene on chromosome 1 account for the majority of JH (type 2A), with homozygosity for G320V accounting for half of cases. JH is rarely associated with *HAMP* gene mutations on chromosome 19 (type 2B). This gene encodes an antimicrobial peptide known as 'hepcidin' which is principally synthesised in hepatocytes and acts as an iron regulatory hormone within the body. An intermediate severity form of haemochromatosis is seen with homozygosity for transferrin receptor 2 (TfR2) mutations (type 3), though this can sometimes explain JH [14].

A specific form of iron overload is associated with mutations in the ferroportin (*SLC40A1*) gene also known as type 4 haemochromatosis. The ferroportin protein controls iron export from a number of cell types including enterocytes and macrophages where it has a role in iron entry from the gut and in iron recycling, respectively. Mutations in *SLC40A1* occur similarly in non-Caucasians unlike HFE. The classical disorder is characterised by a raised ferritin with normal or low transferrin saturation and a tendency towards anaemia following venesection. Iron loading occurs predominantly within the reticulo-endothelial system and splenic iron uptake may be observed on MRI. At a microscopic level the distribution of iron in the liver is different to HH with Kupffer cell iron deposition occurring early. The clinical significance of iron loading and the benefit of venesection remain unclear. The differential diagnosis includes hereditary hyperferritinaemia with or without cataracts which requires sequencing of the ferritin light chain (*FTL*) gene [15].

Discovery of additional iron regulatory genes has considerably advanced our understanding of the molecular control of iron homeostasis. Until then, it was known that C282Y abrogates the binding of beta2-microglobulin to HFE thus preventing cell surface expression and interaction with transferrin receptors. This provided a ready explanation for how HFE might interfere with iron entry into cells but did not explain how HFE influences whole body iron control. The hepcidin peptide acts a negative regulator of iron absorption.

In the iron deficient state, hepcidin synthesis is reduced in order to stimulate gastrointestinal uptake but in the setting of secondary iron overload, hepcidin expression is increased to suppress iron absorption. Recessive mutations in *HFE*, *HJV* and *TfR2* all cause paradoxical suppression of hepcidin synthesis with subsequent iron overload (Fig. 12.4). Ferroportin is directly inhibited by hepcidin, preventing release of iron from enterocytes and macrophages [16]. Thus when hepcidin levels are low, in the context of haemochromatosis, ferroportin is readily expressed and releases iron into the circulation from the gut and from macrophages. As hepcidin appears central to the molecular control of iron balance, modulating its activity may represent a future viable therapy for disorders of iron loading. For example, interfering RNAs targeting

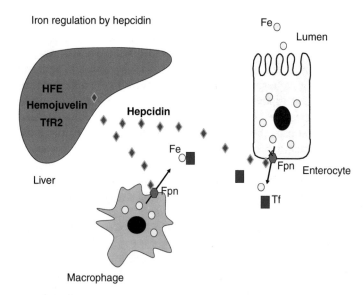

FIGURE 12.4 This schema illustrates how hepcidin synthesis is coordinated by a number of haemochromatosis-related genes in the liver. Hepcidin exerts its downstream effect on ferroportin which is located on the cell surface of macrophages and enterocytes and which is internalised following hepcidin binding. In haemochromatosis hepcidin synthesis is reduced which allows ferroportin to export iron freely into the circulation

TMPRSS6 (the gene product of which inhibits hepcidin production by hepatocytes) have been shown to increase hepcidin expression and ameliorate iron overload in mouse models of haemochromatosis.

Conclusion

The discovery of *HFE* 25 years ago provided a simple tool for diagnosis and improved our understanding of the natural history of what is the commonest autosomal genetic disorder in Caucasians. HH is entirely preventable but as yet population screening has not been advocated. Therefore, a low index of suspicion for HH in both primary and secondary care is needed for timely diagnosis and further reduction of the morbidity and mortality historically linked with this disorder. Cascade screening for *HFE* homozygosity is an important consideration after a diagnosis of HH. Although venesection is the mainstay for iron depletion, patients with HH can on the whole donate blood safely and enhance the donor pool for the benefit of others. For those intolerant of venesection alternative therapies are emerging including oral iron chelation and ultimately molecular correction of iron homeostasis. Finally, we are now in an era where patients with unexplained iron overload can be diagnosed via an exome or indeed whole genome panel approach.

Answers
1. (c) The initial step is to check the transferrin saturation (preferably fasting). If this is raised, then an *HFE* gene test should be performed. A raised ferritin with normal transferrin saturation might relate to obesity/insulin resistance for example.
2. (b) and (d) Given the patient has a raised ferritin and is symptomatic, therapeutic venesection should be initiated. First degree relatives require *HFE* genotyping in order to identify homozygotes. Serum ferritin is reasonable to check at the same time but gene testing is the priority.

References

1. Niederau C, Fischer R, Sonnenberg A, et al. Survival and causes of death in cirrhotic and in noncirrhotic patients with primary hemochromatosis. N Engl J Med. 1985;313:1256–62.
2. Feder JN, Gnirke A, Thomas W, et al. A novel MHC class I-like gene is mutated in patients with hereditary haemochromatosis. Nat Genet. 1996;13:399–408.
3. Merryweather-Clarke AT, Pointon JJ, Shearman JD, Robson KJ. Global prevalence of putative haemochromatosis mutations. J Med Genet. 1997;34:275–8.
4. Pilling LC, Tamosauskaite J, Jones G, et al. Common conditions associated with hereditary haemochromatosis genetic variants: cohort study in UK Biobank. BMJ. 2019;364:k5222.
5. Buch S, Sharma A, Ryan E, et al. Variants in PCSK7, PNPLA3 and TM6SF2 are risk factors for the development of cirrhosis in hereditary haemochromatosis. Aliment Pharmacol Ther. 2021;53(7):830–43.
6. EASL Clinical Practice Guidelines on haemochromatosis. European association for the study of the liver. J Hepatol. 2022;77:479–502.
7. Guyader D, Jazquelinet C, Moirand R, et al. Noninvasive prediction of fibrosis in C282Y homozygous hemochromatosis. Gastroenterology. 1998;115:929–36.
8. Legros L, Bardou-Jacquet E, Latournerie M, et al. Non-invasive assessment of liver fibrosis in C282Y homoyzgous HFE hemochromatosis. Liver Int. 2015;35:1731–8.
9. Bardo-Jacquet E, Laine F, Guggenbuhi P, et al. Worse outcomes of patients with HFE hemochromatosis with persistent increases in transferrin saturation during maintenance therapy. Clin Gastroenterol Hepatol. 2017;15:1620–7.
10. Fitzsimons EJ, Cullis JO, Thomas DW, et al. Diagnosis and therapy of genetic haemochromatosis (review and 2017 update). Br J Haematol. 2018;181:293–303.
11. Falize L, Guillygomarc'h A, Perrin M, et al. Reversibility of hepatic fibrosis in treated genetic hemochromatosis: a study of 36 cases. Hepatology. 2006;44:472–7.
12. Gurrin LC, Osborne NJ, Constantine CC, et al. The natural history of serum iron indices for HFE C282Y homozygosity associated with hereditary hemochromatosis. Gastroenterology. 2008;135:1945–52.

13. Phatak P, Brissot P, Wurster M, et al. A phase 1/2, dose-escalation trial of deferasirox for the treatment of iron overload in HFE-related hereditary hemochromatosis. Hepatology. 2010;52:1671–779.
14. Griffiths WJH, Besser M, Bowden DJ, Kelly DA. Juvenile haemochromatosis. Lancet Child Adolesc Health. 2021;5:524–30.
15. Bhuva M, Sen S, Elsey T, et al. Sequence analysis of exon 1 of the ferritin light chain (FTL) gene can reveal the rare disorder 'hereditary hyperferritinaemia without cataracts'. Br J Haematol. 2019;184:1037–40.
16. Nemeth E, Tuttle MS, Powelson J, et al. Hepcidin regulates cellular iron efflux by binding to ferroportin and inducing its internalization. Science. 2004;306:2090–3.

Chapter 13
Pregnancy and Liver Disease

Hamish M. Miller and Rachel H. Westbrook

Key Learning Points
- Pregnancy related liver disease occurs in 3% of pregnancies.
- Intrahepatic cholestasis of pregnancy (ICP) with serum bile acid measurements exceeding 100 µmol/L are associated with an significantly increased risk of stillbirth [1].
- The HELLP (haemolysis, elevated liver enzymes and low platelets) syndrome represents a severe form of pre-eclampsia and immediate preparation for delivery of the foetus must be made.
- AFLP is a rare but life threatening complication of pregnancy. These patients should be managed in a High Dependency Unit/Intensive Care Unit setting.
- Treatment of acute variceal bleeding in pregnancy is managed as per the non-pregnant patient with resuscitation, antibiotic use and endoscopic haemostasis. However, caution is advised with the use of vasopressin or synthetic analogues due to an association with uterine ischaemia.

H. M. Miller · R. H. Westbrook (✉)
Sheila Sherlock Liver Centre, Royal Free Hospital, London, UK
e-mail: hamish.miller@nhs.net; rachel.westbrook@nhs.net

© Springer Nature Switzerland AG 2022 261
T. Cross (ed.), *Liver Disease in Clinical Practice*, In Clinical Practice, https://doi.org/10.1007/978-3-031-10012-3_13

Case Study

A 31-year-old female presents day 1 post forceps delivery. She is noticeably jaundiced and confused. Admission bloods show the following: Haemoglobin 88, WCC 22.88, Platelets 45, INR 3.4, Sodium 120, Potassium 7.2, Creatinine 291, Urea 10.7, Bilirubin 135, ALT 73, AST 77, ALP 260, gamma GT 125, albumin 20, CRP 34, Lactate 3.9. Her blood pressure was 200/120.

Questions

1. What are the differential diagnoses?
2. What further investigations would you order?
3. How and where would you manage this patient?

Introduction

Abnormalities in liver function tests can be related or unrelated to pregnancy. Pregnancy related liver disease affects up to 3% of pregnancies and can be associated with significant morbidity and mortality for both mother and foetus [2]. A focused evaluation is required to distinguish the liver diseases specific to the pregnant state from pre-existing liver disease or liver disease occurring de novo in pregnancy (Table 13.1). Rapid and correct evaluation allows correct and timely management for the mother and baby; thus limiting risk of an adverse outcome.

TABLE 13.1 List of commonly occurring liver conditions in pregnancy, along with clinical presentation, liver biochemistry and recommended investigations

Pregnancy related liver disease

	Presentation	Liver function tests	Investigations
Hyperemesis Gravidarum	Vomiting, dehydration, weight loss	Raised transaminases (2–5× upper limit of normal (ULN)). Normal bilirubin	
Intrahepatic cholestasis of pregnancy	Pruritus (typically worse on palms and soles)	Transaminases 2–5× ULN. Normal bilirubin. Increased bile acids	
Acute fatty liver of pregnancy	Nausea/vomiting, abdominal pain, malaise, anorexia. Can have jaundice and encephalopathy if severe	Transaminases 3–15× ULN. Can have raised bilirubin if severe, mostly conjugated	Ultrasound or CT to exclude other differentials including hepatic haematoma. Liver biopsy

(continued)

TABLE 13.1 (continued)

		Presentation	Liver function tests	Investigations
Hypertension-related liver diseases	Pre-eclampsia/eclampsia	Abdominal pain, headache, visual disturbance, nausea and vomiting. Seizures in eclampsia	Transaminases 2–5× ULN. Normal bilirubin	
	HELLP syndrome	Right upper quadrant pain, nausea and vomiting, headache, rarely can have bleeding and jaundice	Transaminases 2–30× ULN normal. Bilirubin 1.5–10× ULN	
	Liver infarction/rupture	Abdominal pain (from vague to constant sharper pain with referral to shoulder tip), hypotension, abdominal distension, shock	Markedly raised transaminases	CT or MRI

Non-pregnancy related liver disease

Pre-existing liver disease	Cirrhosis with portal hypertension	Can present with variceal bleeding.		Endoscopic surveillance
	Viral			
	Post liver transplant			
	Autoimmune			
Co-incidentally with pregnancy	Viral	Jaundice, can present with fulminant hepatic failure (particularly with HEV)	Raised bilirubin	Viral screen including viral hepatitis, HSV, EBV, CMV.
	Autoimmune			
	Vascular	Budd-Chiari: Right upper quadrant pain, jaundice, ascites.		Abdominal ultrasound including dopplers of the liver and portal system
	Drug			
	Gallstones		Cholestatic pattern — Raised ALP and bilirubin.	

[25]

Normal Physiology in Pregnancy

Physiological changes seen in pregnancy can mimic those seen in liver disease. In the second and third trimester a hyper-dynamic circulation develops with expansion of circulating blood volume, an increase cardiac output and a reduction in peripheral vascular resistance, as is common in cirrhosis. The hyper-oestrogenic state of pregnancy also occurs in patients with cirrhosis secondary to impaired hepatic metabolism of oestrogen. These physiological similarities result in clinical signs including: palmar erythema and spider naevi, which are physiological and not pathological, in pregnancy. Clinically insignificant oesophageal varices are found in up to 50% of pregnant women due to a reduction of venous return from compression of the inferior vena cava (IVC) by the gravid uterus [3].

Biochemical and haematological indices taken during pregnancy need to be interpreted in the light of the altered normal ranges for test results. The majorities of indices remain unchanged or slightly reduced secondary to haemodilution. Of note the maternal alkaline phosphatase (ALP) increases in the third trimester when ALP is produced both from the placenta and as a result of foetal bone development; a biliary source can be excluded by a normal gamma-glutamyl transpeptidase (GGT) level. The alpha fetoprotein (AFP) level increases in pregnancy as AFP is produced by the foetal liver. There is an increase in serum proteins such as the pro-coagulant factors I (fibrinogen), II, VIII, IX and XII, with a decrease in protein S. Elevations in transaminases, bilirubin or the prothrombin time are abnormal and indicate a pathological state which requires rapid further evaluation.

Gallbladder motility is decreased in pregnancy, with an increase fasting and residual gallbladder volume after contraction seen on ultrasound. Both pregnancy and the oral contraceptive pill increases cholesterol saturation of bile salts contributing to lithogenicity. Biliary sludge is a common asymptomatic finding, which often resolves after pregnancy. Cholecystitis is not uncommon and a cholecystectomy is the second commonest operation performed in pregnant women (after appendicectomy) [4].

Pregnancy Related Liver Diseases

Hyperemesis Gravidarum

Hyperemesis gravidarum (HG) is a clinical syndrome consisting of intractable nausea, vomiting, dehydration, ketogenesis and weight loss (>5%) complicating between 0.3% and 3.6% [5] of pregnancies. Its pathogenesis is incompletely understood but is thought to be related to peak human chorionic gonadotrophin (hCG) levels. HG typically occurs before 9 weeks of gestation and is more common amongst those with multiple or molar pregnancies, and those with a previous history of HG. Two genes, GDF15 and IGFBP7, have been implicated in HG but a causal relationship has not yet been proven [6]. Abnormalities in aminotransferases, particularly alanine aminotransferase occur in 50% of patients admitted for HG and indicate severe disease [7]. Management is supportive (after excluding alternative causes for abnormal liver function tests) with anti-emetics, vitamin B6 supplementation, intravenous fluids, electrolyte correction and thromboprophylaxis is essential as HG still accounts for one maternal death per annum. HG is a fully reversible condition and elevation in aminotransferases should return to normal with resolution of symptoms. Persistent abnormal liver biochemistry after vomiting has ceased should prompt investigation for an alternative diagnosis.

Intrahepatic Cholestasis of Pregnancy

Intrahepatic cholestasis of pregnancy (ICP) or obstetric cholestasis is the most common pregnancy related liver disease with an incidence of between 0.2% and 2% of all pregnancies [8]. ICP most commonly affects women in the third trimester but has been reported in as early as 7-week gestation. It is a reversible form of cholestasis and presents with intense pruritis (often worse on palms and soles) with raised serum bile acids (BA) (>11 μmol/L), which typically resolves within 6 weeks of delivery. (Typical laboratory abnormalities are detailed in Table 13.1.)

The pathogenesis is complex, however, it is likely that elevated oestrogen and progesterone metabolites in pregnancy unmask the disease in genetically susceptible women. One study has shown a link between mutations in the ATP-binding subfamily member 4 (ABCB4) gene and ICP. In this study, 16% of Caucasian patients with ICP had mutations in the ABCB4 gene [9]. It has also been suggested that mutations in Farnesoid X receptors may increase the risk of developing ICP [10].

The main risk is to the foetus. Prospective cohort studies of perinatal outcomes in ICP suggest that serum bile acid measurements exceeding 100 μmol/L are associated with an increased risk of still birth. The risk of still birth also increases as gestation advances in this cohort [11].

The management of intrahepatic cholestasis of pregnancy was reviewed recently as part of the PITCHES trial. This study included 604 women, of which 144 had severe ICP and BA >40 and concluded that there is no significant difference between ursodeoxycholic acid (UDCA) and placebo for most of the adverse perinatal outcomes including perinatal death, preterm delivery or admission to the neonatal unit. Therefore, they concluded that UDCA should no longer be considered first line in the management of ICP. However, the most recent guidance from the AASLD still recommends UDCA at a dose of 10–15 mg/kg as first line management. Another option that has been trialled is the combination of rifampicin and UDCA. One trial showed a decrease in serum bile acids in 54% of patients whose serum bile acids remained high whilst on just UDCA. A further study is being carried out comparing the use of rifampicin versus UDCA but the results are yet to be published [12].

Parenteral Vitamin K should be given in those who have elevation in prothrombin time secondary to cholestasis and impairment of fat soluble vitamin absorption as this will correct coagulation and reduce risk of peri-partum and neonatal haemorrhage. Aqueous cream with 1–2% menthol cream can be effective in reducing pruritus [8].

Women with ICP should be counselled for a recurrence rate of up to 90% [13] in subsequent pregnancies and an increased risk of pruritus or cholestatic impairment when taking the combined oral contraceptive pill. Repeat liver function tests are essential post-delivery to ensure resolution of abnormalities. Ongoing symptoms or biochemical impairment beyond 3-months postpartum should prompt further investigations for alternative/concurrent diagnoses.

Finally, there is data to suggest that ICP is not a benign condition and is associated with (via bile acid transport deficits) an increased risk of biliary issues in later life. No recommendations exist as yet with regards the benefit of follow up of such patients [14].

Pre-eclampsia/Eclampsia/HELLP Syndrome

Pre-eclampsia is a multisystem manifestation of abnormal placentation and placental insufficiency in pregnancy characterised typically by hypertension (>140/90), proteinuria (>300 mg/day) with renal, liver, neurological or haematological dysfunction after 20 weeks of gestation. Pre-eclampsia affects 3–8% of pregnancies between 20 weeks gestation and 4 weeks postpartum [15]. The presence of seizures differentiates pre-eclampsia from eclampsia. Major risk factors include chronic kidney disease, previous episodes of pre-eclampsia or hypertension, diabetes and autoimmune disorders [15]. Presenting symptoms are non-specific and may mimic viral infections—and consist of abdominal pain, headache, visual disturbance, nausea and vomiting; thus a high index of suspicion is needed for further evaluation. Peripheral oedema and hyper-reflexia are common. On laboratory evaluation, raised creatinine and thrombocytopenia are often present. However, a platelet count of less than 100×10^9/L, serum creatinine and serum albumin are not good predictors of complications [15]. The presence of elevated serum aminotransferases indicate severe disease and should prompt a multidisciplinary team discussion regarding delivery because if rapid hypertensive control and delivery is not achieved, women are at risk of renal dysfunction, cerebral haemorrhage, hepatic infarction, hepatic haematomas or hepatic rupture with consequent markedly increased perinatal mortality and morbidity.

The HELLP (haemolysis, elevated liver enzymes and low platelets) syndrome represents a severe form of pre-eclampsia and complicates up to 20% of cases and should be seen as part of the same disease spectrum [16]. Hypertension is evident in up to 85% and proteinuria is common. However, it is important to recognise that HELLP syndrome can occur in the absence of hypertension and proteinuria, reflecting the multisystem nature of pre-eclampsia and related disorders. It typically presents between 28 and 36 weeks of gestation, but can present up to 1-week postpartum. The diagnosis is based mainly on clinical features and the presence of haemolysis, thrombocytopenia and transaminitis on biochemical evaluation. The presenting symptoms are varied and include right upper quadrant or epigastric pain in approximately (40–86)% of cases, nausea and vomiting (36–84% of cases), headache (33–61% of cases) and rarely bleeding and jaundice [17]. A significant number of patients are asymptomatic. Classical laboratory indices are detailed in Table 13.1.

In HELLP, it is postulated that endothelial damage secondary to placental insufficiency results in inappropriate coagulation cascade activation with the formation of microcirculatory fibrin cross-linked networks, a microangiopathic haemolytic anaemia and a consumptive thrombocytopaenia. Hepatic ischaemia follows microvascular thrombosis in the sinusoids resulting in elevated aminotransferases and a disseminated intravascular coagulopathy can occur with evidence of raised fibrin degradation products, low fibrinogen and secondary increase in the prothrombin time.

The only cure for pre-eclampsia and HELLP syndrome is delivery of the placenta. Hypertension should be treated with nifedipine, labetalol or hydralazine. Magnesium sulphate should be given to prevent maternal seizures and glucocorticoids to promote foetal lung maturity if gestation is less than 34 weeks. Following delivery maternal features of pre-eclampsia/HELLP resolve within 48 h in the majority. Women should be monitored in a high dependence setting due to the small but recognised risk postpartum worsening of maternal symptoms.

A recent landmark paper published in the New England Journal of Medicine has identified that women with a high risk of pre-eclampsia (>1 in 100) benefit from taking low dose aspirin started between weeks 11 and 14 of gestation and continued until week 36. In the aspirin group, there was a significantly lower incidence of pre-eclampsia but there was no significant difference between the incidence of other complications, either for the foetus or the mother [18].

Serious maternal morbidity is associated with the development of disseminated intravascular coagulation (DIC; 21%), placental abruption (16%), acute renal failure (8%), pulmonary oedema (6%), parenchymal/subcapsular hepatic haematoma and rupture (1%). The maternal mortality of severe pre-eclampsia which is complicated by HELLP syndrome can be as high as 24% [19]. Neonatal outcomes range from prematurity with up to 70% affected, to a perinatal mortality rate between 7% and 20%. Neonatal outcome is more strongly associated with gestational age and birthweight than severity of HELLP syndrome [16].

Acute Fatty Liver of Pregnancy (AFLP)

AFLP is a rare but serious metabolic complication of pregnancy arising due to microvesicular fatty infiltration of hepatocytes. It has an incidence of 5 per 100,000 pregnancies with multi-parity and reduced BMI being recognised risk factors in a large UK population based study [20]. AFLP is thought to be secondary to an inherited defect of mitochondrial beta-oxidation. This results in a build-up of long-chain fatty acids which ultimately return into the maternal circulation, deposit in the maternal liver and manifest as maternal liver disease. In 20% of patients with AFLP, there is evidence of long-chain 3-hydroxyacyl CoA dehydrogenase (LCHAD) deficiency in their offspring [21]. These children are at risk of developing fatal non-ketotic hypoglycaemic attacks and therefore all babies born from women with AFLP should be considered for genetic testing for LCHAD and other defects in fatty oxidation.

AFLP mostly presents in the third trimester and always before delivery, but is often diagnosed postpartum. The most frequent symptoms are nausea or vomiting, abdominal pain, malaise and anorexia, with jaundice and encephalopathy in the more severely affected. Pre-eclampsia is present in about half. Common laboratory changes are detailed in Table 13.1. They include hyperbilirubinaemia, variable serum transaminase rises (up to 500 IU/L), acute renal dysfunction, a leucocytosis above normal pregnancy levels and thrombocytopaenia. Coagulopathy in AFLP can reflect both hepatic dysfunction and or the presence of DIC (affecting up to 10% with AFLP) [22] with reduced fibrinogen levels. Ultrasound or CT is useful in excluding other differentials such as a hepatic haematoma and often reveals fatty infiltration, which can be useful retrospectively when compared to imaging months postpartum.

A definitive diagnosis is made on liver histology, however, this is rarely performed due to the emergent progression of the disease and need to stabilise and deliver affected women. In the absence of confounding aetiology, clinical diagnostic criteria have been developed and validated for AFLP (Table 13.2) [23]. An abbreviated method of diagnosing AFLP using only gastrointestinal symptoms, aminotransferases, bile acids, activated partial prothrombin time (APTT)/ prothrombin time (PT) and bilirubin has shown promising initial results but has not yet been replicated in larger studies [24]. If clarity is lacking regarding the diagnosis, a liver biopsy can always take place postpartum as changes persist for several weeks.

TABLE 13.2 Swansea criteria for acute fatty liver of pregnancy

Six or more of features below in absence of other aetiology

- Vomiting

- Abdominal pain

- Polydypsia/polyuria

- Encephalopathy

- Raised bilirubin (>14 µmol/L)

- Hypoglycaemia (<4 mmol/L)

- Leucocytosis (>11 × 10^6/L)

- Raised uric acid (>340 µmol/L)

- Elevated ammonia (>42 IU/L)

- Ascites or hyperechoic liver on US

- Elevated transaminases (>42 IU/L)

- Renal impairment (creatinine >150 µmol/L)

- Coagulopathy (PT >14 s or APTT >34 s)

- Microvesicular steatosis on biopsy

Management involves early recognition, resuscitation of the mother and rapid delivery of foetus regardless of gestational age. Consequently, maternal mortality has improved from 92% in the 1970s to between 7% and 18% [25]. True hepatic synthetic failure often manifests with hypoglycaemia, lactic acidosis and raised serum ammonia levels. Due to the risk of fulminant hepatic failure, such patients must be discussed with and then subsequently managed in a liver transplant centre. Maternal resuscitation involves correction of hypoglycaemia, hypovolaemia and aggressive reversal of coagulopathy with blood products to reduce bleeding complications during and following delivery. Plasma exchange can improve maternal outcomes postpartum. There is a possibility of AFLP recurrence in subsequent pregnancies even in the absence of known beta-oxidation defects thought the exact rates are unknown.

Hepatic Haemorrhage and Rupture

Spontaneous hepatic haemorrhage and rupture can complicate pre-eclampsia, HELLP and AFLP, but rarely occurs in their apparent absence. Mortality is extremely high (up to 50%) [16]. Marked rises in the transaminases are not typical of HELLP and suggest hepatic infarction, haematoma, rupture or unrelated cause of inflammation (e.g. viral hepatitis). Additionally, changes in the character of abdominal pain, particularly from an intermittent vague diffuse visceral pain to a constant sharper pain, with referral to the shoulder tip, may herald a growing subcapsular hepatic haematoma and impending rupture. However, hepatic haematomas can also present covertly with pyrexia, modest liver transaminases derangement, anaemia and neutrophil leucocytosis or rapidly manifesting as haemoperitoneum with abdominal distention, hypovolemic shock and collapse when ruptured.

Computed tomography or magnetic resonance is the investigation of choice and discussion with a hepatobiliary surgeon is mandatory. Contained haematomas can be managed conservatively with volume replacement, aggressive coagulation support, prophylactic antibiotics and blood product transfusion. In contrast, hepatic rupture requires urgent angiography with hepatic artery embolisation and/or surgical intervention involving packing, arterial ligation and hepatic resection if haemodynamically unstable.

Non-pregnancy Related Liver Diseases

Cirrhosis and Portal Hypertension

Women with cirrhosis have a disruption in their hypothalamic-pituitary axis and abnormal oestrogen metabolism. Pregnancy is thus rare due to a combination of anovulation, amenorrhoea, reduced fertility and libido [26]. When pregnancy does occur there is a high rate of spontaneous foetal loss, preterm delivery, need for intensive neonatal support for the foetus and an increased risk of hepatic decompensation and death for the mother [27]. Maternal mortality for pregnant women with cirrhosis was reported to be as high as 10.5% in the early 1980s, but encouragingly more recent series have reported reduced mortality rates of 1.8% with a decompensation rate of around 15% [28]. Outcomes of pregnancy in women with cirrhosis are related to the severity of the underlying maternal liver disease. Utilisation of prognostic scoring systems such as MELD or UKELD, typically used to predict mortality in patients with cirrhosis undergoing procedures or to guide need for liver transplantation, can help predict likely maternal outcomes in pregnancy. Specifically, a preconception MELD score ≥10 had an 83% sensitivity and specificity for predicting hepatic decompensation, whereas women with a preconception MELD ≤6 are unlikely to have any significant maternal complications [27].

Maternal mortality in cirrhotic women is in part due to a four-fold increase in occurrence of variceal bleeding compared to non-pregnant counterparts. Due to an increased circulating volume and caval compression by the gravid uterus, portal hypertension worsens in pregnancy with its risks of variceal bleeding peaking late in the second trimester where circulating blood volume is increased but vasodilatation seen in third trimester is yet to occur. Further risk occurs during the second stage of labour with the prolonged Valsalva manoeuver.

Preconception screening and eradication of oesophageal varices would seem appropriate. AASLD recommends endoscopic surveillance at the start of the second trimester. If small varices are found at endoscopy, then propranolol is recommended but if the varices are medium to large then management options are either propranolol or variceal ligation. Variceal ligation is the recommended option if there are high risk features [22].

Treatment of acute variceal bleeding in pregnancy is managed emergently like in the non-pregnant population with resuscitation, early antibiotic prophylaxis (cephalosporins are recommended [22]) and timely endoscopic haemostasis. The strong vasoconstrictive effects of vasopressin or synthetic analogues are associated with uterine ischaemia and are generally avoided. However, limited data currently suggests no adverse foetal effects with somatostatin or octreotide and therefore their used can be considered as an alternative where available to terlipressin. Transjugular intrahepatic portosystemic shunts (TIPSS) are also a rescue option in refractory variceal bleeding in pregnancy [29].

Hepatitis B and C Virus Infection and Pregnancy

Hepatitis B virus (HBV) infection is usually associated with good prognosis except in those with established cirrhosis and in fulminant hepatitis. From a foetal transmission perspective, the risk of developing chronic HBV infection is inversely proportional to the age at exposure with up to 90% of babies exposed perinatally developing chronic HBV infection. Therefore, a key consideration is the prevention of perinatal transmission to reduce the prevalence of chronic hepatitis B carriers, half of which can be attributed to vertical transmission worldwide.

All pregnant women in the UK are tested for Hepatitis B surface antigen (HBsAg) in early pregnancy, followed by HBV DNA if this is found to be positive [30]. Pregnancy itself has little or no effect on the natural history of HBV infection from the maternal perspective. All infants born to HBsAg positive mothers should receive a course of hepatitis B vaccination and HB immunoglobulin within 24 h [31]. Such neonatal vaccination is highly efficacious (preventing vertical transmission in 95%) and suggests that transmission mainly occurs intrapartum rather than during pregnancy. Risk factors for vertical transmission, in spite of prophylaxis, are maternal eAg positivity and high HBV viral load (>10^7 IU/mL). In this instance, oral nucleotide analogues such as tenofovir, in addition to active immunisation have been shown to reduce perinatal transmission. It is recommended that antiviral therapy is started between weeks 28 and 32 if the HBV DNA is greater than 200,000 IU/mL and can be ceased either at delivery or up to 3 months afterwards [22]. Tenofovir has an established role in the prevention of HIV transmission in utero and the Antiretroviral Pregnancy Registry also reports no increase in teratogenicity. There is no proven role for cae-sarean sections in preventing mother to child transmission. Breast feeding should be encouraged, providing immunopro-phylaxis is given at birth.

Like chronic HBV infection, Hepatitis C (HCV) infection in pregnancy confers minimal risk to mother except in the context of cirrhosis. Detectable HCV RNA levels in newborn infants suggest that unlike HBV infection, neonatal transmis-sion predominates with a transmission rate of 5.8% of HCV RNA positive mothers [32]. Due to passive transfer of mater-nal anti-HCV antibodies diagnosis of vertical transmission is made when HCV RNA is detected on two consecutive sam-ples 3 months apart, or when antibodies are detected after 18 months of age. Risk factors for vertical transmission are co-infection with HIV, maternal HCV viral load and active intravenous drug use. Co-infection with HIV increases rates of vertical transmission to 10.8% [32]. There is no evidence that the mode of delivery influences the risk of vertical trans-mission, and breast feeding is not contraindicated in women with HCV infection.

Autoimmune Hepatitis and Pregnancy

Similar to other autoimmune diseases in pregnancy, autoim-mune hepatitis control usually improves during pregnancy due to the immune-tolerant state pregnancy confers and flares of disease activity are seen in up to 80% of women postpartum [33]. Patients with stable AIH on immunosup-pression are often concerned about the potential risk of tera-togenicity secondary to their immunosuppressive medication. Clear data now exists showing that flares in disease activity are more likely in patients off immunosuppression and, more-over, those patients are more likely to develop hepatic decompensation. Prednisolone is considered safe and should be used for AIH in pregnancy [33]. Azathioprine has been associated with and increased risk of cleft palate and skeletal anomalies in mice but there is no proven association between azathioprine use during pregnancy and adverse foetal outcomes [22, 34]. Transient lymphopaenias, hypogammaglobulinaemia and thymic hypoplasias have been reported in neonates born to mothers on azathioprine but are reversed after birth. Guidance from AASLD suggests a strategy of minimal adjustment to prednisolone/azathioprine during pregnancy and postpartum. Finally, it should be noted that AIH hepatitis can present de novo in pregnancy and testing for immunoglobulins and autoantibodies should be routine in any women who presents with elevated aminotransferases during pregnancy.

Liver Transplantation

Following liver transplantation, women can regain their fertility often as early as 1-month post transplantation. However, it is recommended that pregnancy is delayed until at least 1 year after liver transplantation as this allows stabilisation of immunosuppression and the risk of acute cellular rejection reduces after 1 year [35]. Outcomes of pregnancy in LT patients are good overall, but with an increased incidence of preterm delivery, hypertension/pre-eclampsia, infections, gestational diabetes and rejection of the graft. Hypertensive complications and pre-eclampsia are attributed to the increase in renal dysfunction and hypertension secondary to the use of immunosuppressive calcineurin inhibitors (cyclosporine and tacrolimus). Gestational diabetes is induced by long term use of steroid immunosuppression and tacrolimus therapy. Acute cellular rejection (ACR) can complicate up to 17% of LT patients in pregnancy and there is data to support delaying pregnancy for 1 year following LT significantly reduces this risk. Preterm delivery may be needed because of the need to manage pre-eclampsia and episodes of ACR during pregnancy [36].

Immunosupression should not be discontinued for pregnancy. Tacrolimus, Cyclosporine, azathioprine and steroids should all be continued as benefit far outweighs potential risk of teratogenicity. Mycophenolate is contraindicated as it has been shown to have a high rate of spontaneous abortion and structural abnormalities as well as an increased risk of stillbirth [35]. It should be discontinued in both males and females with a 6 month washout prior to conception and alternative immunosuppression considered.

Liver Disease De Novo in Pregnancy

Acute Viral Infections and Pregnancy

Acute viral hepatitis is the most common cause of jaundice in pregnancy worldwide. Both hepatitis A and E are transmitted by the faeco-oral route and are associated with poor hygiene. In pregnancy, Hepatitis A (HAV) infection has a similar clinical course to the non-pregnant population. Severity of disease is associated with advanced maternal age and infection in the third trimester where there is an increased risk of prematurity.

In contrast, pregnant women are more vulnerable to hepatitis E (HEV) infection, and it is the most prevalent viral cause of acute liver failure in pregnancy. The risk of fulminant hepatic failure in HEV and pregnancy is between 15% and 20% and in certain areas, such as the Indian subcontinent, the risk is greater [37]. Fulminant hepatitis due to HEV may resemble liver failure from AFLP, HELLP or HSV hepatitis and should be considered in pregnant women with acute hepatitis living in or travelling from endemic areas. The fatality rate from HEV infection is much higher in pregnant women compared to the rest of the population (15–25% as opposed to 0.5–4%) [38]. Poor maternal outcomes are associated with presence of encephalopathy, irrespective of delivery. Management is supportive, although liver transplantation has been reported for this indication [39].

Herpes simplex virus (HSV) hepatitis although rare, has a predilection for the immunocompromised and therefore pregnant women are more susceptible. It can be caused by primary or latent disease and present with mucocutaneous lesions in 50%, raised aminotransferases, thrombocytopaenia and coagulopathy, commonly in the absence of jaundice. Maternal mortality is reported at around 40% [40]. CT shows multiple sub-centimetre low-density areas of liver necrosis and diagnosis can be confirmed on histology. Treatment with aciclovir is associated with a survival benefit and should be started prior to confirmatory test if the diagnosis is suspected [40].

Pregnancy and Thrombosis

Budd-Chiari syndrome (BCS) or hepatic venous outflow tract obstruction can present de novo in pregnancy or consequent to thrombus extension resulting in an acute presentation. The prevalence of pregnancy related BCS is estimated to make up around 6.8% of all BCS presentations [41]. If a patient is known to have a prothrombotic state in pregnancy, low molecular weight heparin is advocated over vitamin K antagonists (due to concerns of a risk of miscarriage and congenital malformations). In pregnancy, presentation is typically right upper quadrant pain, jaundice and ascites. Management involves diagnosis with ultrasound, early anticoagulation and consideration of a transjugular intrahepatic portosystemic shunt. Budd-Chiari syndrome often has a multifactorial thrombotic aetiology and so evidence of thrombophilia's and myeloproliferative neoplasms should be sought after. Pregnancy is very rarely the sole prothrombotic risk factor. Maternal outcomes are good provided patients have stable disease although recurrence of disease can occur if anticoagulation is discontinued. Foetal outcomes vary but pregnancies reaching 20 weeks of gestation (despite a 76% prematurity rate) have good outcomes.

Gallstones in Pregnancy

Pregnancy is a lithogenic state and is associated with increased risk for cholelithiasis with around 10% of pregnant women developing gallstones or viscous biliary sludge. Between 0.05% and 0.8% of pregnant women have gallstones which cause symptoms [42]. Cholecystectomy (open or laparoscopic) can be done safely in the second trimester, while ERCP and sphincterotomy is feasible if required. A large study has shown that there was no significant difference with regards preterm birth or foetal mortality between pregnant women who were either managed conservatively or surgically for gallstone disease. However, the same study did show that surgically managed gallstone disease did decrease the rate of maternal readmission to hospital [42]. Epidemiological studies have suggested that the risks of cholelithiasis remain for 5 years postpartum following which returns to baseline.

Summary

Liver diseases in pregnancy are clinically important because of the increased morbidity and mortality for both the mother and baby. The spectrum of disease and presentation is variable making evaluation, diagnosis and the early instigation of correct management challenging, but vital to achieving a good outcome. Patients benefit form multidisciplinary input by experienced hepatologists and obstetricians. Maternal and foetal outcomes are improving due to ongoing research, improved guidelines and our better understanding of preconception risk factors, disease stratification, disease mechanisms and therapeutic options.

Answers to Case Study

1. The differential at this stage is wide. See Table 13.1 for classification of liver disease in pregnancy. Important differentials in this patient would include acute fatty liver of pregnancy, pre-eclampsia or acute liver failure of another aetiology such as paracetamol overdose.

2. Investigations would include a non-invasive liver screen including a blood film and a paracetamol level. Imaging would include a liver ultrasound scan with doppler and if necessary, a CT scan. A liver biopsy would also help with diagnosis (Fig. 13.1).

3. This patient should be managed in a high dependency/intensive care setting and ideally would be managed at a tertiary hepatology centre. They would require supportive care and input from the multidisciplinary team. This patient requires correction of the hyperkalaemia and hypoglycaemia and to consider empirical antibiotics. Specifically for acute fatty liver of pregnancy, the offspring should be screened for long-chain 3-hydroxyacyl CoA dehydrogenase (LCHAD) deficiency. It is also worth noting that this particular patient is postpartum, though had she still been pregnant, delivery of the foetus should be considered.

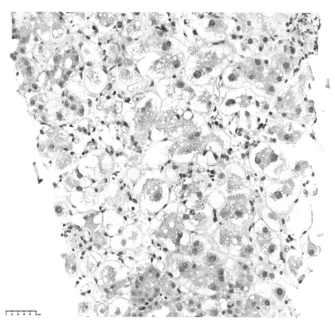

FIGURE 13.1 Liver Biopsy of the patient discussed in the case study. Hepatocytes show ballooning and fine vacuolation of their cytoplasm along with larger steatotic droplets in places. H&E 400×. (Courtesy of Prof Alberto Quaglia, Consultant Histopathologist)

References

1. Chappell LC, et al. Ursodeoxycholic acid versus placebo in women with intrahepatic cholestasis of pregnancy (PITCHES): a randomised controlled trial. Lancet. 2019;394(10201):849–60. https://doi.org/10.1016/S0140-6736(19)31270-X.
2. Westbrook RH, Dusheiko G, Williamson C. Pregnancy and liver disease. J Hepatol. 2016;64:933–45.
3. Joshi D, James A, Quaglia A, Westbrook RH, Heneghan MA. Liver disease in pregnancy. Lancet. 2010;375(9714):594–605. https://doi.org/10.1016/S0140-6736(09)61495-1.
4. Juhasz-Böss I, Solomayer E, Strik M, Raspé C. Abdominaleingriffe in der schwangerschaft—Eine interdisziplinäre herausforderung. Dtsch Arztebl Int. 2014;111:465–72.
5. The Royal College of Obstetricians and Gynaecologist. The management of nausea and vomiting of pregnancy and hyper-emesis gravidarum: green-top guideline no. 69. RCOG Green-top Guidel. No. 69; 2016. p. 1–27.
6. Fejzo MS, et al. Placenta and appetite genes GDF15 and IGFBP7 are associated with hyperemesis gravidarum. Nat Commun. 2018;9(1):1178.
7. Conchillo JM, et al. Liver enzyme elevation induced by hyper-emesis gravidarum: aetiology, diagnosis and treatment. Neth J Med. 2002;60:374–8.
8. Williamson C, Geenes V. Intrahepatic cholestasis of pregnancy. Obstet Gynecol. 2014;124(1):120–33. https://doi.org/10.1097/AOG.0000000000000346.
9. Bacq Y, et al. ABCB4 gene mutations and single-nucleotide polymorphisms in women with intrahepatic cholestasis of pregnancy. J Med Genet. 2009;46(10):711–5. https://doi.org/10.1136/jmg.2009.067397.
10. van Mil SWC, et al. Functional variants of the central bile acid sensor FXR identified in intrahepatic cholestasis of pregnancy. Gastroenterology. 2007;133(2):507–16. https://doi.org/10.1053/j.gastro.2007.05.015.
11. Ovadia C, et al. Association of adverse perinatal outcomes of intrahepatic cholestasis of pregnancy with biochemical markers: results of aggregate and individual patient data meta-analyses. Lancet. 2019;393:899–909.
12. Hague WM, et al. A multi-centre, open label, randomised, parallel-group, superiority Trial to compare the efficacy of

URsodeoxycholic acid with RIFampicin in the management of women with severe early onset Intrahepatic Cholestasis of pregnancy: the TURRIFIC randomised trial. BMC Pregnancy Childbirth. 2021;21(1):51. https://doi.org/10.1186/s12884-020-03481-y.

13. Piechota J, Jelski W. Intrahepatic cholestasis in pregnancy: review of the literature. J Clin Med. 2020;9:1361.

14. Marschall HU, Wikström Shemer E, Ludvigsson JF, Stephansson O. Intrahepatic cholestasis of pregnancy and associated hepatobiliary disease: a population-based cohort study. Hepatology. 2013;58:1385–91.

15. Mol BWJ, et al. Pre-eclampsia. Lancet. 2016;387(10022):999–1011. https://doi.org/10.1016/S0140-6736(15)00070-7.

16. Sibai BM, et al. Maternal morbidity and mortality in 442 pregnancies with hemolysis, elevated liver enzymes, and low platelets (HELLP syndrome). Am J Obstet Gynecol. 1993;169(4):1000–6. https://doi.org/10.1016/0002-9378(93)90043-I.

17. Sibai BM. Diagnosis, controversies, and management of the syndrome of hemolysis, elevated liver enzymes, and low platelet count. Obstet Gynecol. 2004;103:981–91.

18. Rolnik DL, et al. Aspirin versus placebo in pregnancies at high risk for preterm preeclampsia. N Engl J Med. 2017;377:613–22.

19. Turgut A, Demirci O, Demirci E, Uludoğan M. Comparison of maternal and neonatal outcomes in women with HELLP syndrome and women with severe preeclampsia without HELLP syndrome. J Prenat Med. 2010;4:51–8.

20. Knight M, Nelson-Piercy C, Kurinczuk JJ, Spark P, Brocklehurst P. A prospective national study of acute fatty liver of pregnancy in the UK. Gut. 2008;57(7):951–6. https://doi.org/10.1136/gut.2008.148676.

21. Browning MF, Levy HL, Wilkins-Haug LE, Larson C, Shih VE. Fetal fatty acid oxidation defects and maternal liver disease in pregnancy. Obstet Gynecol. 2006;107:115–20.

22. Sarkar M, et al. Reproductive health and liver disease: practice guidance by the American Association for the Study of Liver Diseases. Hepatology. 2021;73(1):318–65.

23. Ch'ng CL, Morgan M, Hainsworth I, Kingham JGC. Prospective study of liver dysfunction in pregnancy in Southwest Wales. Gut. 2002;51(6):876–80. https://doi.org/10.1136/gut.51.6.876.

24. Zhong Y, Zhu F, Ding Y. Early diagnostic test for acute fatty liver of pregnancy: a retrospective case control study. BMC Pregnancy Childbirth. 2020;4:1–6.

25. Katarey D, Westbrook RH. Pregnancy-specific liver diseases. Best Pract Res Clin Obstet Gynaecol. 2020;68:12–22.
26. Hagström H, et al. Outcomes of pregnancy in mothers with cirrhosis: a national population-based cohort study of 1.3 million pregnancies. Hepatol Commun. 2018;2(11):1299–305. https://doi.org/10.1002/hep4.1255.
27. Westbrook RH, et al. Model for end-stage liver disease score predicts outcome in cirrhotic patients during pregnancy. Clin Gastroenterol Hepatol. 2011;9(8):694–9. https://doi.org/10.1016/j.cgh.2011.03.036.
28. Shaheen AAM, Myers RP. The outcomes of pregnancy in patients with cirrhosis: a population-based study. Liver Int. 2010;30:275–83.
29. Rahim MN, Pirani T, Williamson C, Heneghan MA. Management of pregnancy in women with cirrhosis. United Eur Gastroenterol J. 2021;9:110–9.
30. Terrault NA, et al. Update on prevention, diagnosis, and treatment of chronic hepatitis B: AASLD 2018 hepatitis B guidance. Hepatology. 2018;67(4):1560–99. https://doi.org/10.1002/hep.29800.
31. Dionne-Odom J, Tita ATN, Silverman NS. #38: Hepatitis B in pregnancy screening, treatment, and prevention of vertical transmission. Am J Obstet Gynecol. 2016;214(1):6–14. https://doi.org/10.1016/j.ajog.2015.09.100.
32. Benova L, Mohamoud YA, Calvert C, Abu-Raddad LJ. Vertical transmission of hepatitis C virus: systematic review and meta-analysis. Clin Infect Dis. 2014;59:765–73.
33. Braga A, Vasconcelos C, Braga J. Autoimmune hepatitis and pregnancy. Best Pract Res Clin Obstet Gynaecol. 2020;68:23–31.
34. Rosenkrantz JG, Githens JH, Cox SM, Kellum DL. Azathioprine (Imuran) and pregnancy. Am J Obstet Gynecol. 1967;97(3):387–94. https://doi.org/10.1016/0002-9378(67)90503-0.
35. Rahim MN, et al. Pregnancy in liver transplantation. Liver Transplant. 2020;26:564–81.
36. Armenti VT, Herrine SK, Radomski JS, Moritz MJ. Pregnancy after liver transplantation. Liver Transplant. 2000;6(6):671–85. https://doi.org/10.1053/jlts.2000.18703.
37. Patra S, Kumar A, Trivedi SS, Puri M, Sarin SK. Maternal and fetal outcomes in pregnant women with acute hepatitis E virus infection. Ann Intern Med. 2007;147(1):28–33. https://doi.org/10.7326/0003-4819-147-1-200707030-00005.

38. Kourtis AP, Read JS, Jamieson DJ. Pregnancy and severity of infection. N Engl J Med. 2014;370:2211–8.
39. Shalimar E, Acharya SK. Hepatitis E and acute liver failure in pregnancy. J Clin Exp Hepatol. 2013;3:213–24.
40. Kang AH, Graves CR. Herpes simplex hepatitis in pregnancy: a case report and review of the literature. Obstet Gynecol Surv. 1999;54(7):463–8. https://doi.org/10.1097/00006254-199907000-00026.
41. Ren W, et al. Prevalence of Budd-Chiari syndrome during pregnancy or puerperium: a systematic review and meta-analysis. Gastroenterol Res Pract. 2015;2015:839875.
42. Ibiebele I, Schnitzler M, Nippita T, Ford JB. Outcomes of gallstone disease during pregnancy: a population-based data linkage study. Paediatr Perinat Epidemiol. 2017;31:522–30.

Chapter 14
The Orphan Liver Disease

Reenam Khan and Philip Newsome

Key Learning Points

Porphyria
- Porphyrias are disorders of haem biosynthesis. They are classified as erythropoietic or hepatic based on the primary site of enzyme deficiency.
- Patients have neurovisceral or cutaneous symptoms or both, depending on which metabolites accumulate. Aminolevulinic acid (ALA) is neurotoxic, whilst porphyrins are associated with cutaneous symptoms. In patients with neurovisceral symptoms, check urine ALA and porphobilinogen (PBG) levels. In patients with cutaneous symptoms, check the plasma and urine porphyrin profile.
- Treatment depends on the type of porphyria. Patients should be advised to avoid triggers. Specific treatments include the use of haem and glucose in acute intermittent

R. Khan
Liver Unit, Queen Elizabeth Hospital, Birmingham, UK
e-mail: khanrs@bham.ac.uk

P. Newsome (✉)
Institute of Biomedical Research, The Medical School, University of Birmingham, Birmingham, UK
e-mail: p.n.newsome@bham.ac.uk

© Springer Nature Switzerland AG 2022   287
T. Cross (ed.), *Liver Disease in Clinical Practice*, In Clinical Practice, https://doi.org/10.1007/978-3-031-10012-3_14

porphyria and the use of venesection and low-dose chloroquine in porphyria cutanea tarda. Givosiran, an ALA synthase I directed small interfering RNA, has now been approved in the USA for treatment of acute intermittent porphyria.

Alpha-1-Antitrypsin (A1AT) Deficiency

- A1AT is a serine protease inhibitor. A1AT deficiency is an inherited metabolic disorder in which A1AT cannot be exported from the liver. In the lungs, this causes emphysema, whilst accumulation of the abnormal protein in the liver causes hepatocyte apoptosis, inflammation and cirrhosis.
- Consider A1AT deficiency in patients who develop emphysema at a young age, or without a smoking history. It should be screened for in patients: (a) with unexplained deranged liver function tests, (b) with bronchiectasis of unclear aetiology, (c) with a family history of liver disease, bronchiectasis or emphysema.
- Serum A1AT can be quantified but the gold standard for diagnosis of A1AT deficiency is phenotyping using isoelectric focusing.
- Although pooled human plasma A1AT is used to treat associated pulmonary disease, there is currently no licensed specific treatment available for A1AT disease affecting the liver. Patients with advanced liver disease should be considered for liver transplant.
- Treatments under investigation include the use of siRNA to downregulate production of the mutant protein and use of carbamazepine to promote degradation of abnormal A1AT.

Cystic Fibrosis Liver Disease (CFLD)

- Around one-third of patients with cystic fibrosis develop liver disease, which is most commonly hepatic steatosis.
- Patients with CF secrete bile which is more viscous and less alkaline than normal. This can predispose to obstruction of the biliary tree and injury to the cholangiocytes and

hepatocytes. This can ultimately trigger fibrosis and then cirrhosis with portal hypertension.

- Assessment of patients with CFLD should involve annual review, including examination for hepatosplenomegaly, blood tests to assess liver function and abdominal ultrasound.
- Ursodeoxycholic acid can be used to treat patients with CFLD. Liver transplant can be considered in advanced liver disease but survival outcomes are worse than those undergoing liver transplant for other reasons.
- The disease modifying drug, Kaftrio, has recently been licensed in the UK for certain subgroups of patients with CF. Whilst it is associated with improvements in lung function (FEV1), it can have hepatobiliary side effects. Patients on Kaftrio should have regular monitoring of liver function tests, and use of Kaftrio should be avoided in patients with severe hepatic impairment (Child-Pugh C).

Case

A 46-year-old Caucasian male was referred to the gastroenterology clinic with abdominal distension and jaundice. His medical history included chronic obstructive pulmonary disease. He had a five pack-year smoking history and was a teetotaller. He had three brothers who died of liver failure aged in their 50s.

On cardiorespiratory examination, he had a prolonged expiratory phase and widespread wheeze. FEV1 on spirometry was 40%. Further examination revealed scleral icterus, asterixis and palmar erythema. His abdomen was soft and non-tender, with splenomegaly of 2 cm below the left costal margin. Below are the results of blood tests:

Hb 9.3 g/dL	Urea 5.5 mmol/L	Platelets 110×10^9/L
Bilirubin 56 μmol/L	Albumin 31 mmol/L	ALT 150 IU/L
Creatinine 69 μmol/L	INR 1.7	AST 110 IU/L

US abdomen showed a cirrhotic liver with 13 cm spleno-megaly. A liver screen was performed. Ferritin, caeruloplas-min and AFP were normal. Viral screen (including hepatitis A, B and C, CMV and EBV) was unremarkable, and autoan-tibody screen was negative. Serum A1AT was reduced at 5 μmol/L.

Questions
1. What is the likely diagnosis?
2. How would you confirm the diagnosis?
3. What is 'augmentation therapy'?

'Orphan' diseases are rare conditions in which there is often reluctance by general physicians to manage the diseases because the diagnosis and management are relatively poorly understood. This chapter focuses on three orphan diseases of the liver: porphyria, alpha-1-antitrypsin deficiency and cystic fibrosis.

Porphyria

Overview

The porphyrias are eight inborn disorders of metabolism characterised by defective haem biosynthesis (Fig. 14.1). Haem is an important component of vital proteins including haemoglobin, myoglobin, cytochrome p450 enzymes and respiratory cytochromes. Approximately 80% of haem is syn-thesised in erythroid precursor cells in the bone marrow. Most of the rest is synthesised by hepatocytes in the liver. Haem synthesis is a multistep process that involves eight enzymes. The first reaction in this pathway, mediated by ALA synthase, is the rate-limiting step. ALA synthase has two iso-forms: ALAS1 in non-erythroid cells and ALAS2 in erythroid cells. ALAS1 activity is inhibited by haem and high glucose levels, whereas activity is increased by cytochrome p450 inducers.

Abnormalities in haem biosynthesis can result in accumu-lation of pathway intermediates, such as 5-aminolevulinic

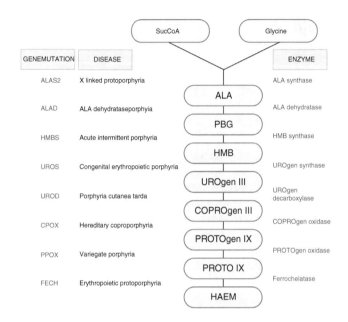

FIGURE 14.1 An overview of the haem biosynthesis pathway, and the enzyme and genetic defects associated with the eight porphyrias. *ALA* δ-aminolevulinic acid, *ALAD* ALA dehydratase, *CPOX* coproporphyrinogen oxidase, *FECH* ferrochelatase, *HMB* hydroxymethylbilane, *HMBS* hydroxymethylbilane synthase, *PBG* porphobilinogen, *SucCoA* Succinyl-CoA, *UROD* uroporphyrinogen decarboxylase, *UROgen* uroporphyrinogen, *COPROgen* coproporphyrinogen, *PPOX* protoporphyrinogen oxidase, *PROTOgen* protoporphyrinogen, *PROTO* protoporphyrin

acid (ALA), porphobilinogen (PBG) and porphyrins, which bring about the clinical manifestations of the porphyrias. ALA is neurotoxic, whereas porphyrinogens cause photosensitivity.

The enzymatic defects can be inherited, with a variety of modes of inheritance. However, haem biosynthesis depends on interplay between both genetic and environmental factors. Therefore, patients with inherited enzymatic defects may never have any clinical disease manifestations.

Classification of Porphyrias

Porphyrias can be classified according to the primary site of enzyme deficiency (i.e. hepatic or erythropoietic) or clinical features (i.e. acute vs chronic, and whether symptoms are neurovisceral vs cutaneous, or a mixture). If porphyria is suspected, determine if the symptoms are neurovisceral or cutaneous. Then biochemical analysis can help to identify which step in haem biosynthesis is abnormal. Subsequently, analysis of gene mutations allows confirmation of the diagnosis (Fig. 14.2). Following diagnosis, screening relatives at risk enables counselling for asymptomatic patients on the importance of avoiding triggers.

There are **four acute hepatic porphyrias (AHP)**: acute intermittent porphyria (AIP), hereditary coproporphyria (HCP), variegate porphyria (VP) and ALA dehydratase defi-

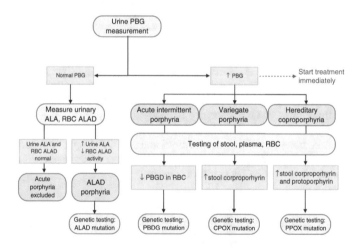

FIGURE 14.2 An algorithm for diagnosing acute porphyrias in patients with neurovisceral symptoms. Using a combination of urine, stool and blood testing for characteristic biochemical abnormalities, it is possible to determine the likely underlying porphyria. *ALA* δ-aminolevulinic acid, *ALAD* ALA dehydratase, *CPOX* coproporphyrinogen oxidase, *PBDG* porphobilinogen deaminase, *PBG* porphobilinogen, *PPOX* protoporphyrinogen oxidase, *RBC* red blood cell

ciency porphyria (ADP). AIP is the most common and severe of these. Symptoms include neurologic attacks, cramping abdominal pain, constipation, abdominal or bladder distension, nausea, vomiting, hypertension, headache, tremors, dysuria and muscle weakness. There are no cutaneous symptoms. Attacks are precipitated when ALAS1 activity is induced, for example, by alcohol, certain drugs, steroids, low calorie intake and stress. Approximately 3–5% of patients with AHP suffer from severe or recurrent acute attacks, associated with impaired quality of life. Long-term complications of AHP, especially AIP, include hepatocellular carcinoma, chronic pain and chronic renal failure.

Management of acute hepatic porphyrias involves avoiding known triggers and treating symptoms, for example, using analgesics for abdominal pain, and phenothiazines for nausea and vomiting. In mild attacks, intravenous glucose should be given. For patients who do not respond, or who have a moderate/severe attack, intravenous hemin therapy should be administered. In patients with frequent attacks, which are unresponsive to treatment, treatment options include off-label use of prophylactic haemin infusions and hormonal suppression therapy. Liver transplant can be considered as a last resort. The drug 'Givosiran' is an aminolevulinate synthase 1 (ALAS1)-directed small interfering RNA (siRNA) covalently linked to a ligand that enables targeted delivery to hepatocytes. It has recently been approved in the USA for the treatment of AIP, based on findings in a phase III (ENVISION) clinical trial [1]. In this trial, Givosiran treatment was associated with significantly reduced frequency of attacks in patients with AIP, although this was accompanied by an increased risk of hepatic and renal adverse events [1]. Other strategies are aimed at enhancing expression of the deficient protein; for example, through administration of porphobilinogen deaminase (PBDG) mRNA packaged into nanoparticles [2], or via adenovirus-mediated transfer of PBGD cDNA [3].

In the cutaneous porphyrias, excess porphyrins and porphyrinogens are deposited in the upper dermal capillary walls. Porphyria cutanea tarda (PCT) is a hepatic cutaneous porphyria, characterised by cutaneous symptoms without neurological features. Patients develop vesicles on sun-exposed areas of the skin, with crusting, superficial scarring, hypertrichosis and hyperpigmentation. Whilst severe liver disease is unusual in PCT, mild abnormalities of liver function tests are common, with 50% of patients demonstrating raised serum transaminases [4]. Up to 90% of patients with PCT have mild-moderate iron overload with hepatic siderosis, and this is implicated in the disease pathogenesis [4]. Management of PCT includes avoidance of risk factors, such as sunlight, alcohol, oestrogens and iron supplements. Repeated venesection to reduce hepatic iron almost always achieves a good response. Oral iron chelating agents can be considered in patients with anaemia or those who do not tolerate venesection; however, their efficacy is inferior to venesection, and they are associated with hepatic and renal side effects. Alternatively, use of low-dose chloroquine can be used to promote porphyrin excretion (as high doses of chloroquine are hepatotoxic). This is of similar efficacy to venesection [5]; although more costly. There is a very rare condition called hepatoerythropoietic porphyria (HEP), also caused by a mutation in the UROD (uroporphyrinogen decarboxylase) gene. HEP does not typically respond to low-dose chloroquine or phlebotomy, and therefore the priority of management is photoprotection.

There are **three erythropoietic cutaneous porphyrias**: congenital erythropoietic porphyria (CEP), X-linked protoporphyria (XLP) and erythropoietic porphyria (EPP). These usually present with cutaneous photosensitivity in childhood. In CEP, patients develop bullae, vesicles, altered skin pigmentation and hypertrichosis. The increase in erythrocyte porphyrins causes haemolysis and splenomegaly. Regular blood transfusions to suppress erythropoiesis can reduce porphyrin accumulation, but are associated with iron overload. Patients should also be advised to avoid sunlight. XLP and EPP have similar clinical features, with severe pain, erythema and itching following exposure to sunlight. Vesicles and bullae are uncommon in these conditions, and haemolytic anaemia is mild or absent. Because protoporphyrins are lipid soluble, they can be taken up by the liver and excreted in bile, with potential for causing hepatic parenchymal damage and biliary stones. In around 5% of patients, protoporphyrin accumulation causes severe liver disease, which may progress to cholestatic liver failure. Treatment includes avoiding sunlight. There is limited benefit with use of oral beta-carotene. In patients with liver disease, cholestyramine may promote faecal excretion, and plasmapheresis is sometimes helpful. In patients who have liver transplantation for EPP-mediated liver failure, overall survival is comparable to patients having liver transplant for other diseases. However, as the source of the excess protoporphyrins is the bone marrow rather than the liver, disease recurrence is common (69%), and the increased risk of post-operative biliary complications may cause graft damage. In such patients, bone marrow transplant should also be considered to reduce the incidence of graft loss.

Novel treatment strategies under investigation for erythropoietic porphyrias include the use of afamelanotide, an alpha-melanocyte stimulating hormone analogue, which is a melanin inducer. In phase III trials (NCT01605136), afamelanotide was associated with reduced photosensitivity, fewer phototoxic reactions and improved quality of life, although there was no change in protoporphyrin or hepatic enzyme levels. Pre-clinical studies are also investigating the potential of anti-sense oligonucleotides to restore normal activity of the hypomorphic FECH allele (IVS3-48C), which is implicated in >95% of cases of EPP [6].

Alpha-1-Antitrypsin Deficiency

Overview

Alpha-1-antitrypsin (A1AT) is a large glycoprotein produced mainly by hepatocytes. It is a serine protease inhibitor and is the predominant inhibitor of neutrophil elastase in the lungs.

A1AT is also an acute phase protein, and therefore levels are elevated in inflammatory states. A1AT deficiency is the most common genetic cause of metabolic liver disease in neonates and children [7]. It is caused by a mutation on the SERPINA1 gene (previously known as the Pi gene), which has been localised to chromosome 14q32. The abnormal A1AT undergoes spontaneous polymerisation and thus cannot be exported from hepatocytes. The resulting A1AT deficiency in the lungs causes proteolytic connective tissue damage, predisposing to early-onset panlobular emphysema. In the liver, accumulation of A1AT causes cell apoptosis, hepatic inflammation and cirrhosis.

Genetics and Epidemiology

A1AT deficiency is an autosomal recessive disorder with codominant expression. Whilst over 100 alleles have been identified, only some of these cause liver disease. Based on migration properties on isoelectric testing, the normal allele is identified M, which accounts for 95% of alleles. Common abnormal variants include S (with 50–60% protein activity) and Z (with 10–20% protein activity), which account for 2–3% and 1% of alleles, respectively. It is estimated that 1:10 individuals are carriers of the 'S' or the 'Z' variant. The ZZ genotype is associated with severe A1AT deficiency and occurs in 1:3500 births, being more common in Europeans and North Americans and very rare amongst Asian and Mexican Americans [7]. In mutations where there is absence of A1AT production, there is lung disease without associated liver disease.

Clinical Presentation

In patients with the ZZ genotype, there is a bimodal distribution in the clinical presentation, with one peak in infancy and another in adults aged in their 50s. In infancy, presentation is usually with jaundice secondary to acute cholestasis or neonatal hepatitis. Around 10% of infants with A1AT deficiency develop neonatal hepatitis, but most make a clinical recovery.

When the rate of accumulation of abnormal folded protein in the hepatic endoplasmic reticulum exceeds the liver's capacity to degrade/remove it, this can trigger a series of reactions that ultimately result in the development of liver fibrosis, cirrhosis and HCC [8]. Only 2–3% of ZZ infants develop cirrhosis requiring transplantation in childhood [9].

Around one-third of adult patients with the ZZ genotype develop liver cirrhosis [10]. Risk factors for disease progression include male sex, age >50 years, viral hepatitis and diabetes. Unfortunately, adults often present late in the course of their disease, frequently due to a lack of symptoms or misdiagnosis [11]. Heterozygotes for A1AT deficiency are often asymptomatic, but heterozygosity can be a co-factor in development of chronic liver disease [12]. Indeed, retrospective studies have revealed that a large number of patients undergoing liver transplant for A1AT were in fact heterozygotes, who had a 'second hit' that accelerated progression to end-stage liver disease [13].

Diagnosis

Summarised in Box 14.1 are clinical features which should prompt suspicion of A1AT deficiency, as recommended by guidelines from the American Thoracic Society [14].

Abdominal examination may reveal signs of end-stage liver disease, and ultrasound can assess liver structure. Although changes in serum transaminases may be seen, the degree of liver injury is often out of proportion to the level of transaminitis. Diagnosis of A1AT deficiency can involve quantification of A1AT, phenotyping or genotyping. Initial testing usually involves measuring serum A1AT, using nephelometry. Serum A1AT concentration <10–20%

Box 14.1 Conditions in Which Alpha-1-Antitrypsin Deficiency Should Be Suspected [14]

- Early-onset emphysema (aged 45 years or less)
- Emphysema in the absence of a recognised risk factor (smoking, occupational dust exposure, etc.)
- Emphysema with prominent basilar hyperlucency
- Otherwise unexplained liver disease
- Necrotising panniculitis
- Antiproteinase-3 positive vasculitis
- Family history of: emphysema, bronchiectasis, liver disease or panniculitis
- Bronchiectasis without evident aetiology

of normal is suggestive of A1AT deficiency. Current methods of A1AT quantification tend to overestimate A1AT levels. Transiently higher levels A1AT levels are associated with systemic inflammation, because A1AT is an acute phase protein. In heterozygotes, A1AT levels may even be normal and therefore cannot be used to exclude A1AT deficiency. Phenotyping using isoelectric focusing migration patterns is the gold standard for diagnosis. However, results can be challenging to interpret, because of the variety of existing alleles. Genotyping can provide definitive diagnosis of known phenotypic variations. Liver biopsy is not necessary for diagnosis but the A1AT aggregates give rise to the hallmark findings of PAS-positive diastase resistant granules in patients with the Z alleles and some other alleles. Liver biopsy may be used for staging disease severity in establishing liver disease secondary to A1AT deficiency.

Treatment

Unfortunately, currently there is no specific treatment available for A1AT deficiency affecting the liver. In patients with end-stage liver disease, liver transplantation can correct the underlying disorder as well as replacing the diseased liver. In children, A1AT deficiency is the leading metabolic cause for liver transplant, with 3 year survival rates of around 85% [15, 16]. In adults, A1AT deficiency represents only 1% of transplants performed, but 5-year graft and patient survival rates are excellent [17]. Although liver transplant recipients have normalisation of A1AT levels, it is unclear whether this can delay progression of lung disease.

According to American Thoracic Society guidelines, patients with A1AT related liver disease should have regular follow-up for assessment of symptoms, examination, liver function tests and ultrasound to screen for the presence of fibrosis or HCC [14]. Patients should be advised to avoid alcohol, eat a healthy diet, lose weight if necessary, avoid NSAIDs and get vaccinated against hepatitis. In the absence of liver disease, patients with A1AT deficiency should have regular blood tests to monitor liver function tests.

Supportive treatments for patients with lung disease secondary to A1AT deficiency include avoidance of smoking, use of bronchodilators, pulmonary rehabilitation, nutritional support, consideration of supplementation oxygen, vaccination against influenza and pneumococcus, and prompt treatment of exacerbations with steroids and antibiotics. Whilst IV 'augmentation' therapy with pooled human plasma has been shown to raise serum A1AT levels, there is less evidence that it causes a significant reduction in decline of FEV1 [18].

A number of novel treatment approaches are currently under investigation. Some approaches have focused on preventing accumulation of the abnormal A1AT. For example, current phase I and II trials are investigating the ability of siRNA to downregulate production of the Z mutant A1AT, and the use of adenoviral vectors to transfer normal A1AT to muscle cells. Other studies have focused on using chemicals, such as 4-phenylbutyric acid, to stabilise the abnormal A1AT to promote its excretion; although results from animal studies were promising, this failed to demonstrate efficacy in clinical trials. A third approach is to enhance degradation of abnormal A1AT via autophagy. In this regard, carbamazepine has shown promise in a mouse model of hepatic fibrosis and is now in phase II clinical trials.

Cystic Fibrosis and Liver Disease

Overview

Cystic fibrosis is the most commonly occurring genetic disease in the Caucasian population. It is caused by abnormalities in the cystic fibrosis transmembrane regulator (CFTR) gene. This affects chloride and sodium transport across membranes, which results in difficulty in efflux of water, causing dehydrated secretions. Over 2000 mutations have been identified, but the delta F508 mutation is responsible in around two-thirds of cases.

Mild CFLD is common and usually asymptomatic. It is estimated that up to 45% of patients with CD have asymptomatic raised serum transaminases and up to 60% of patients have hepatic steatosis [19]. Around one-third of patients with cystic fibrosis develop clinically significant cystic fibrosis liver disease (CFLD). It has been estimated that 2–4% of patients with cystic fibrosis die from CFLD, making it the third most common cause of mortality in CF, after lung disease and complications of liver transplant [20]. The development of liver disease in cystic fibrosis is not related to the severity of cystic fibrosis or the underlying mutation, which suggests that other factors must influence risk. These include male sex, severe lung disease, Hispanic ethnicity, heterozygosity for the PiZ allele of alpha-1 antitrypsin, neonatal meconium ileus and pancreatic insufficiency [21, 22].

There is a range of clinical presentations of CFLD, including cholelithiasis, neonatal cholestasis, hepatitis, hepatic steatosis, hepatic fibrosis or cirrhosis with or without portal hypertension.

The most common manifestation is hepatic steatosis, occurring in approximately 67% of patients with cystic fibrosis, although the mechanism of this is not clearly understood [23]. Even in cases of widespread steatosis, features of steatohepatitis are normally absent. Neonatal cholestasis occurs in less than 10% of infants with CF, presenting with prolonged conjugated hyperbilirubinaemia. The clinical features tend to regress during the first few months of life, and this condition is not a predictor of cirrhosis in later life [19].

However, the most clinically significant manifestation of CFLD is biliary cirrhosis with portal hypertension. CFTR genes are expressed on epithelial cells lining the intrahepatic and extrahepatic bile ducts and the gallbladder. In cystic fibrosis, bile is more viscous and less alkaline. The dehydrated secretions can block bile ducts, predisposing to gallstones, infection and damage from toxins. This process also causes injury to cholangiocytes and hepatocytes, thus triggering periductal inflammation and fibrosis and eventually multilobular cirrhosis with portal hypertension. Patients with cirrhosis and portal hypertension usually present in childhood. In a large cohort of 561 patients with CFLD with cirrhosis and portal hypertension, the mean age of presentation was only 10 years of age, with 90% of patients presenting by 18 years [24]. Once patients develop liver failure, transplant is the only curative option. Non-cirrhotic portal hypertension is also recognised in CFLD. This is characterised by nodular hypoplasia and is associated with microscopic obliterative portal venopathy, although the detailed mechanisms of this condition are not completely understood [25]. Other biliary problems include development of gallstones in 12–24% of patients, which are relatively more common in adults. The majority of transplants performed for CFLD are in children. Approximately 25–30% of patients with CF have microgallbladder, which is defined as a gallbladder measuring <35 mm in the longest axis [19].

Investigations

In suspected CFLD, patients require examination for hepato-splenomegaly, abdominal ultrasound and measurement of liver enzymes. There may be asymmetrical hepatomegaly in CFLD due to the presence of focal regenerative nodules. Clinical signs of advanced liver disease, such as splenomegaly or caput medusae, are usually subtle or present at a very late stage of disease. Significant liver disease is considered if any liver enzyme is over 1.5 times the upper limit of normal on at least two occasions 6 months apart. However, changes in biochemical parameters have a low sensitivity and specificity for CFLD with cirrhosis. Thrombocytopaenia should be monitored closely as it may suggest splenic sequestration.

Ultrasound can demonstrate any hepatomegaly, steatosis, hepatic texture, splenomegaly and gallbladder problems. Combined with Doppler, ultrasound allows assessment of portal hypertension. Although a significantly abnormal ultrasound has a 84% positive predictive value for advanced CFLD, it is less useful for excluding CFLD when it is normal. Non-invasive liver elastography (Fibroscan) is useful for diagnosing CFLD and establishing its severity. MRI offers high quality images of the pancreatic and hepatobiliary structures and is less operator-dependent than ultrasound. If there is any doubt about the diagnosis, liver biopsy can help to assess whether the predominant problem is steatosis or biliary disease, the severity of the disease and response to treatment. It should also be used to confirm the presence of cirrhosis prior to liver transplant. However, it is important to consider that lesions in CFLD tend to be distributed non-uniformly across the liver; therefore, liver biopsy may underestimate disease severity.

Patients with established CFLD also require regular follow-up. This includes using annual examination for hepato-splenomegaly and biochemical assessment (liver enzymes, prothrombin time and platelet count) and abdominal US. Due to the presence of regenerative nodules, hepatomegaly in CFLD may be asymmetric.

Treatment

In terms of general supportive measures, for patients with CFLD it is important to optimise nutrition. Patients with CFLD may require higher doses of fat-soluble vitamins than those without, due to abnormalities in bile acid quantity/function in the intestine. Patients should be advised to be vaccinated against hepatitis A and B and to avoid alcohol and medications with hepatotoxic effects.

Patients with abnormal ultrasound findings or persistently deranged LFTs are commenced on ursodeoxycholic acid (UDCA) at 20 mg/kg/day in two or three divided doses. This is a hydrophilic bile acid, which stimulates bile flow and displaces toxic hydrophobic bile acids. The main side effect of UDCA is diarrhoea, which usually responds to dose reduction. Its use is controversial, whilst some studies suggest that it improves biochemical parameters, there is little evidence that it influences the likelihood of needing a liver transplant.

CF patients with portal hypertension should have endoscopic screening for the presence of oesophageal varices and band ligation considered if needed. Beta-blockers should not be given in adults with varices, due to their potential to cause bronchoconstriction.

In patients with end-stage liver disease liver transplant can be considered. The 5-year survival rate for children and adults is 85.8% and 72.7%, respectively [26]. Compared with patients having liver transplant for other reasons, patients with CFLD have a lower post-operative survival. This may be because CF patients are more likely to have poor nutrition status and concomitant lung disease. The prognosis of combined lung and liver transplant is poor, with a 5 year survival of only 49% [27].

Recently, the drug 'Kaftrio' has recently been licensed in the UK for treatment of patients with cystic fibrosis. It is indicated in patients who are aged 12 and over, and homozygotes for the delta F508 mutation, or heterozygotes for F508 with a minimal function mutation. In these groups of patients, phase III clinical trials showed improvements in lung function (FEV1) of 10% and 14%, respectively [28, 29]. Kaftrio is a combination of ivacaftor, tezacaftor and elexacaftor and should be taken together with another medicine containing ivacaftor alone. Elexacaftor and tezacaftor work to increase the number of CFTR proteins on the cell surface, whilst Ivacaftor enhances the activity of the defective CFTR protein.

Abnormalities in liver function tests, particularly serum transaminases, are common during Kaftrio treatment. Therefore, patients need regular monitoring of liver function tests. Kaftrio can be used in patients with mild hepatic impairment (Child's Pugh A). In patients with severe hepatic impairment (Child's Pugh C), Kaftrio should be avoided. In patients with moderate hepatic impairment (Child's Pugh B), Katrio should only be used if there is a clear medical need, and the expected benefit outweighs the risks.

Answers to Case Study Questions

1. Alpha-1-antitrypsin deficiency, with liver failure
2. Serum phenotyping and genotyping
3. The use of purified human alpha antitrypsin for treatment of pulmonary disease associated with alpha-1-antitrypsin deficiency

References

1. Balwani M, et al. Phase 3 trial of RNAi therapeutic givosiran for acute intermittent porphyria. N Engl J Med. 2020;382(24):2289–301.
2. D'Avola D, et al. Phase I open label liver-directed gene therapy clinical trial for acute intermittent porphyria. J Hepatol. 2016;65(4):776–83.
3. Jiang L, et al. Systemic messenger RNA as an etiological treatment for acute intermittent porphyria. Nat Med. 2018;24(12):1899–909.
4. Singal AK. Porphyria cutanea tarda: Recent update. Mol Genet Metab. 2019;128(3):271–81.
5. Singal AK, et al. Low-dose hydroxychloroquine is as effective as phlebotomy in treatment of patients with porphyria cutanea tarda. Clin Gastroenterol Hepatol. 2012;10(12):1402–9.

6. Oustric V, et al. Antisense oligonucleotide-based therapy in human erythropoietic protoporphyria. Am J Hum Genet. 2014;94(4):611–7.

7. de Serres FJ, Blanco I, Fernandez-Bustillo E. Genetic epidemiology of alpha-1 antitrypsin deficiency in North America and Australia/New Zealand: Australia, Canada, New Zealand and the United States of America. Clin Genet. 2003;64(5):382–97.

8. Fairbanks KD, Tavill AS. Liver disease in alpha 1-antitrypsin deficiency: a review. Am J Gastroenterol. 2008;103(8):2136–41; quiz 2142.

9. Sveger T. The natural history of liver disease in alpha 1-antitrypsin deficient children. Acta Paediatr Scand. 1988;77(6):847–51.

10. Eriksson S, Carlson J, Velez R. Risk of cirrhosis and primary liver cancer in alpha 1-antitrypsin deficiency. N Engl J Med. 1986;314(12):736–9.

11. de Serres F, Blanco I. Role of alpha-1 antitrypsin in human health and disease. J Intern Med. 2014;276(4):311–35.

12. Kok KF, et al. Heterozygous alpha-I antitrypsin deficiency as a co-factor in the development of chronic liver disease: a review. Neth J Med. 2007;65(5):160–6.

13. Bartlett JR, et al. Genetic modifiers of liver disease in cystic fibrosis. JAMA. 2009;302(10):1076–83.

14. American Thoracic Society, European Respiratory Society. American Thoracic Society/European Respiratory Society statement: standards for the diagnosis and management of individuals with alpha-1 antitrypsin deficiency. Am J Respir Crit Care Med. 2003;168(7):818–900.

15. Esquivel CO, et al. Indications for pediatric liver transplantation. J Pediatr. 1987;111(6 Pt 2):1039–45.

16. Prachalias AA, et al. Liver transplantation for alpha-1-antitrypsin deficiency in children. Transpl Int. 2000;13(3):207–10.

17. Greene CM, et al. alpha1-Antitrypsin deficiency. Nat Rev Dis Primers. 2016;2:16051.

18. Stoller JK, Aboussouan LS. Alpha1-antitrypsin deficiency. Lancet. 2005;365(9478):2225–36.

19. Debray D, et al. Best practice guidance for the diagnosis and management of cystic fibrosis-associated liver disease. J Cyst Fibros. 2011;10(Suppl 2):S29–36.

20. Siano M, et al. Ursodeoxycholic acid treatment in patients with cystic fibrosis at risk for liver disease. Dig Liver Dis. 2010;42(6):428–31.

21. Lewindon PJ, et al. The role of hepatic stellate cells and transforming growth factor-beta(1) in cystic fibrosis liver disease. Am J Pathol. 2002;160(5):1705–15.

22. Salvatore F, Scudiero O, Castaldo G. Genotype-phenotype correlation in cystic fibrosis: the role of modifier genes. Am J Med Genet. 2002;111(1):88–95.

23. Herrmann U, Dockter G, Lammert F. Cystic fibrosis-associated liver disease. Best Pract Res Clin Gastroenterol. 2010;24(5):585–92.

24. Stonebraker JR, et al. Features of severe liver disease with portal hypertension in patients with cystic fibrosis. Clin Gastroenterol Hepatol. 2016;14(8):1207–15.e3.

25. Hillaire S, et al. Liver transplantation in adult cystic fibrosis: clinical, imaging, and pathological evidence of obliterative portal venopathy. Liver Transpl. 2017;23(10):1342–7.

26. Mendizabal M, et al. Liver transplantation in patients with cystic fibrosis: analysis of United Network for Organ Sharing data. Liver Transpl. 2011;17(3):243–50.

27. Milkiewicz P, et al. Transplantation for cystic fibrosis: outcome following early liver transplantation. J Gastroenterol Hepatol. 2002;17(2):208–13.

28. Heijerman HGM, et al. Efficacy and safety of the elexacaftor plus tezacaftor plus ivacaftor combination regimen in people with cystic fibrosis homozygous for the F508del mutation: a double-blind, randomised, phase 3 trial. Lancet. 2019;394(10212):1940–8.

29. Middleton PG, et al. Elexacaftor-tezacaftor-ivacaftor for cystic fibrosis with a single Phe508del allele. N Engl J Med. 2019;381(19):1809–19.

Chapter 15
Fontan-Associated Liver Disease (FALD)

Hera Asad, Tehreem P. Chaudhry, and Petra Jenkins

Key Learning Points
- FALD is a complication of the Fontan circulation and is increasing in frequency.
- The aetiology of FALD is likely multifactorial.
- Risk factors for FALD are high Fontan pressure, duration of Fontan and underlying viral hepatitis, alcohol and hepatotoxic drugs.
- Surveillance should commence in advanced FALD because of the increased risk of HCC.
- There is no agreed standard in how best to assess the fibrosis stage in these patients at neither a national nor international level.

Chapter Review Questions
1. What is FALD?

 (a) A hepatic complication of the Fontan procedure seen in a minority of patients.

———
H. Asad · T. P. Chaudhry (✉)
Department of Gastroenterology and Hepatology, Royal Liverpool University Hospital, Liverpool, UK
e-mail: tehreem.chaudhry@liverpoolft.nhs.uk

P. Jenkins
Liverpool Heart and Chest Hospital, Liverpool, UK
e-mail: petra.jenkins@lhch.nhs.uk

© Springer Nature Switzerland AG 2022   307
T. Cross (ed.), *Liver Disease in Clinical Practice*, In Clinical Practice, https://doi.org/10.1007/978-3-031-10012-3_15

(b) A spectrum of liver disease from mild fibrosis to cirrhosis, portal hypertension and HCC.

(c) Liver cirrhosis secondary to venous congestion.

2. Why is FALD important?

(a) FALD is an indication for consideration of liver transplantation.

(b) FALD is considered one of the major determinants of morbidity and mortality in the adult Fontan population.

(c) FALD is the leading cause of liver cirrhosis.

3. What are the 10-, 20- and 30-year post-Fontan incidence of FALD?

(a) 1%, 6% and 43%
(b) 5%, 10% and 50%
(c) 2%, 6% and 40%

4. Which non-invasive composite score of liver disease is the most helpful in FALD?

(a) VAST
(b) MELD-XI
(c) APRI

5. Which radiological imaging modality best positively correlates with total fibrosis score, time from Fontan, Fontan pressure, GGT, MELD score, pulmonary vascular resistance index and inversely with catheter derived cardiac index?

(a) Ultrasound
(b) Contrast CT
(c) MRE (magnetic resonance elastography)

Chapter Review Answers

1. (b)
2. (b)
3. (a)
4. (b)
5. (c)

The Evolving Fontan Procedure

First described in 1968, the Fontan procedure is a palliative surgery to improve survival in those with single ventricle congenital heart disease, whereby biventricular repair is therefore not possible. The procedure aims to divert systemic venous return from the superior and inferior venae cavae directly into the pulmonary arteries. This principle remains unchanged, but the procedure itself has evolved over time.

The original atriopulmonary connection (APC) involved directly connecting the right atrium to the left pulmonary artery, whilst the superior vena cava (SVC) was connected to the right pulmonary artery. However, this led to atrial dilatation which subsequently increased the risk of atrial arrhythmias and atrial thrombi leading to significant morbidity and mortality. Thus the procedure was modified to minimise involvement of the right atrium in the circulation.

This is achieved in the total cavopulmonary connection (TCPC), of which there are two variants. The lateral tunnel (LT)-TCPC is where an intra-atrial wall is created, to direct blood flow from the inferior vena cava (IVC) directly to the pulmonary arteries via this channel. Alternatively, the extra-cardiac conduit (EC)-TCPC describes a connection between the IVC and the pulmonary arteries outside of the heart, thus the right atrium is bypassed altogether. A fenestration is sometimes created to allow blood flow between the lateral tunnel/conduit and the right atrium to enable some right-to-left shunting of deoxygenated blood into the systemic circulation which improves the cardiac output and survival rates.

As the success of this procedure continues, so does the growth of the Fontan population, with one prediction that this cohort will double in size over the next 20 years.

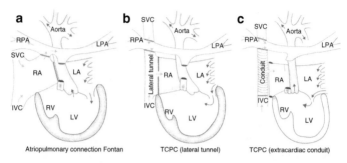

(**a**) Atriopulmonary connection Fontan showing the right atrium directly connected to the pulmonary arteries. (**b**) Lateral tunnel Fontan showing the IVC blood flow being directed to the pulmonary arteries in a right atrium lateral tunnel. (**c**) Extracardiac conduit Fontan showing the IVC being connected to the pulmonary arteries outside the right atrium. (**b** and **c**) Also show a fenestration between the total cavopulmonary connection pathway and the right atrium. *RPA* right pulmonary artery, *LPA* left pulmonary artery, *SVC* superior vena cava, *RA* right atrium, *LA* left atrium, *IVC* inferior vena cava, *RV* right ventricle, *LV* left ventricle

Defining Fontan-Associated Liver Disease

FALD refers to the hepatic effects of the Fontan circulation, seen in almost all patients postprocedure. It encompasses a spectrum of diseases from mild fibrosis to cirrhosis and hepatocellular carcinoma (HCC), usually progressing over time. FALD is also considered one of the major extracardiac determinants of mortality in adult Fontan patients.

Fontan Circulatory Dynamics

The Fontan circulation has different haemodynamic characteristics to normal. This is due to the systemic and pulmonary circulations running in series rather than in parallel, and both circuits being powered by a single ventricle.

Cardiac output is invariably reduced due to limited pre-load filling in the absence of a pulmonary ventricle. This leads to venous congestion and increases the venous volume, in turn raising the central venous pressure (CVP). Systemic venous hypertension through venous constriction means a decrease in venous compliance which also raises the CVP. Raised CVP and non-pulsatile flow lead to a state of passive venous congestion secondary to increased afterload. Due to low cardiac output, zone 3 hepatocytes may be compromised by reducing oxygen delivery to centrilobular cells. Chronic congestion stresses hepatic vasculature which results in fibrogenesis due to centrilobular hepatocyte atrophy, sinusoidal fibrosis, bridging fibrosis and finally cirrhosis. Additional mechanisms include staged operations and cardiopulmonary bypass, as well as abnormal lymphatic drainage.

The Timescale of Events

Both the severity and incidence of hepatic damage increase with time, thus necessitating the need for routine liver surveillance in these patients.

One study which collected follow-up data found the 10-, 20- and 30-year post-Fontan incidence of cirrhosis increased from 1% to 6% to 43%, respectively. The study also reported the mean time of diagnosis of cirrhosis was 23.4 ± 6.3 years after the Fontan procedure. This was very similar to the mean time of diagnosis of HCC at 20 ± 2.9 years post-Fontan.

Clinical Presentation

Most Fontan patients, even with biopsy findings of marked fibrosis and architectural distortion, appear to be asymptomatic from their liver disease though some complain of generalised symptoms of anorexia, weight loss and lethargy. Physical examination may reveal signs of chronic liver disease (Table 15.1). Those with decompensated liver disease

TABLE 15.1 Clinical and biochemical correlates of FALD

Category	Modality	Findings
Clinical evaluation	Symptoms assessment	Anorexia Fatigue Weight loss
	Physical examination	Hepatomegaly Splenomegaly Ascites Peripheral oedema Caput medusa Jaundice Palmar erythema Asterixis Spider naevi Clubbing Gynaecomastia
Laboratory evaluation	Transaminases (ALT, AST)	Rarely elevated Do not correlate with degree of fibrosis in FALD
	ALP, bilirubin, GGT	
	Platelets	Platelets $<150 \times 10^9/L$ correlate with degree of fibrosis
	PT/INR	Raised PT/INR correlates with degree of fibrosis
	AFP	Does not correlate with disease severity in FALD
	Albumin	Can be low due to PLE
Non-invasive scores	VAST	VAST ≥ 2 correlates with incidence of major adverse events
	MELD-XI	Correlates with degree of fibrosis

Table adapted [1, 2]

can present with jaundice, encephalopathy, ascites and variceal haemorrhage.

Important distinctions between FALD and hepatic congestion caused either acutely or by other forms heart disease such as cardiomyopathy, cor pulmonale or tricuspid regurgitation are listed as follows:

- Lack of a pulsatile liver: This is due to the absence of a subpulmonary ventricle.
- Lack of hepatojugular reflux: Again, due to lack of normal jugular venous pulsatility.
- Lack of right upper quadrant pain: This can occur due to stretching of the liver capsule but in Fontan patients, hepatic congestion is chronic and does not cause this.

Diagnosing Cirrhosis in FALD

The gold standard for quantifying liver fibrosis and diagnosing cirrhosis is liver biopsy. Percutaneous liver biopsy provides the best quality liver cores aiding more accurate diagnosis of liver disease. Where this is not possible, due to coagulopathy or ascites, a transjugular liver biopsy can be performed. The smaller liver cores obtained can then be combined with haemodynamic measurements to aid diagnosis.

However, in practice most diagnoses of cirrhosis in Fontan patients are made by correlating imaging findings from CT, MRI, MRE or liver ultrasound with clinical assessment made by a hepatologist. The role for such non-invasive strategies is important given that biopsy imposes procedural risks (Table 15.2). Specifically, there is an increased risk of bleeding due to elevated CVP and the increased use of oral anticoagulants in this population. Furthermore, biopsy is susceptible to sampling error as liver changes in FALD are not uniformly distributed. In addition, conventional scoring systems (METAVIR, ISHAK) cannot be completely used in Fontan patients as fibrosis is centrilobular/sinusoidal. Hence biopsy is usually performed in symptomatic patients or those being assessed for heart transplant rather than as a screening tool.

TABLE 15.2 Imaging in FALD

Modality	Use	Limitations
Ultrasound	• Screening for FALD • Evaluates for ascites, liver nodules and vascular patency	• Limited use in patients with ascites • Non-specific findings • Difficult to detect small lesions due to heterogenous parenchyma
Contrast CT/MRI	• Assesses liver morphology and vascular patency • Evaluates for and characterises liver nodules including HCC • Evaluation for surgical planning for liver transplantation	• Radiation exposure with CT • MRI may be contraindicated if pacemaker in situ • Nephrotoxic contrast agent • Both CT and MRI are poor at detecting morphological changes with early cirrhosis • Can be difficult to distinguish benign focal lesions and vascular anomalies from HCC, necessitating biopsy
Elastography	• Assesses liver stiffness • Perform serial studies to evaluate for progression • MRE may be a potential screening tool for HCC	• Does not distinguish between passive congestion and fibrosis • Limited use in patients with ascites • Cut-off scores for liver stiffness not established in Fontan patients

TABLE 15.2 (continued)

Modality	Use	Limitations
Liver biopsy	• Gold standard tool for quantifying fibrosis and diagnosing cirrhosis	• Invasive with procedural complications, e.g. bleeding, infection, perforation • Higher risk procedure due to underlying coagulopathy and increased use of vitamin K antagonist therapy • Sampling error due to patchy fibrotic changes • No validated scoring system for screening for FALD • Early central fibrosis is not evaluated

Table adapted [1, 2]

Biochemical Markers

Using serum markers of hepatic function to screen asymptomatic Fontan patients or to stage liver fibrosis is of limited value, as liver function testing is often normal or may only be mildly deranged and not correlate with radiological findings.

The typical pattern seen is of mild cholestasis with raised GGT, ALP and bilirubin. If aminotransferases are elevated, then ALT is more commonly raised but usually by no more than two to three times the upper limit of normal. If reduced total protein and/or albumin levels are seen, then this could be related more to protein-losing enteropathy than it is to impaired liver synthetic function.

Thrombocytopaenia, known to be a marker of portal hypertension and hypersplenism, has also been shown to correlate with a greater degree of portal fibrosis. Elevated prothrombin time (PT/international normalised ratio [INR]) has been shown to correlate with high-grade Metavir (F3-F4) and sinusoidal fibrosis (2–3) scores. Lymphopenia is also common in adult Fontan cohort and is associated with portal hypertension (Table 15.1).

Non-invasive Composite Scores of Liver Disease

Multiple composite scoring systems are applied to chronic liver diseases. These include serum AST/ALT ratio (AAR), fibrosis-4 score (FIB-4), AST to platelet index (APRI), model for end-stage liver disease (MELD) score, Child-Pugh score and enhanced liver fibrosis (ELF) score.

Most Fontan patients are anticoagulated; therefore, the **MELD-XI** score which excludes the INR is used instead. Multiple studies have found a statistically significant positive correlation between MELD-XI scores and biopsy derived hepatic fibrosis scores. However, a specific MELD-XI threshold predictive of hepatic fibrosis with high sensitivity and specificity has not been identified.

The **VAST** (Varices, Ascites, Splenomegaly and Thrombocytopaenia) score evaluates features of portal hypertension. 1 point is given for each of the aforementioned features. A VAST score ≥2 was found to be associated with a significantly increased incidence of major adverse events, defined as death, heart transplant or listing for transplant, or HCC.

Despite numerous composite scoring systems, any is yet to be validated for use in FALD and many have undetermined diagnostic cut-off values for cirrhosis in FALD or even a correlation with biopsy findings (Table 15.1).

Radiological Imaging

Several imaging modalities have been studied to determine their ability to diagnose advanced FALD (Table 15.2). There remains inconsistency in the correlations between radiological findings and the progression of liver disease seen on histology. Owing to this, and a lack of guidelines, institutional practices of radiological monitoring remain inconsistent as well.

Ultrasound is valuable to screen for features of FALD and may be useful for identifying the progression of FALD before biochemical markers of hepatic function. The liver may be normal or slightly hypoechoic on ultrasound at the early stage of congestive hepatopathy, but as fibrosis develops, the most common findings seen are heterogenous parenchymal echotexture, surface nodularity, hyperechoic lesions and caudate lobe hypertrophy. In FALD a nodular liver surface is a common feature and does not necessarily imply underlying cirrhosis.

Contrast-enhanced CT and MRI are superior to ultrasound in detecting detailed liver architecture and liver masses. A common finding is of heterogenous liver enhancement with mosaic or reticular patterns, and this is associated with increased liver fibrosis. If arterially enhancing nodules are seen, then this may represent as either HCC or areas of focal nodular hyperplasia (FNH). The disadvantages of CT are the exposure to ionising radiation and risk of contrast nephropathy to young patients. Meanwhile MR imaging may be contraindicated in some FALD patients who have incompatible pacemakers.

MR with **diffusion-weighted imaging (DWI)** may be helpful in evaluating liver fibrosis and liver micro-perfusion, as well as showing regions of abnormal signal intensity that correlate with findings from contrast enhancement. MR with DWI has shown that the apparent diffusion coefficients (ADC) decrease as duration post-Fontan increases, indicative of progressive fibrotic and cirrhotic change with time.

Elastography

Elastography measures liver stiffness in one of the three ways: MRI elastography (known as MRE), shear wave elastography and transient elastography. Liver stiffness increases as hepatic fibrosis progresses, hence it acts as a surrogate marker of fibrosis. However, congestion from hepatic venous outflow obstruction also contributes to liver stiffness. This makes liver stiffness non-specific as it is difficult to determine the relative contributions of hepatic congestion and fibrosis. There is also limited data correlating liver stiffness scores to histology and cardiac haemodynamic prospectively over time. This confounding variable therefore makes it difficult to devise standardised liver stiffness scores. One way around this is to assess serial changes in liver stiffness rather than taking single elastography measurements which has shown to correlate with clinical deterioration and may be useful in monitoring progression over time (Table 15.2).

Studies show increased liver stiffness from MRE correlate with total fibrosis score, time since Fontan operation, Fontan pressure, GGT, MELD score, creatinine and pulmonary vascular resistance index and an inverse correlation with catheterisation derived cardiac index. In addition, MRE is useful in characterising liver nodules, as studies shows malignant nodules have elevated mean stiffness values compared to benign nodules.

Portal Hypertension

Portal hypertension can develop due to increased resistance to hepatic blood flow. This is likely due to multiple mechanisms including raised hepatic afterload, hepatic fibrosis and potential thrombus formation within the intrahepatic sinusoids. Invasive catheter-based haemodynamic studies are the gold standard for diagnosing portal hypertension; however, the pressure measurements made in Fontan physiology are not as expected.

The hepatic venous pressure gradient (HVPG) reflects the intrahepatic contribution to portal pressure. It is the difference between the wedged hepatic vein pressure and the free hepatic vein pressure. In Fontan physiology, it is difficult to assess the true hepatic vein wedge pressure due to intrahepatic macro or micro veno-venous collaterals. This leads to only small transhepatic pressure gradient measurements, rarely >2–3 mmHg, when typically, an elevated HVPG >5 mmHg is suggestive of parenchymal liver disease.

As portal hypertension increases in severity, classic radiological findings of ascites, splenomegaly and portosystemic collateral vessels (varices) can be seen. However, these findings should be interpreted with caution. For instance, venovenous collaterals between the systemic and pulmonary venous systems are frequently seen without a significant transhepatic pressure gradient, hence varices may not be definitively indicative of a raised gradient. Furthermore, ascites may be indicative of lymphatic overflow, protein-losing enteropathy and decompressing collaterals to the peritoneal cavity.

Hepatocellular Carcinoma

Liver cirrhosis is the single most important risk factor for the development of HCC. HCC is increasingly recognised in the Fontan population and has been reported in patients as young as 16 years old. Although rare in Fontan patients, the mechanisms responsible for its development, its natural history in Fontan patients, its delayed recognition and limited therapeutic options all contribute to the high mortality HCC carries in this cohort. HCC in Fontan patients has a 1-year survival rate of only 50%, decreasing to 30% once the tumour becomes symptomatic and/or reaches a size of >4 cm, and even lower in the presence of metastases.

Once advanced FALD is identified, patients should commence HCC surveillance which entails 6-monthly ultrasound. However, there are significant limitations. The diagnosis of HCC is based on imaging criteria or biopsy. The radiological hallmark of HCC is contrast uptake in the arterial phase and washout in the portal venous or delayed phase. Where there is uncertainty or atypical radiological findings, then the diagnosis should be confirmed by biopsy. In Fontan patients there is an increased incidence of vascular anomalies and benign focal lesions that are frequently detected as hyper enhancing nodules. These can mimic HCC leading to increased false-positive rates. Conversely, the radiological findings of HCC may be obscured in the presence of cardiac failure and intra-hepatic vascular shunts. This diagnostic confusion necessitates serial imaging and biopsy. The caveats of biopsy have been discussed earlier, with the additional small but notable risk of biopsy tract seeding in relation with biopsy of tumour nodules. The role of AFP alongside this is undetermined, given that cut-off values with good specificity and sensitivity have not been established, and up to 26% of Fontan patients with HCC have been found to have normal AFP levels.

Evidence to support the optimal treatment strategy for HCC in FALD patients remains limited. Options include surgical resection, which is limited by underlying cirrhosis and circulatory characteristics, radiofrequency ablation which is limited by the high incidence of pacemakers in this cohort, and transarterial chemo-embolisation (TACE) which is limited by the presence of abnormal vasculature. This leaves behind transplantation.

Transplantation: Heart Versus Combined Heart–Liver Transplant

Although transplant-free survival following Fontan surgery exceeds 80% at 20 years, eventual ventricular failure is inevitable for most, necessitating referral and consideration of orthotopic heart transplantation (OHT). Cardiac transplant alone is suitable for Fontan patients with no evidence of cirrhosis or in those with well-compensated cirrhosis. However, Fontan patients who undergo OHT will continue to be at risk for HCC, hence require ongoing screening.

Liver transplantation is indicated in patients with FALD and decompensated cirrhosis or localised HCC. However, given that the underlying Fontan physiology precludes liver transplantation alone, these patients generally require CHLT. There have been several small studies showing good outcomes for CHLT. Although it has a higher early mortality rate compared to heart or liver transplantation alone, it does have a lower cardiac graft rejection rate in the longer term.

FALD Screening

All Fontan patients require screening for FALD. The aim of screening is to diagnose FALD at an early stage. This enables interventions to be considered to optimise the Fontan circulation and prevent or slow the progression to advanced cirrhosis. Patients that do develop cirrhosis should be diagnosed in a timely manner and enrolled into HCC and portal hypertension surveillance.

Currently there are no agreed guidelines for follow up of Fontan patients at either a national or international level. The optimal time and type of screening for hepatic function and complications is also undecided. At 10 years post-Fontan, there is general agreement that the intensity of FALD surveillance should increase since this is when the clinically significant endpoints of cirrhosis and HCC have been consistently described.

Most clinical reviews recommend baseline liver function assessment, followed by annual liver review consisting of clinical examination, blood tests (including LFTs) and abdominal ultrasound. The routine use of any single non-invasive score for assessment of liver fibrosis remains unsupported given the limited data. Furthermore, the routine use of cross-sectional imaging (CT, MR) and elastography is variably deployed amongst centres. American College of Cardiology Stakeholders Meeting in 2017 recommend that imaging studies should be no less frequent than every 1–3 years, suggest the need to devise MRI or CT liver imaging protocols that can be performed in conjunction with cardiac imaging and also support the usefulness of MR or US elastography.

If significant liver disease is suspected in the context of a failing Fontan circulation, then invasive haemodynamic assessment and intervention need to be considered. Fontan patients should also be screened for other risk factors such as viral hepatitis (A, B and C), alcohol, raised BMI and hepatotoxic drugs.

Ultimately, FALD screening pathways will evolve over the coming years as higher-quality evidence emerges to guide selection and timing of the most appropriate tests to undertake. Meanwhile, to some extent, screening should be individualised and determined by the patients' signs, symptoms and quality of life.

Recommended Therapeutic Approaches

There are currently no established medical therapies for treatment of FALD. The prevention of FALD can be divided into optimisation of the Fontan circulation and prevention of liver injury. This is further explained in Tables 15.3 and 15.4. Other more novel therapies include a potential benefit of nitrates.

TABLE 15.3 Optimise Fontan circulation

Optimise anatomy	Optimise physiology
• Identify and treat anatomical abnormalities that adversely affect physiology, e.g. pulmonary artery stenosis, Fontan baffle stenosis, arch obstruction • Consider invasive haemodynamic studies (with intervention if indicated) if imaging studies are inconclusive • The impact of fenestration on risk of liver disease is currently unclear so should not be routinely performed with the intent to treat FALD	• Consider invasive and 'stress' haemodynamic studies in symptomatic patients and those with advanced liver disease, tailoring medical therapy accordingly • Treat systolic heart failure with appropriate medical therapies as used in acquired systolic heart failure • Pacemaker insertion if appropriate • Compression stockings for venous insufficiency • Manage other conditions that affect pulmonary vascular resistance (PVR), e.g. obesity, obstructive sleep apnoea and abnormal chest wall or diaphragm mechanics

TABLE 15.4 Prevent liver injury

Pre-Fontan	Post-Fontan
• Pre-natal diagnosis of cardiac abnormalities to avoid low output/shock presentation in newborns • Specialist anaesthetic/intensive care input during cardiac intervention to avoid low output/hypotensive insults • Hepatitis A and B immunisation	• Avoid alcohol and hepatotoxic medications • Screen and treat co-existing liver disease, e.g. viral hepatitis • Advise against and treat obesity as could promote non-alcoholic fatty liver disease • HCC surveillance in patients with suspected cirrhosis

References

1. Diamond T, Ovchinsky N. Fontan-associated liver disease: monitoring progression of liver fibrosis. Clin Liver Dis. 2018;11(1):1. https://doi.org/10.1002/cld.681. https://pubmed.ncbi.nlm.nih.gov/30992779/.
2. Emamaullee J, Zaidi AN, Schiano T, Kahn J, Valentino PL, Hofer RE, Taner T, Wald JW, Olthoff KM, Bucuvalas J, Fischer R. Fontan-associated liver disease: screening, management, and transplant considerations. Circulation. 2020;142(6):591–604. https://doi.org/10.1161/circulationaha.120.045597.

Further Readings

1. Clift P, Celermajer D. Managing adult Fontan patients: where do we stand? Eur Respir Rev. 2016;25(142):438–50.
2. Pundi K, Pundi KN, Kamath PS, Cetta F, Li Z, Poterucha JT, Driscoll DJ, Johnson JN. Liver disease in patients after the Fontan operation. Am J Cardiol. 2016;117(3):456–60.
3. Rychik J, Veldtman G, Rand E, Russo P, Rome JJ, Krok K, Goldberg DJ, Cahill AM, Wells RG. The precarious state of the liver after a Fontan operation: summary of a multidisciplinary symposium. Pediatr Cardiol. 2012;33(7):1001–12.

4. Simpson KE, Esmaeeli A, Khanna G, White F, Turnmelle Y, Eghtesady P, Boston U, Canter CE. Liver cirrhosis in Fontan patients does not affect 1-year post-heart transplant mortality or markers of liver function. J Heart Lung Transplant. 2014;33(2):170–7.

5. Nandwana SB, Olaiya B, Cox K, Sahu A, Mittal P. Abdominal imaging surveillance in adult patients after Fontan procedure: risk of chronic liver disease and hepatocellular carcinoma. Curr Probl Diagn Radiol. 2018;47(1):19–22.

6. Gordon-Walker TT, Bove K, Veldtman G. Fontan-associated liver disease: a review. J Cardiol. 2019;74(3):223–32.

7. Wu FM, Ukomadu C, Odze RD, Valente AM, Mayer JE Jr, Earing MG. Liver disease in the patient with Fontan circulation. Congenit Heart Dis. 2011;6(3):190–201.

8. Baek JS, Bae EJ, Ko JS, Kim GB, Kwon BS, Lee SY, Noh CI, Park EA, Lee W. Late hepatic complications after Fontan operation; non-invasive markers of hepatic fibrosis and risk factors. Heart. 2010;96(21):1750–5.

9. Elder RW, McCabe NM, Hebson C, Veledar E, Romero R, Ford RM, Mahle WT, Kogon BE, Sahu A, Jokhadar M, McConnell ME. Features of portal hypertension are associated with major adverse events in Fontan patients: the VAST study. Int J Cardiol. 2013;168(4):3764–9.

10. Bae JM, Jeon TY, Kim JS, Kim S, Hwang SM, Yoo SY, Kim JH. Fontan-associated liver disease: spectrum of US findings. Eur J Radiol. 2016;85(4):850–6.

11. Surrey LF, Russo P, Rychik J, Goldberg DJ, Dodds K, O'Byrne ML, Glatz AC, Rand EB, Lin HC. Prevalence and characterization of fibrosis in surveillance liver biopsies of patients with Fontan circulation. Hum Pathol. 2016;57:106–15.

12. Wells ML, Fenstad ER, Poterucha JT, Hough DM, Young PM, Araoz PA, Ehman RL, Venkatesh SK. Imaging findings of congestive hepatopathy. Radiographics. 2016;36(4):1024–37.

13. Dijkstra H, Wolff D, van Melle JP, Bartelds B, Willems TP, Oudkerk M, Hillege H, van den Berg AP, Ebels T, Berger RM, Sijens PE. Diminished liver microperfusion in Fontan patients: a biexponential DWI study. PLoS One. 2017;12(3):e0173149.

14. Poterucha JT, Johnson JN, Qureshi MY, O'Leary PW, Kamath PS, Lennon RJ, Bonnichsen CR, Young PM, Venkatesh SK, Ehman RL, Gupta S. Magnetic resonance elastography: a novel technique for the detection of hepatic fibrosis and hepatocel-

lular carcinoma after the Fontan operation. Mayo Clin Proc. 2015;90(7):882–94.

15. Myers RP, Cerini R, Sayegh R, Moreau R, Degott C, Lebrec D, Lee SS. Cardiac hepatopathy: clinical, hemodynamic, and histologic characteristics and correlations. Hepatology. 2003;37(2):393–400.

16. European Association For The Study Of The Liver. EASL–EORTC clinical practice guidelines: management of hepatocellular carcinoma. J Hepatol. 2012;56(4):908–43.

17. Possner M, Gordon-Walker T, Egbe AC, Poterucha JT, Warnes CA, Connolly HM, Ginde S, Clift P, Kogon B, Book WM, Walker N. Hepatocellular carcinoma and the Fontan circulation: clinical presentation and outcomes. Int J Cardiol. 2021;322:142–8.

18. Daniels CJ, Bradley EA, Landzberg MJ, Aboulhosn J, Beekman RH, Book W, Gurvitz M, John A, John B, Marelli A, Marino BS. Fontan-associated liver disease: proceedings from the American College of Cardiology Stakeholders Meeting, October 1 to 2, 2015, Washington DC. J Am Coll Cardiol. 2017;70(25):3173–94.

Chapter 16
Diagnosis and Management of Hepatocellular Carcinoma

Elizabeth Sweeney and Tim Cross

Key Learning Points
- HCC is the sixth commonest cancer worldwide and the third commonest cause of cancer death.
- HCC is associated with cirrhosis in western populations, but can occur in non-cirrhotics especially in eastern populations with chronic hepatitis B infection.
- The role of surveillance remains controversial, although meta-analyses and international liver organizations support its use.
- The BCLC classification is used by most western centres to stage disease and to guide the most appropriate therapy.
- Potentially curative treatments are commonly defined as liver resection, ablation and liver transplantation.
- Stereotactic body radiotherapy (SBRT) is likely to gain greater use in the future across multiple disease stages, e.g. BCLC 0-C.
- Non-curative disease is classically defined as treatment with transarterial chemo/bland embolization, radioemboli-

E. Sweeney · T. Cross (✉)
Royal Liverpool University Hospital, Liverpool, UK
e-mail: tim.cross@liverpoolft.nhs.uk

© Springer Nature Switzerland AG 2022   327
T. Cross (ed.), *Liver Disease in Clinical Practice*, In Clinical Practice, https://doi.org/10.1007/978-3-031-10012-3_16

zation for intermediate (BCLC B) and sorafenib, lenvatinib or immunotherapy for advanced (BCLC C disease).

- The introduction of immune-oncology is likely to revolutionize the management of patients with advanced HCC and may find a role in intermediate stage disease.
- Expanding the criteria for liver transplant and the role of downstaging to within transplant criteria is a source of ongoing exploration.

Case Study

A 67-year old man with cirrhotic genetic haemochromatosis (GH) and a history of alcohol excess attends the radiology department for his 6-monthly liver ultrasound scan. The scan shows two lesions which had not previously been seen measuring 20 and 29 mm, respectively. He is otherwise well and has no other co-morbidities. His blood results are as follows: albumin 44 g/dL, AST 36 IU/L, bilirubin 15 μmol/L, creatinine 87 μmol/L, sodium 143 mmol/L, alpha-fetoprotein 4 μmol/L, platelet count 67×10^9/L and PT 12 s. He is fit and well and exercises regularly. He has taken no alcohol for 10 years once he was diagnosed with cirrhosis.

An MRI is organized and this confirms the presence of two liver lesions with arterialization in the arterial phase and washout in the portal venous phase.

1. Which of the following statements are true?

   (a) Genetic haemochromatosis is not associated with HCC.
   (b) HCC can develop in the absence of cirrhosis.
   (c) Alpha-fetoprotein is a good screening test for patients at risk of HCC.
   (d) Staging CT Chest, abdomen is mandated to exclude extra-hepatic disease.
   (e) Cardiovascular disease should be excluded.

2. Which of the following treatments would be appropriate (true) in this case?

   (a) Liver resection
   (b) Immuno-oncology
   (c) Transarterial chemoembolization
   (d) Liver transplantation
   (e) Ablation of HCC (microwave, radiofrequency, cryoablation).

Introduction

Hepatocellular carcinoma (HCC) is the sixth commonest form of cancer and is the third commonest form of cancer related death worldwide [1]. The development of HCC is closely related with the presence of cirrhosis. In African and Asian populations HCC may be seen in the absence of cirrhosis. It is a disease with a worldwide distribution, but is more prevalent in regions where both chronic hepatitis B (CHB) and chronic hepatitis C infections (CHC) are endemic [2]. This means that HCC is more common in parts of Africa, South East Asia and the Far East. The existence of viral co-infections (human immunodeficiency virus (HIV) and hepatitis delta infection (HDV)) further heightens the risk of HCC [1, 3]. In Europe and North America there has been a rise in the prevalence of HCC caused by alcohol, non-alcoholic steatohepatitis (NASH) and CHC infection. The introduction of universal vaccination for the prevention of CHB infection was recommended by the World Health Organization in 1990 and would have an impact on the number of future cases of HCC. Studies have indicated that treating both CHB and CHV reduces the risk of the future development of HCC [4].

Diagnosis of Hepatocellular Carcinoma

HCC is either diagnosed as a first clinical presentation where it may be suspected from clinical imaging or it may be found during ultrasound surveillance. Ultrasound scanning is used in surveillance for HCC. Six-monthly scans are recommended in patients with cirrhosis or patients with CHB infection in whom there is a family history of HCC [5]. The role of PET imaging in HCC diagnosis and staging is currently not recommended in the standard clinical work-up for these patients.

Once a lesion has been identified the diagnosis of HCC is made on the presence of characteristic features of a HCC using dynamic imaging in a patient deemed to be at risk of the disease. Dual phase CT and contrast MRI using gadolinium or primovist contrast agents are used, although diffusion weighted imaging is increasingly utilized [6, 7]. The classical HCC nodule demonstrates arterialization during the arterial phase of the scan with subsequent washout observed in the lesion during the porto-venous phase of the scan (Fig. 16.1). In cases where the lesions are small (≤ 1 cm) an interval scan using the same modality in 3–4 months is often recommended to determine if there is any change in size or if the lesion takes on features more suggestive of a HCC. In cases where the nature of the abnormality is still unclear a lesional biopsy is recommended to secure a histological diagnosis [8].

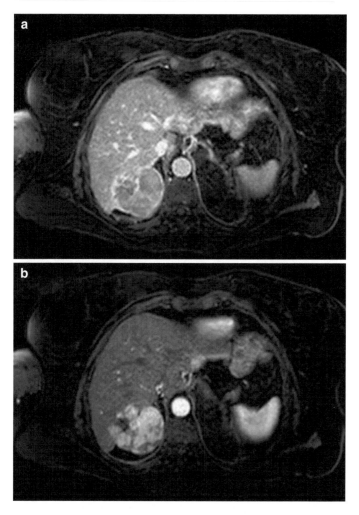

FIGURE 16.1 MRI liver with gadolinium enhancement. (a) A large hypovascular lesion is seen in segment 7 on the delayed phase imaging. This shows arterialization in the arterial phase (b) and then shows washout in the portal venous phase and venous phase (c). This lesion demonstrates the classical hallmarks of a HCC

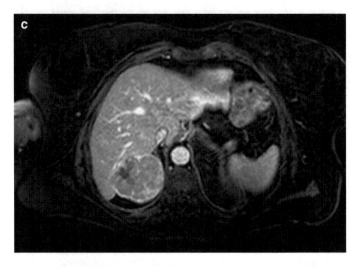

Figure 16.1 (continued)

Current Treatment Modalities for Treatment of Hepatocellular Carcinoma

Treatment for HCC broadly falls into three categories: curative, non-curative and palliative. A framework is required to help clinicians decide on the optimal treatment for their patients. It is possible to divide this approach into tumour characteristics (i.e. tumour size, number of nodules, AFP, the presence of metastases and portal vein invasion) and the patient characteristics (e.g. Child-Pugh score, co-morbidities, age, frailty, ascites, jaundice). Most clinicians use the Barcelona Clinic Liver Cancer (BCLC) staging system [9] (Fig. 16.2). Briefly, disease is categorized into five groups: Stage 0 a single small lesion ≤2 cm in a non-cirrhotic liver (optimal treatment—liver resection); Stage A—a solitary lesion ≥2 cm but ≤4.5 cm or three lesions the largest of which is 3 cm, in the absence of extra-hepatic disease or where there are features of portal hypertension (optimal treatment liver transplantation); Stage B—a solitary lesion >5.5 cm or >3 liver lesions, the largest of which is >3 cm (optimal treatment loco-regional

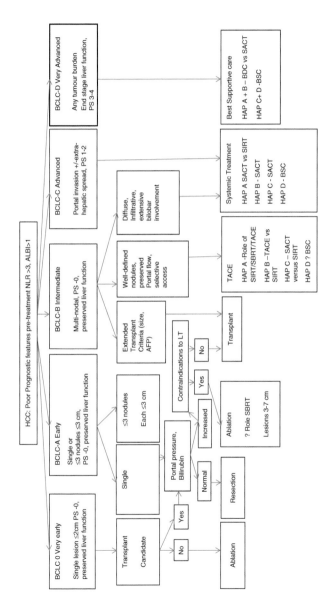

Figure 16.2 The proposed modification of the current BCLC staging system. The modified liverpool BCLC algorithm for the management of patients with hepatocellular carcinoma [4]

therapies, e.g. transarterial chemo/radioembolization (TACE/TARE) and ablative techniques (for lesions ≤3 cm)); Stage C—liver nodules of any size but in the presence of tumour thrombus in the portal venous system or extra-hepatic disease, e.g. lymph nodes, lung, bone metastases (optimal treatment immune-oncology, Sorafenib, lenvatinib, etc.). Stage D—HCC in the presence of decompensated liver disease, e.g. ascites, liver dysfunction (optimal treatment—best supportive care).

These stages only act as a guide and there is some fluidity between them. Other staging methods include the CLIP [10], the Milan criteria [11] and recent the Hong Kong Liver cancer staging system [12]. The Milan criteria identified a group of patients who would benefit from liver transplantation (LT). Mazzaferro and colleagues systematically reviewed outcomes from LT in a cohort of Italian HCC patients and discovered that the outcomes from LT were good in patients with single lesions ≤4.5 cm or when there are three lesions the largest of which is no bigger than 3 cm. This landmark study has formed the basis of LT practice for nearly 20 years. Other groups have tried to see if those boundaries for liver size can be pushed a little further by assessing outcomes in larger tumours or where more than three HCC nodules are present, e.g. UCSF criteria [13, 14], metroticket [15]. In reality, the majority of patients are not candidates for LT and LT is certainly not going to address the underlying causes of HCC and the diseases that lead to its development. Thus, attention has been re-focused on methods to better select patients who will derive benefit from loco-regional therapies and to predict who is at greater risk of disease recurrence after LT, or who could be managed to provide good life expectancy in the absence of LT. These additional methods include The ART strategy [16], the HAP score [17] and the Duvoux score [18] (Table 16.1).

TABLE 16.1 Prognostic models used to guide the management of hepatocellular carcinoma

Author	Score	Parameters
Bruix et al. [6]	Barcelona Clinic Liver Cancer stage	See Fig. 16.2
	Hong Kong Liver Cancer	

A more complicated version of BCLC derived from a large cohort from Hong Kong aiming to identify patients who may benefit from more radical treatments that considered under BCLC. Needs validation outside of Asia

Mazzaferro et al. [11]	The Milan Criteria	×1 HCC ≤5 cm
		Or ×3 lesions ≤3 cm

If within criteria good results from LT, i.e. 5 year survival ~70%

Yao et al. [13]	The UCSF criteria	×1 lesion ≤6.5 cm
		×3 lesions largest <4.5 cm
		Total tumour diameter <8.5 cm

Able to achieve LT results comparable with Milan criteria with expanded access

Mazzaferro et al. [15]	The Metroticket score	Diameter of largest nodule
		Sum of hepatic malignant nodules
		"Up to seven criteria"

If sum of diameter of largest lesion and number nodules <7–5 year survival ~70% for LT

TABLE 16.1 (continued)

Author	Score	Parameters
Duvoux et al. [18]	The Duvoux score	Tumour diameter
		≤3 cm = 0, 3–6 cm = 1 points
		>6 cm = 4 points
		Number of nodules
		1–3 = 0 points
		≥4 = 2 points
		AFP
		≤100 = 0 points, 100–1000 = 2 points
		>1000 = 3 points

Score > 2 associated with greater risk of disease recurrence post LT

Author	Score	Parameters
Kadalayil et al. [17]	The HAP score	AFP >400 ng/ mL = 1
		Tumour >7 cm = 1
		Albumin <36 g/ dL = 1
		Bilirubin >17 µmol/L = 1

Sum of scores HAP A = 0, HAP B = 1, HAP C = 2, HAP D > 2 allows identification of patients of risk of decompensation after TACE. Median survivals HAP A 27.6 months, HAP B 18.5 months, HAP C 9 months, HAP D 3.8 months

TABLE 16.1 (continued)

Author	Score	Parameters
Hucke et al. [16]	The ART strategy	Radiologic tumour response
		Present = 0, absent = 1 point
		AST rise >25%
		Present = 4 points, absent = 0
		Child-Pugh score increase
		1 point rise = 1.5 points
		≥2 points = 3 points
		Absent = 0 points

Used to identify patients who will not benefit from TACE. A score of >2.5 identifies patients who do not benefit from further TACE

The Role of HCC Surveillance in at Risk Patients

The rationale for screening and surveillance is simple. If one looks for a particular disease in a population at risk for that condition at regular intervals, it is more likely that, should that disease arise, it will be detected at an earlier stage at which point curative treatment would be possible. It is known that patients who develop HCC tend to have liver cirrhosis and are older [19]. The recommendations from EASL, AASLD, are that a liver ultrasound examination should be performed on a 6-monthly basis for all patients with cirrhosis or patients with CHB where there is a family history of HCC. AFP is no longer recommended as a screening tool [1].

For surveillance programmes to be effective the test used must be accurate, cost-effective, readily available and targeted to the right population. Liver ultrasound is readily available in many health care systems, but does have problems. The technique is user dependent, and for a programme to work best it would be preferred to have dedicated practitioners who just do USS HCC surveillance. Ultrasound is less good in patients who are obese and those with narrow rib spaces. It is also challenging in patients with dysplastic or regenerative nodules, at which point further imaging is mandated and then subsequent follow-up imaging becomes more problematic (and expensive). In a UK study it was discovered that the provision, organization and uptake of ultrasound surveillance for HCC were poor [19].

A meta-analysis of 32 studies comprising 13,367 patients concluded that ultrasound has a low sensitivity of 47% (95% CI 33–61%) to detect early-stage HCC in patients with cirrhosis [20]. Therefore, more work needs to be done in order to define the best surveillance strategies for different patient cohorts.

Are there ways in which the accuracy of surveillance could be improved? A statistical model called the GALAD score has been proposed as a tool for determining the risk of HCC in individuals with chronic liver disease. The score comprises gender, age and serological tumour markers including AFP-L3, α fetoprotein (AFP) and des-carboxy-prothrombin. The score has been validated in a large multicentre, multicontinent study comprising 6834 patients. The AUC for GALAD in all cohorts examined was greater than 0.90 [21].

The use of cross-sectional imaging modalities such as CT or MRI is not recommended for surveillance due a lack of data on efficacy and concerns regarding cost-effectiveness and potential harm related to radiation and contrast exposure. Although the role of non-contrast MRI is an imaging modality under investigation as a possible alternative to patients who are not optimal candidates for USS.

Other potential biomarkers related to HCC have been identified and have the potential to be utilized as HCC surveillance markers. However, few have yet been evaluated in phase 2 studies [22].

Further work is required until a more tailored approach to HCC surveillance is possible. The emergence of reliable novel disease biomarkers would also be a significant step forward.

The Role of Liver Transplantation in the Management of HCC

The definitive treatment for the majority of HCC cases is LT. This is because transplantation removes both the cancer and the cirrhotic liver that is susceptible to further tumours and decompensation. The role of LT in the management of HCC is well-defined, but some areas require further investigation.

The Role of Downstaging

Is it possible to downstage a tumour such that it would then fall within transplantable range? This is a question that has puzzled transplant clinicians since the advent of LT as a meaningful treatment modality. If a lesion(s) is outside criteria but can be brought within criteria by a treatment, e.g. transarterial chemoembolization, are the outcomes similar to those patients who do not require "downstaging"? A meeting of international experts on the role of LT for the management for HCC proposed three statements on this matter: (1) the criteria for successful downstaging should include tumour size and the number of viable tumours; (2) AFP concentrations before and after downstaging might add further information and (3) based on existing evidence, no recommendations can be made for preferring a specific loco-regional therapy for downstaging over others [23].

There is a growing body of evidence that liver transplant for HCC beyond Milan criteria is not associated with worse outcomes. Several different models exist with expanded criteria for cadaveric liver transplantation for HCC. The University of California San Francisco (UCSF) criteria describes a solitary tumour ≤6.5 cm or ≤3 tumours with the largest ≤4.5 cm. The "up to seven" criteria include a combination of tumour maximum size and number of lesions in patients without microvascular invasion. The Clinic of Universidad of Navarra (CUN) criteria describes 1 tumour ≤6 cm or ≤3 tumours with the largest ≤5 cm. The criteria described by Toso et al. includes total tumour volume and AFP. The criteria of the University of Hangzhou involve total tumour diameter, histological grade and AFP. Onaca et al. describe criteria of a solitary tumour ≤6 cm or 2–4 tumours ≤5 cm.

All of these criteria have been shown to have favourable outcomes that are comparable to patients transplanted within Milan criteria [24].

Treatment on the Waiting List

The anxiety with any malignant process is that, if left alone, the cancer will continue to grow and progress. If the tumour grows beyond a certain size or number of tumour nodules curative therapy will no longer be possible. An additional problem is that, under the current system of organ donation and allocation, the wait time for a LT is unpredictable and is influenced by factors such as recipient and donor blood group, weight and height. Interestingly, some authors have said that wait time does not influence outcomes [25]. Patients who do well after a long wait list time may be those with the less aggressive tumour biology. In order to maintain patients within criteria some liver transplant centres will offer locoregional therapy by way of ablative techniques (microwave, radiofrequency ablation) or embolic approaches (transarterial embolization, transarterial radio-embolization). The aim is to maintain patients within transplant criteria whilst awaiting the operation. An ablation technique will have no impact on availability of for LT but for patients who undergo chemoembolization patients are suspended from the wait list for 4 weeks after treatment because of the impact on white cells and the perceived increased risk of infections at the time of LT. There is also a concern that TACE may cause hepatic decompensation and make patients too unfit for surgery. It is for this reason that some centres are reluctant to give TACE to patients on the waitlist. But, in the face of unpredictable wait times for cadaveric organs or deceased non-heart beating donors, other centres have felt compelled to offer loco-regional treatment to optimize their patients' chances of progressing onto the liver transplant. International experts concede that treatment may be appropriate where wait times are likely to be in excess of 6 months [23, 26].

Liver Transplantation as Salvage Therapy

Given the continuing rise in the number of patients being considered for LT with only a modest increase in the donor pool, there has been a call to optimize the use of available organs. The reason behind this is due to the increasing number of HCC patients who occupy places on the liver transplant waitlist. This is felt to be disproportionate in comparison to the actual disease burden presented by HCC. Some clinicians feel that increasing the number of transplants performed for HCC may have a deleterious impact on other patients awaiting LT, particularly in medical systems where HCC patients are given some prioritization. In a model where LT and liver resection were at one time regarded as the only effective (curative) treatment, the advent of new techniques such as ablative therapies potentially offer good treatment for small HCCs. The 1-year mortality from liver transplant of 9% at 1 year, for frail patients, the risks of major surgery may outweigh the risks. Thus, patient selection is a vital. For small HCCs (i.e. ≤2 cm), in the absence of cirrhosis or significant portal hypertension (<10 mmHg), these patients can be offered liver resection, an ablation technique and if unfit for anaesthetic could be considered for stereotactic body radiotherapy (SBRT). Unfortunately, despite small lesions being present surgery is not often possible, but ablation is possible for the majority of these patients. Ablation approaches have only provided an effective treatment zone of up to 3 cm. If there is well-preserved liver function, there is no barrier for more than one lesion being treated. Newer ablative techniques may allow a treatment zone for lesions up to 5 cm in maximum diameter.

Alpha-fetoprotein is a tumour marker that is elevated in some cases of HCC. It is no longer used as a screening tool but a useful prognostic tool. Very high levels of AFP portend a poor outcome and studies have suggested that levels >400 IU/L at the time of liver transplant are associated with a higher risk of disease recurrence post-transplant [27, 28]. So in terms of creating a model that helps identify patients who may or may not benefit from LT it can be seen that a system consisting of tumour size, number of tumour nodules and AFP level might have some utility. Duvoux and colleagues devised a scoring system consisting of these three variables and assigned different scores according to tumour size, number of nodules and AFP [18]. It is possible that using this approach, patients could be stratified to loco-regional treatment before liver transplantation, and that this could be used to help reduce the number of LTs performed for HCC where survival might be comparable with loco-regional techniques.

Delisting HCC Patients

One of the most difficult decisions transplant clinicians need to make is to decide when LT is no longer in the interest of the patient. The patient is delisted if the HCC acquires unfavourable characteristics that are incompatible with long term survival (i.e. <50% chance of 5 year survival). This includes all the poor prognostic indicators that are assessed prior to listing, i.e. increase in tumour size beyond accepted listing criteria, tumour invasion of the portal vasculature and extra-hepatic disease (lymph nodes, lung and bone metastases). Other factors include factors that are not directly due to the tumour, e.g. cardio-respiratory illness, frailty, the development of additional malignancies and factors that would make anaesthesia and surgery too high risk, e.g. morbid obesity.

Improving Existing Therapies

The majority of patients with HCC are not candidates for LT and it is natural that the pressure for new therapies has been for this group of patients (BCLC B and C). The advent of transarterial embolization techniques was a step forward and for some time there was a debate over whether there was any survival benefit conferred by administering a chemoembolization over a bland embolization technique (i.e. embolization of feeding vessel to the tumour). The demonstration by Llovet and Bruix suggesting the benefits of TACE has led investigators to seek ways of improving the efficacy of this treatment [29]. Initially, the chemotherapeutic agents (doxorubicin, cisplatin) were mixed with lipiodol and administered as a mixture. More recently drug-eluting beads have been manufactured. Interestingly there is no study to demonstrate which chemotherapeutic agent is the best in HCC. The optimal timing and selection of patients is important. Techniques such as the ART strategy and the HAP score have been introduced to help identify those patients who will derive less benefit from treatment. Researchers have also been exploring ways in which to increase the impact of treatment. Pre-treatment with systemic doxorubicin has been suggested as one way to enhance the lethality of chemoembolization and a recent paper suggested that metformin may have a role in reducing the risk of developing HCC in patients with NASH and alcohol-related cirrhosis and may aid in improving the efficacy of future treatment [30]. There has also been more interest in the use of transarterial radio-embolization (TARE). Recent studies with TARE have been promising and it has the benefit of being applicable in patients with portal vein thrombosis, in whom conventional TACE would be contra-indicated. The effect of the treatment is delivered locally and appears to have a sustained effect. This means that a single, rather than multiple, treatment, is possible. Yet, TARE is time-consuming and requires interventional radiology support. Treatment requires two radiology sessions, the first, to plan treatment and to look for parasitic supplies that might take some of the radioactivity away from the tumour zone and towards healthy tissue in the lungs, stomach and small intestine. This can lead to a debilitating radiation pneumonitis or gastritis that can lead to significant morbidity and even death. As such, assessing for parasitic supplies and shunting (with the aid of nuclear medicine) is an essential part of the work-up. A parasitic supply is defined as tumour vascularizations and new vessels derived from neighbouring organs or structures, and supplemental to the normal blood supply of the diseased organ. Only once shunts have been excluded, or are below a certain level, can treatment be given.

Selective internal radiation therapy (SIRT) is now approved by NICE for the treatment of unresectable HCC in patients with compensated liver disease for whom TACE is not appropriate. Both the SARAH trial and the SIRveNIB trial were phase 3, multicentre, open label investigator lead trials comparing SIRT with sorafenib in patients with BCLC C disease. Patients with recurrent disease after surgery or thermoablative therapy and patients who have failed TACE were also included in the SARAH trial. Both trials showed no survival difference between sorafenib and SIRT. However, there were fewer adverse events in patients treated with SIRT which may make this the preferable choice [31, 32]. More work needs to be done in order to define the relevant population that will have maximum benefit from SIRT over other systemic treatment options.

Stereotactic body radiation therapy (SBRT) is a non-invasive technique for delivering high doses of radiotherapy to a lesion whilst minimizing damage to surrounding structures and organs. This technique might be preferred for lesions in close proximity to structures such as blood vessels, bile ducts, the diaphragm, etc. There is emerging evidence for the use of SBRT in patients with early-stage HCC who are not fit for surgical resection or ablative therapies as well as in patients with advanced disease who have failed other treatments, e.g. TACE [33]. SBRT is thus a further tool in the clinicians armamentarium. However, more work needs to be done to better define the patient cohorts that will confer the most benefit from this treatment option.

Systemic Therapy

Up until recently the only treatment option for patients with advanced metastatic HCC (BCLC C), in the absence of liver decompensation, was sorafenib. The SHARP trial demonstrated a median survival with sorafenib of 10.7 months versus 7.9 months with placebo (hazard ratio 0.69, 95% CI 0.55 0.88 $P = 0.00058$) [34].

There are now other treatment options for this group of patients. An open label, phase 3, multicentre trial comparing lenvatinib with sorafenib in first line treatment of unresectable HCC demonstrated non-inferiority of lenvatinib [35].

Both treatments are now recommended by NICE as options for patients with Child-Pugh A cirrhosis and an ECOG performance status of 0 or 1, who have not received prior systemic therapy for HCC.

Patients who have previously been treated with sorafenib can be offered cabozantinib, a vascular endothelial growth factor (VEGF) inhibitor. A double-blind, placebo controlled, randomized phase 3 trial demonstrated an improved overall and progression free survival for patients receiving cabozantinib compared to placebo. Median overall survival was 10.2 months with cabozantinib and 8.0 months with placebo (hazard ratio for death 0.76, 95% CI 0.63–0.92, $P = 0.005$) [36].

The era of immunotherapy has now extended to hepatocellular carcinoma and is yet another option for first line systemic therapy in patients with advanced disease. A global, open label, phase 3 trial compared Atezolizumab plus Bevacizumab (n = 336) with sorafenib (n = 165) in patients with unresectable HCC, who had not previously received systemic therapy. The immunotherapy regime resulted in improved overall and progression free survival compared with sorafenib. Overall survival at 12 months was 67.2% (95% CI 61.3–73.1) with atezolizumab-bevacizumab and 54.6% (95% CI 45.2–64.0) with sorafenib [37].

Early results from a phase 1b study have shown promise for the addition of lenvatinib to the immunotherapy agent Pembrolizumab for patients with unresectable HCC [38] and this was later followed up in the Keynote 240 study [39]. In the study 413 patients were randomly assigned. These patients had been previously treated with sorafenib. As of January 2, 2019, median follow-up was 13.8 months for Pembrolizumab and 10.6 months for placebo. Median OS was 13.9 months (95% CI, 11.6–16.0 months) for pembrolizumab versus 10.6 months (95% CI, 8.3–13.5 months) for placebo (hazard ratio [HR], 0.781; 95% CI, 0.611–0.998; P = 0.0238). In this study, OS and PFS did not reach statistical significance per specified criteria. The results are consistent with those of KEYNOTE-224, supporting a favourable risk-to-benefit ratio for pembrolizumab in this population.

The important consideration with any treatment is the prospect of adverse effects of treatment. The clinical trials of immuno-oncology (IO) have highlighted some issues.

1. Bleeding: In the IMBrave 250 study there was an increased risk of variceal bleeding in the IO arm versus Sorafenib (25% versus 15%), even though both groups had 26% variceal rate in both arms. Most clinicians would advise a recent oesophago-gastro-duodenoscopy (OGD) prior to treatment. Some clinicians will not give IO if the patient has had a variceal bleed in the preceding 6 months, although others suggest that treatment could start from 14 days post bleed. Some groups have tried to determine guidance. The London HOB oncology group came up with the following guidance before commencing Atezo/Bev: (a). Variceal bleed last 6 months not for Atexo/Bev, (b). OGD within 6–12 months and no varices or on B-Blockade—start Atezo/Bev, (c). No varices start Atezo/Bev. It is likely that this guidance will evolve. In addition to bleeding some patients may also develop thrombosis, e.g. portal vein thrombosis (PVT). The bleeding and clot formation have been blamed mainly on the Bevacizumab and so some clinicians would consider a switch from dual to monotherapy

with Atezolizumab alone, but this decision should best be made within a MDT/cancer board meeting.

2. Hypertension and Proteinuria: Patients at increased risk of kidney disease, e.g. diabetes, and patients with chronic viral hepatitis should be screened for proteinuria and have baseline renal function assessed. If renal dysfunction or proteinuria is found a referral to the renal team is mandated. Where hypertension does exist treatment with angiotensin converting enzyme inhibitors or angiotensin II blockers is often effective.

3. Diarrhoea: Mainly of the IO treatments can instigate immune mediated colitis and occasionally hepatitis. Infective causes of diarrhoea should be excluded as should inflammatory bowel disease or malignancy. One should consider the most common causes. If a diarrhoea screen is negative, a flexible sigmoidoscopy or colonoscopy is needed and biopsies taken to elicit the cause. An immune mediated colitis (and hepatitis) often resolves with high dose corticosteroids and occasional may need the addition of other immunosuppressive agents, e.g. mycophenolate mofetil, tacrolimus. The IO drug may need to be reduced or even stopped in some circumstances, but can sometimes be re-introduced.

Getting More from Sorafenib

Clinicians have wondered if adding sorafenib to patients undergoing loco-regional therapies such as ablation or chemoembolization might confer a survival advantage. However, the evidence so far does not support this theory.

The STORM trial was a phase 3, randomized, double-blind, placebo controlled trial assessing the use of sorafenib as adjuvant treatment following surgical resection or ablation. The data failed to show any benefit from sorafenib compared with placebo in recurrence free survival following these treatments [40].

TACE II was a multicentre, randomized, placebo controlled, double-blind phase 3 trial looking at adjuvant sorafenib following TACE in patients with unresectable HCC confined to the liver. The results showed no benefit from sorafenib in progression free survival [41].

Researchers have wondered if drug combinations might exacerbate the efficacy of sorafenib. But using sorafenib with erlotinib, everolimus and BIIB IGFR mAb, has produced disappointing results, with problems due to toxicity or because no benefit was proven with combination.

Stereotactic body radiation therapy (SBRT) is a non-invasive technique for delivering high doses of radiotherapy to a lesion whilst minimizing damage to surrounding structures and organs. This technique might be preferred for lesions in close proximity to structures such as blood vessels, bile ducts, the diaphragm, etc. There is emerging evidence for the use of SBRT in patients with early-stage HCC who are not fit for surgical resection or ablative therapies as well as in patients with advanced disease who have failed other treatments [42]. However, more work needs to be done to better define the patient cohorts that will confer the most benefit from this treatment option.

Conclusion

In the future clearer targets will need to be derived from our understanding of the biology of these tumours. This will help inform the best treatment for each patient based upon knowledge of the patient and their tumour. There remain lots of unanswered questions. Improved methods of surveillance and diseases stratification are needed, and given the problems with ultrasound as a surveillance tool it might be useful to have biomarkers built in to trial design to allow identification of new surveillance tools (and markers of tumour biology). Immunotherapy is an exciting prospect that is in its infancy but is currently an additional option for patients with advanced disease. The best therapy may be required in combination and with greater understanding of genetics and risk profiling it may be possible in the future to tailor the best treatment for each patient. In addition, with new therapies more questions shall arise such as how should these new treatments be used in the context of liver resection, liver transplantation (pre-and post-surgery), and what role in loco-regional therapies. There is much to do, but this is an exciting time to be involved in the treatment of patients with HCC.

Answers to Questions

1. Which of the following statements are true?

   (a) Genetic haemochromatosis is not associated with HCC. **False—there is a strong association with HCC**
   (b) HCC can develop in the absence of cirrhosis. **True**
   (c) Alpha-fetoprotein is a good screening test for all patients at risk of HCC. **False—only 30% of cases of HCC secrete alpha-fetoprotein. It is a poor screening tool but can be used as a prognostic indicator and marker of aggressive tumour biology**.
   (d) Staging CT chest, abdomen is mandated to exclude extra-hepatic disease. **True—the presence of extra-hepatic disease would preclude liver resection and transplantation and is therefore an important test to do**.
   (e) Cardiovascular disease should be excluded. **True—GH is associated with cardiovascular disease (possible because of the association with diabetes mellitus) and must be actively sought in a transplant assessment process**.

2. Which of the following treatments would be appropriate (true) in this case?

   (a) Liver resection. False—The low platelet count suggests portal hypertension and thus resection may be best avoided. Given the high risk of diseases recurrence in the remnant liver and the multifocal nature of diseases (particularly if disease in different lobes), liver transplantation would be a better choice.

(b) Immuno-oncology. **False—This treatment is reserved for patients with extra-hepatic disease in the absence of hepatic decompensation (BCLC C).**

(c) Transarterial chemoembolization. **False—This is reserved for patients with hepatic disease who are outside resection or liver transplant criteria (BCLC B). Although this modality may be used if thermal ablations are considered too hazardous (e.g. challenging anatomical location) or if the patient is not fit for an ablation, e.g. not fit for general anaesthetic.**

(d) Liver transplantation. **True—This is the optimal treatment.**

(e) Ablation of HCC (microwave, radiofrequency, cryoablation). **True—given that the wait time for transplant may be beyond 6 months ablation is recommended as a bridge to transplant in these cases.**

References

1. EASL-EORTC clinical practice guidelines: management of hepatocellular carcinoma. J Hepatol. 2012;56(4):908–43.
2. Parkin DM, Bray F, Ferlay J, Pisani P. Global cancer statistics, 2002. CA Cancer J Clin. 2005;55(2):74–108.
3. Cross TJ, Rizzi P, Horner M, Jolly A, Hussain MJ, Smith HM, et al. The increasing prevalence of hepatitis delta virus (HDV) infection in South London. J Med Virol. 2008;80(2):277–82.
4. Russo FP, Zanetto A, Pinto E, Battistella S, Penzo B, Burra P, Farinati F. Hepatocellular carcinoma in chronic viral hepatitis: where do we stand? Int J Mol Sci. 2022;23(1):500. https://doi.org/10.3390/ijms23010500.
5. Singal A, Volk ML, Waljee A, Salgia R, Higgins P, Rogers MA, et al. Meta-analysis: surveillance with ultrasound for early-stage hepatocellular carcinoma in patients with cirrhosis. Aliment Pharmacol Ther. 2009;30(1):37–47.
6. Bruix J, Sherman M. Management of hepatocellular carcinoma: an update. Hepatology. 2011;53(3):1020–2.
7. Bruix J, Sherman M. Management of hepatocellular carcinoma. Hepatology. 2005;42(5):1208–36.

8. International Consensus Group for Hepatocellular NeoplasiaThe International Consensus Group for Hepatocellular Neoplasia. Pathologic diagnosis of early hepatocellular carcinoma: a report of the international consensus group for hepatocellular neoplasia. Hepatology. 2009;49(2):658–64.

9. Bruix J, Sherman M, Llovet JM, Beaugrand M, Lencioni R, Burroughs AK, et al. Clinical management of hepatocellular carcinoma. Conclusions of the Barcelona-2000 EASL conference. European Association for the Study of the Liver. J Hepatol. 2001;35(3):421–30.

10. A new prognostic system for hepatocellular carcinoma: a retrospective study of 435 patients: the Cancer of the Liver Italian Program (CLIP) investigators. Hepatology. 1998;28(3):751–5.

11. Mazzaferro V, Regalia E, Doci R, Andreola S, Pulvirenti A, Bozzetti F, et al. Liver transplantation for the treatment of small hepatocellular carcinomas in patients with cirrhosis. N Engl J Med. 1996;334(11):693–9.

12. Yau T, Tang VY, Yao TJ, Fan ST, Lo CM, Poon RT. Development of Hong Kong Liver Cancer staging system with treatment stratification for patients with hepatocellular carcinoma. Gastroenterology. 2014;146(7):1691–700.e3.

13. Yao FY, Ferrell L, Bass NM, Watson JJ, Bacchetti P, Venook A, et al. Liver transplantation for hepatocellular carcinoma: expansion of the tumor size limits does not adversely impact survival. Hepatology. 2001;33(6):1394–403.

14. Yao FY, Xiao L, Bass NM, Kerlan R, Ascher NL, Roberts JP. Liver transplantation for hepatocellular carcinoma: validation of the UCSF-expanded criteria based on preoperative imaging. Am J Transplant. 2007;7(11):2587–96.

15. Mazzaferro V, Llovet JM, Miceli R, Bhoori S, Schiavo M, Mariani L, et al. Predicting survival after liver transplantation in patients with hepatocellular carcinoma beyond the Milan criteria: a retrospective, exploratory analysis. Lancet Oncol. 2009;10(1):35–43.

16. Hucke F, Sieghart W, Pinter M, Graziadei I, Vogel W, Muller C, et al. The ART-strategy: sequential assessment of the ART score predicts outcome of patients with hepatocellular carcinoma retreated with TACE. J Hepatol. 2014;60(1):118–26.

17. Kadalayil L, Benini R, Pallan L, O'Beirne J, Marelli L, Yu D, et al. A simple prognostic scoring system for patients receiving transarterial embolisation for hepatocellular cancer. Ann Oncol. 2013;24(10):2565–70.

18. Duvoux C, Roudot-Thoraval F, Decaens T, Pessione F, Badran H, Piardi T, et al. Liver transplantation for hepatocellular carcinoma: a model including alpha-fetoprotein improves the performance of Milan criteria. Gastroenterology. 2012;143(4):986–94. e3; quiz e14–5.

19. Cross TJS, Villaneuva A, Shetty S, Wilkes E, Reeves H, et al. A national survey of the provision of ultrasound surveillance for the detection of hepatocellular carcinoma. Frontline Gastroenterol. 2016;7:82–9.

20. Tzartzeva K, Obi J, Rich NE, et al. Surveillance imaging and alpha fetoprotein for early detection of hepatocellular carcinoma in patients with cirrhosis: a meta-analysis. Gastroenterology. 2018;154(6):1706–17.

21. Berhane S, Toyoda H, Tada T, et al. Role of the GALAD and BALAD-2 serologic models in diagnosis of hepatocellular carcinoma and prediction of survival in patients. Clin Gastroenterol Hepatol. 2016;14(6):875–88.

22. Kanwal F, Singal AG. Surveillance for hepatocellular carcinoma: current best practice and future direction. Gastroenterology. 2019;157(1):54–64.

23. Clavien PA, Lesurtel M, Bossuyt PM, Gores GJ, Langer B, Perrier A. Recommendations for liver transplantation for hepatocellular carcinoma: an international consensus conference report. Lancet Oncol. 2012;13(1):e11–22.

24. Pavel MC, Fuster J. Expansion of the hepatocellular carcinoma Milan criteria in liver transplantation: future directions. World J Gastroenterol. 2018;24(32):3626–36.

25. Samoylova ML, Dodge JL, Yao FY, Roberts JP. Time to transplantation as a predictor of hepatocellular carcinoma recurrence after liver transplantation. Liver Transpl. 2014;20(8):937–44.

26. Majno P, Lencioni R, Mornex F, Girard N, Poon RT, Cherqui D. Is the treatment of hepatocellular carcinoma on the waiting list necessary? Liver Transpl. 2011;17(Suppl 2):S98–108.

27. Merani S, Majno P, Kneteman NM, Berney T, Morel P, Mentha G, et al. The impact of waiting list alpha-fetoprotein changes on the outcome of liver transplant for hepatocellular carcinoma. J Hepatol. 2011;55(4):814–9.

28. Hameed B, Mehta N, Sapisochin G, Roberts JP, Yao FY. Alpha-fetoprotein level > 1000 ng/mL as an exclusion criterion for liver transplantation in patients with hepatocellular carcinoma meeting the Milan criteria. Liver Transpl. 2014;20(8):945–51.

29. Llovet JM, Bruix J. Systematic review of randomized trials for unresectable hepatocellular carcinoma: chemoembolization improves survival. Hepatology. 2003;37(2):429–42.

30. Chen HP, Shieh JJ, Chang CC, Chen TT, Lin JT, Wu MS, et al. Metformin decreases hepatocellular carcinoma risk in a dose-dependent manner: population-based and in vitro studies. Gut. 2013;62(4):606–15.

31. Vilgrain V, Pereira H, Assenat E. Efficacy and safety of selective internal radiotherapy with yttrium-90 resin microspheres compared with sorafenib in locally advanced and inoperable hepatocellular carcinoma (SARAH): an open-label randomised controlled phase 3 trial. Lancet Oncol. 2017;18(12):1624–36.

32. Chow PKH, Gandhi M, Tan SB. SIRveNIB: selective internal radiation therapy versus sorafenib in Asia-Pacific patients with hepatocellular carcinoma. J Clin Oncol. 2018;36(19):1913–21.

33. Shanker MD, Liu HY, Lee YY, et al. Stereotactic radiotherapy for hepatocellular carcinoma: expanding the multidisciplinary armamentarium. J Gastroenterol Hepatol. 2021;36(4):873–84.

34. Llovet JM, Ricci S, Mazzaferro V, Hilgard P, Gane E, Blanc JF, et al. Sorafenib in advanced hepatocellular carcinoma. N Engl J Med. 2008;359(4):378–90.

35. Kudo M. Lenvatanib versus sorafenib in first line treatment of patients with unresectable hepatocellular carcinoma: a randomised phase 3 non-inferiority trial. Lancet. 2018;391(10126):1163–73.

36. Abou-Alfa GK. Cabozantinib in patients with advances and progressing hepatocellular carcinoma. N Engl J Med. 2018;379:54.

37. Finn RS, Qin S, Ikeda M, et al. Atezolizumab plus bevacizumab in unresectable hepatocellular carcinoma. N Engl J Med. 2020;382(20):1894–190.

38. Finn RS, Ikeda M, Zhu AX, et al. Phase Ib study of lenvatinib plus pembrolizumab in patients with unresectable hepatocellular carcinoma. J Clin Oncol. 2020;38(26):2960–70.

39. Finn RS, Ryoo BY, Merle P, et al. Pembrolizumab as second-line therapy in patients with advanced hepatocellular carcinoma in KEYNOTE-240: a randomized, double-blind, phase III trial. J Clin Oncol. 2020;38(3):193–202.

40. Bruix J, Takayama T, Mazzaferro V, et al. Adjuvant sorafenib for hepatocellular carcinoma after resection or ablation (STORM): a phase 3, randomised, double-blind, placebo-controlled trial. Lancet Oncol. 2015;16(13):1344–54.

41. Meyer T, Fox R, Ma YT, et al. Sorafenib in combination with transarterial chemoembolisation in patients with unresectable hepatocellular carcinoma (TACE 2): a randomised placebo-controlled, double-blind, phase 3 trial. Lancet Gastroenterol Hepatol. 2017;2(8):565–75.
42. Thomas HR. Stereotactic body radiation therapy (SBRT) in hepatocellular carcinoma. Curr Hepatol Rep. 2021;20:12–22.

Chapter 17
Liver Transplantation

Rohit Gupta and James O'Beirne

Key Learning Points
- Liver transplantation is a life-saving treatment for selected patients with severe forms of liver disease.
- Models exist to predict the severity of liver disease and need for liver transplantation, e.g. United Kingdom end-stage liver disease score (UKELKD), the model of end-stage liver disease (MELD) these scores can also be used to prioritize patients on the waiting list and in conjunction with donor factors are useful for allocation of organs to maximize transplant benefit.
- Patients with chronic liver disease including acute on chronic liver failure, acute liver failure, hepatocellular carcinoma and variant syndromes have access to liver transplantation.
- Prior to listing a comprehensive assessment of patient fitness, addiction behaviours and psycho-social factors must be performed.
- Patients listed for liver transplant must have a minimum expected survival of 50% at 5 years from transplant.

R. Gupta · J. O'Beirne (✉)
Department of Hepatology, Sunshine Coast University Hospital, Birtinya, QLD, Australia
e-mail: James.OBeirne@health.qld.gov.au

© Springer Nature Switzerland AG 2022   355
T. Cross (ed.), *Liver Disease in Clinical Practice*, In Clinical Practice, https://doi.org/10.1007/978-3-031-10012-3_17

Case Study

A 65-year-old man with non-alcoholic steatohepatitis cirrhosis presented to the outpatient clinic. He had portal vein thrombosis and chronic hepatic encephalopathy with three admissions in the previous year despite lactulose and rifaximin. Laboratory workup was remarkable for INR 1.1, creatinine 105 μmol/L, bilirubin 22.3 μmol/L, sodium 141 and albumin 30 g/L. This patient had Child-Pugh Class B cirrhosis (7 points) and the UKELD and MELD scores were 48 and 10 points, respectively.

Questions

1. Should this patient be referred for liver transplantation based on the severity of his liver disease?
2. What aspects of the patient's medical history should be examined closely during transplant assessment?
3. Is the patients age a barrier to receiving a liver transplant?

Introduction

Thomas Starzl and colleagues performed the first successful liver transplant in humans in 1963 and since then liver transplantation (LT) has revolutionized the care of patients with acute and chronic liver failure of all aetiologies refractory to medical therapy [1]. Currently LT is a common practice worldwide with survival rates reaching 96% at 1 year for elective procedures in low risk patients [2]. As safety and early survival has improved over time, so has the number of indications and candidates who may benefit leading to the current organ shortage.

Despite improvements in early survival rates there has been a less impressive increase in long-term survival reflecting the challenge of long-term management of LT recipients, a population under lifelong immunosuppression with increased risk of renal failure, cardiovascular events and malignancies.

Candidates

Careful patient selection is essential for the short- and long-term success of liver transplantation. LT should be considered in patients with irreversible and progressive liver disease without an alternative therapy in whom it is expected that LT will prolong life. Patients with an anticipated life expectancy without LT of 1 year or less should be considered for LT. As donor organs are scarce, attention must be paid to the expected outcome following LT. Patients should expect to have at least 50% chance of survival at 5 years [3]. A number of different models based on biochemical parameters are used throughout the world to identify candidates with a poor prognosis that might benefit from LT (MELD, UKELD). These scores allow for the establishment of a minimal listing threshold below which LT is not likely to add benefit. They also allow stratification of listed patients such that patients with more severe disease are afforded priority. Increasingly factors related to the donor and graft are considered in allocating organs to recipients in order to maximize 'transplant benefit' [4].

Indications for Liver Transplantation

Potential LT candidates can be broadly divided into five groups:

1. Patients with chronic liver disease (cirrhosis), of any aetiology, who develop a complication, namely ascites, spontaneous bacterial peritonitis (SBP) hepatic encephalopathy, variceal bleeding (particularly after medical therapy failure), synthetic dysfunction (hyperbilirubinaemia and/or coagulopathy) or worsening renal function.
2. Patients with acute liver failure (ALF) of any cause, defined by the development of hepatic encephalopathy within 12 weeks of the onset of acute liver injury and/or jaundice without previously recognized chronic liver disease.

3. Liver tumours, most commonly, patients with early hepato-cellular carcinoma meeting specific criteria who are not candidates for resection.
4. Variant syndromes where mortality risk is not reflected by commonly used prognostic scores such as MELD and UKELD. For example: hepatopulmonary syndrome, recurrent cholangitis, hepatic encephalopathy (requiring two or more hospital admissions within a 6-month period) and diuretic refractory ascites.
5. Metabolic or genetic diseases characterized by near-normal liver architecture and severe extrahepatic manifestations such as familial amyloid polyneuropathy, primary hyperoxaluria and familial hyperlipidaemia.

Increasingly, other indications for liver transplantation are being evaluated such as transplantation for cholangiocarcinoma, colorectal liver metastases and acute on chronic liver failure. These advances have been enabled by better understanding of the natural history of the disease and expanded access to previously unusable organs through the use of machine perfusion technology [5].

In Europe, 148,421 LT were performed between 1988 and June 2020, most of which were due to cirrhosis (54%), followed by cancers (18%) and cholestatic/congenital diseases (7%) [6]. ALF was responsible for 8% of LT performed in this period [6].

Prognostic Scoring Systems for End-Stage Liver Disease

The selection of patients and the timing of transplantation are key determinants for patient outcomes. Patients who are transplanted too early will be exposed to the risks of surgery and immunosuppression, whereas patients referred too late may be too sick for intervention. To help clinicians in this decision process, prognostic scoring systems have been developed to determine the need for transplantation (minimal listing criteria) and prioritize them in the waiting list based on liver disease severity and risk of mortality.

The Model of End-Stage Liver Disease (MELD)

MELD was developed in 2000 to determine the 3-month survival of patients with end-stage liver disease (ESLD) who underwent a TIPS placement after gastrointestinal bleeding. A modification was adapted to predict 90-day mortality of patients waiting for LT and replaced the Child-Pugh scoring system used in the USA since 2002. MELD has now been adopted in most liver transplantation networks to prioritize listed patients. The variables of MELD equation are serum bilirubin, creatinine and INR. Children under the age of 12 are assessed with a different system, the Paediatric End-Stage Liver Disease (PELD) score that does not include creatinine and uses bilirubin and INR (similarly to the MELD score) and albumin, age, growth failure.

MELD is used to prioritize patients for LT. A MELD of 15 is the point at which LT would be expected to improve 1 year survival and naturally, the higher the score the greater chance of dying and thus a higher priority for LT. Of note, this score also predicts mortality after LT in patients with MELD >35.

Modification of MELD (MELD-Na)

Since the adoption of MELD in liver transplant centre, attempts have been undertaken to further optimize the score. The most promising and frequently used score is the MELD-Na. This score incorporates serum sodium level with the MELD score and has shown to improve the prediction of mortality than the standard MELD and may also reduce listing mortality rate.

The United Kingdom Model for End-Stage Liver Disease (UKELD)

UKELD is a mathematical model that predicts mortality from liver cirrhosis. It was created from patients listed for LT at all UK liver transplant units and later validated in an independent prospective cohort. UKELD has now been adopted in all UK centres. The score is derived from serum bilirubin, creatinine, sodium and INR. Patients fulfil minimal listing criteria for LT when the UKELD is ≥49. This cut-off is used because it predicts a 1-year mortality of ≥9% without LT compared to the 9% 1-year mortality after LT. Since there are conditions that benefit from LT, but that are not mirrored by the UKELD score, the UK NHS Blood and Transplant Health Authority defined the variant syndromes that include patients that can be listed for LT even if their UKELD is lower than 49 (Table 17.1).

TABLE 17.1 Potential candidates for liver transplantation

1. Chronic liver disease with MELD ≥15 or UKELD ≥49 points

Alcoholic liver disease

Non-alcoholic fatty liver disease

Chronic viral hepatitis: Hepatitis B, C and D

Autoimmune liver diseases: Autoimmune hepatitis, primary biliary cholangitis, primary sclerosing cholangitis and overlap syndromes

Genetic diseases with predominant liver parenchymal damage: Genetic hemochromatosis, Wilson's disease, alpha-1-tripsin deficiency and tyrosinaemia

Secondary sclerosing cholangitis

Graft versus host disease

Budd-Chiari syndrome

Cryptogenic cirrhosis

2. Acute liver failure

Acetaminophen poisoning

Sero-negative or indeterminate

Amanita phalloides ingestion

Viral infections (e.g. hepatitis B)

Wilson's disease

Acute fatty liver of pregnancy

Autoimmune hepatitis

Primary non-function of liver graft

TABLE 17.1 (continued)

3. Malignant disease
Hepatocellular carcinoma
Epithelioid hemangio-endothelioma (can also be categorized as
a variant syndrome)
Hepatoblastoma
Cholangiocarcinoma

4. Variant syndromes
Diuretic resistant ascites (unresponsive or intolerant to
maximum diuretic dosage and nonresponsive to TIPS or where
TIPS is not feasible)
Chronic hepatic encephalopathy (confirmed by EEG or trail
making tests with at least two related admissions in 1 year not
responsive to medical therapy)
Intractable pruritus (after excluding a contributing psychiatric
co-morbidity)
Hepatopulmonary syndrome
Recurrent cholangitis (refractory to medical, surgical and
endoscopic therapy)
Genetic diseases associated with severe or life-threatening
extrahepatic complications: Crigler Najjar syndrome, urea cycle
disorders, familial amyloid polyneuropathy (FAP), primary
hyperoxaluria type 1, familial hypercholesterolaemia, glycogen
storage disease [2] and atypical haemolytic uremic syndromes
Polycystic liver disease

Adapted from the NHS Blood and Transplant Health Authority
Policy 195/4 Liver transplantation: Selection criteria and Recipient
Registration, March 2015

Super-Urgent LT

The indications and rules for urgent priority LT are similar in
most European centres and include patients with acute liver
failure (ALF) and patients with primary graft non-function of
the liver (PGNF) or graft failure due to vascular complications early after transplant. These patients represent a singu-
lar group of LT candidates compared to patients with chronic
liver disease, with a shorter time frame for (re)assessment
and (re)listing due to high short-term mortality without
transplant.

TABLE 17.2 Absolute and relative contraindications to liver transplantation

Absolute	Relative
– Psychological, physical and social inability to tolerate the procedure and comply with post-transplant treatments – Active and uncontrolled sepsis – Active extrahepatic, metastatic malignancy or cholangiocarcinoma[a] – AIDS – Advanced cardiopulmonary disease – Extensive portal and mesenteric vein thrombosis – Irreversible and severe brain damage – HCC and tumour rupture, extrahepatic spread or AFP >1000 ng/mL	– Age older than 65 and younger than 2 – Portal vein thrombosis – Prior porta-caval shunt – Prior complex hepato-biliary/abdominal surgery – Obesity (BMI ≥40 kg/m²) or malnutrition – HIV – Renal impairment (predictor of post-LT death) – Active alcohol and/or substance abuse – History of cancer <5 years

[a]Absolute contraindication in most centres. In case of perihilar cholangiocarcinoma LT can be offered in specialized centres with clinical research protocols

ALF patient selection for emergent LT is usually based on the King's College Hospital criteria (Table 17.2).

ALF secondary to paracetamol overdose:

1. pH <7.25 (>24 h post overdose) or
2. INR >6.5 (PT >100 s) and serum creatinine >300 μmol/L (>3.4 mg/dL) in patients with grade 3 or 4 hepatic encephalopathy.

Non-paracetamol associated ALF:

1. INR >6.5 (PT >100 s), or
2. Any three of the following:

Age <10 or >40 years; aetiology non-A, non-B hepatitis or idiosyncratic drug reaction; duration of jaundice before hepatic encephalopathy >7 days; INR >3.5 (PT >50 s); serum bilirubin >300 μmol/L (>17.6 mg/dL).

Malignant Liver Disease

Hepatocellular carcinoma (HCC) is the most common malignant cause for LT. It should be considered in patients with early HCC that is not resectable due to its location or concerns related to poor synthetic function and features of portal hypertension (e.g. hepatic venous pressure gradient ≥10 mmHg). Recurrent disease following LT is problematic for patients with advanced disease and hence LT is limited to patients with early HCC. The most widely used are the Milan Criteria. These help define patients with HCC and liver cirrhosis with a low risk of recurrence post-LT [7]. The Milan criteria are: one lesion with a diameter <5 cm or up to three nodules each ≤3 cm and no vascular invasion or metastatic disease. As experience has grown in the use of LT for HCC a number of groups have expanded cautiously on the Milan criteria. For instance, The University of California San Francisco (UCSF) criteria expand the number of patients eligible for LT by including single tumours up to 6.5 cm and several nodules, the largest up to 4.5 cm, as long as the total sum of all diameters is <8 cm. The recurrence free survival is similar when applying the UCSF and Milan criteria and guidelines now recommend that an expansion of the Milan Criteria is acceptable if recurrence free survival is comparable.

In the UK, listing criteria have been expanded beyond the Milan Criteria, since it was shown that some patients who had acceptable rates of recurrence were denied LT using the Milan criteria. The current UK criteria are: alpha feto-protein <1000 ng/mL, a single tumour diameter ≤5 cm, up to 5 nodules all ≤3 cm or a single tumour 5–7 cm without significant progression over 6 months with or without loco-regional therapy. In addition, HCC patients outside these criteria, who have undergone down staging loco-regional therapy may be listed if they fulfil recently defined criteria that reflect 'good' tumour biology [8].

In recent years several institutions have undertaken liver transplantation for the indications of perihilar cholangiocarcinoma. The Mayo protocol has been incorporated in these centres for patient selection. The protocol's inclusion criteria are perihilar cholangiocarcinoma unable to be resected that is less than 3 cm in patients who have no evidence of metastasis. Patients receive neoadjuvant chemotherapy prior to transplantation. Other indications such as strictly selected patients with oligo-metastatic colorectal cancer liver metastases are emerging. Whether these newer indications become established will depend on demonstrating equivalent outcomes to accepted indications and the availability of organs.

Absolute and Relative Contraindications to LT

Absolute contraindications include advanced and uncorrectable cardiopulmonary disease, ongoing infection, active extrahepatic malignancy, irreversible severe brain injury and inability to comply with post-transplantation treatment (Table 17.2).

Relative contraindications include factors related to the candidate fitness, past medical history and liver disease itself, which may increase the risk of LT in that particular patient, and outweigh the expected benefits such as portal vein thrombosis.

Advanced age is not a barrier to LT; however, patients ≥65 years have an increased risk of cardiovascular complications and should only be listed after a thorough assessment to exclude significant medical co-morbidities.

Active alcohol intake and substance abuse is an area of controversy and guidelines vary according to centres and countries. In many centres a 6 month abstinence period is mandated prior to LT. This period is considered beneficial since it identifies patients with a lower risk of relapse to alcohol use post-LT and, importantly, allows time for liver injury to recover such that LT may be avoided. The concept of an enforced period of abstinence can be challenged. For instance, there is limited evidence correlating the length of pre-treatment abstinence with post-transplant abstinence. Furthermore for patients with grade 3 acute on chronic liver failure (ACLF) or alcoholic hepatitis (AH) an enforced period of abstinence is unrealistic given the very high short-term mortality. Many centres worldwide now have protocols in place for transplantation of these very sick patients and report good outcomes (see below). Patients being considered for LT with a background of alcohol or substance misuse should be assessed by specialists in addiction to determine the risk of relapse following LT. Overall, the influence of relative contraindications on suitability for LT depends on the expertise of the transplantation team and should be assessed on a case-by-case basis.

An emerging and likely effective therapy for alcoholic hepatitis is liver transplantation. The seminal work by Mathurin et al. showed a significant 1 year survival benefit with liver transplantation of 77% compared to 23% with current management in the setting of life-threatening alcoholic hepatitis [9]. The average MELD in these patients was 34. The selection criteria for liver transplantation in these patients include: first liver decompensating event in patients, Maddrey discriminant function >32 and classified as a non-responder to corticosteroids with Lille score >0.45. The ACCELERATE-AH consortium in the US has published results of liver transplantation in 147 patients with life-threatening alcohol hepatitis achieving a 1 year survival of 94% and 84% at 3 years [10]. The mortality without transplant in this patient group would usually be 70% in 6 months showing the significant benefit of liver transplantation. Whilst scarcity of organs and patients selections have limited universal acceptance, the results show a clear mortality benefit.

Following assessment, the decision to list a patient for LT is ultimately made after a multidisciplinary discussion at a liver transplant centre involving transplant physicians, surgeons, anaesthetists, intensivists, dieticians and addiction and alcohol specialists. Once on the list patients undergo regular reassessment to ensure that they have developed no contraindications to LT. Patients may be withdrawn from the waiting list if there is a favourable clinical course after listing such that no need a LT criteria.

Pre-transplant Assessment

Pre-LT assessment is a fundamental step that allows the transplant team to identify and correct factors that may have a negative impact on LT outcome and/or bring to light conditions that are contraindications, e.g. extrahepatic malignancies.

Cardiopulmonary Assessment

All candidates should undergo an electrocardiogram and transthoracic echocardiogram. Patients with multiple cardiovascular risk factors should also undergo a cardiopulmonary exercise test (CPET) or a pharmacological stress test (nuclear medicine cardiac ischaemic studies, e.g. myoview, or dobutamine stress test) to rule out asymptomatic ischaemic heart disease. If coronary heart disease (CHD) is suspected a coronary angiogram should follow.

A lung function test and chest X-ray are the first line studies to assess respiratory function. If hepatopulmonary syndrome is suspected the alveolar-arterial oxygen gradient should be calculated and contrast echocardiography should be performed. Patients with evidence of pulmonary hypertension on echocardiography should undergo right heart catheterization to confirm this diagnosis. Moderate (mean pulmonary artery pressure ≥35 mmHg) and severe

(≥45 mmHg) PPHTN are associated with increased mortality after LT and should addressed with pulmonary vasodilators before LT.

Renal Assessment

Renal dysfunction has a negative impact on short-term survival after LT. All patients should have glomerular filtration rate estimated and urinalysis and renal ultrasound are recommended. A renal biopsy may be necessary to clarify the aetiology of renal dysfunction. A combined liver–kidney transplant should be considered in patients with GFR <30 mL/min or hepato-renal syndrome requiring renal replacement therapy for more than 8–12 weeks.

Imaging

A contrast CT scan of the chest and abdomen is mandatory to visualize the splanchnic vasculature, particularly, the hepatic artery and main portal system, in order to plan the surgical procedure. Alternatively, a MRI may be used, especially in patients with renal dysfunction and or HCC. Magnetic resonance cholangio-pancreatography is useful in the assessment of patients with sclerosing cholangitis. Occasionally, diagnostic ERCP may be required in this setting, e.g. patient unable to tolerate MRI.

Nutritional Assessment

An assessment by an experienced dietician is mandatory and malnutrition and sarcopenia should be addressed prior to LT. A bone densitometry is also part of the pre-transplant workup since osteoporosis is common in patients with liver cirrhosis. Frailty and sarcopenia have poor prognostication in the setting of cirrhosis and liver transplantation. The Liver Frailty Index (LFI) involves a simple bedside functional assessment of sarcopenia involving grip strength, chair stands and balance testing. Patients with a LFI of >0.45 defined as frail are recommended to be optimized prior to transplantation.

Finally, social and psychiatric assessment and counselling are vital to address potential risk factors for non-adherence and addictive behaviours prior to LT, including smoking cessation. All patients are strongly advised to stop smoking to reduce the cardiovascular and risk of malignancy that are exacerbated as a consequence of LT.

Liver Graft Allocation

In most organizations, when a deceased donor organ becomes available priority is given to super-urgent cases. If the organ is declined or there is no suitable recipient, then it is directed to elective LT in which organ allocation can be patient-directed or centre directed. In a centre oriented system the organ is allocated to a specific centre, and the decision of which patient will receive the organ is made by the centre's multidisciplinary team based on the internal prioritization system. In a patient-directed allocation system a particular organ is 'matched' to a recipient in order to maximize 'transplant benefit'.

The majority of liver grafts originate from deceased donors and can be further divided into donation after brain death (DBD) and donation after circulatory death (DCD).

In order to address organ shortage additional sources of organs are being used: such as 'marginal donors' and living donors. The so-called marginal donors or extended criteria donors (ECD) are donors with unfavourable features and traditionally associated with poorer graft and patient survival and include individuals with advanced age, significant steatosis, hepatitis B core antibody and HCV positive donors and DCD. DCDs are included in this group because they can associated with severe ischaemia-reperfusion injury, and also primary graft non-function, delayed graft function and biliary ischaemia. Scores have been developed to quantify the risk of graft failure by using these ECD, including the donor index risk and the 'balance of risk' score. In recent years the use of machine perfusion techniques which perfuse the retrieved organ and replenish ATP and other metabolites has been shown to be effective at preventing damage associated with cold storage whilst simultaneously allowing assessment of likely function once implanted. These techniques have increased the utilization and safety of previously unusable grafts and expanded the donor pool.

In live donor transplantation a partial liver graft is obtained usually from a family member or a close friend. The technique was initially used in children but has now been expanded for adults who usually receive the right lobe of the donor. In parts of Asia this is the commonest form of liver transplantation whereas in the USA and Europe live donor transplantation in adults is still infrequent mainly due to the very small risk to the donor.

The donor graft pool could be increased by splitting a cadaveric donor liver for two recipients usually an adult and a child. Partial grafts can also be used in auxiliary LT, in which a partial graft is introduced leaving the native liver in situ. This technique is occasionally used in ALF to support the patient's diseased liver whilst it recovers, and in patients with metabolic defects in which case the grafted liver corrects the metabolic disorder, without the need for a complete LT surgery.

Finally, domino LT is a process whereby a liver from a patient with familial amyloid polyneuropathy (FAP) (in who complications have developed but who otherwise have normal liver function) donate their liver. The recipient should be over 55 years to minimize the risk of the neurological consequences of FAP.

Liver Transplant Surgery

The donor organ is dissected and pre-cooled through the portal vein with Ringer's lactate. Secondly, the liver is perfused with 1000 mL of University of Wisconsin (UW) solution through the aorta and portal vein. The graft is then removed, flushed with 1000 mL of UW solution through the hepatic artery and stored in this solution in a plastic bag, afterwards placed on ice in a portable cooler. This retrieval technique has allowed for the liver preservation time to be extended up to 18 h.

In the recipient, the hilar structures and vena cava above and below the liver are dissected. The native liver is then removed after cross-clamping all the vascular structures and the new liver implanted in the right upper quadrant. Most European centres now use the piggy-back technique that preserves the recipient's inferior vena cava by anastomosing it side-to-side to the donor IVC (Fig. 17.1). The traditional

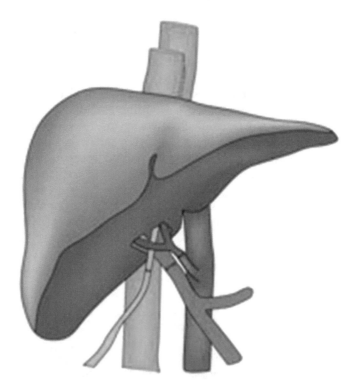

FIGURE 17.1 Piggyback technique

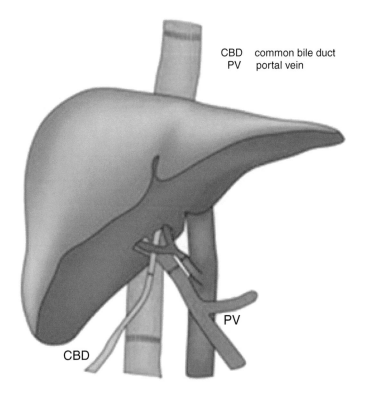

CBD   common bile duct
PV   portal vein

PV

CBD

FIGURE 17.2 Conventional transplant technique

caval reconstruction involves the removal of the recipient's IVC and vascular reconstruction with end-to-end anastomosis between the donor's IVC and the recipient infra and suprahepatic IVC (Fig. 17.2). The piggy-back technique is associated with less transfusion requirements, shorter warm ischemia time and less use of veno-venous bypass. Once vascular anastomoses are completed the preservation fluid is flushed out of the graft and the blood supply opened to the new liver. The bile duct reconstruction can be performed by direct anastomosis or by an end-to-side Roux-en-Y choledocojejunostomy, used in recipients with a diseased or absent bile duct.

Post-transplant Care

The specific major concerns after LT are primary graft non-function, acute cellular rejection, vascular and biliary complications and infections (viral, bacterial and fungal). The time period following LT will aid in the differential diagnosis of these conditions (Table 17.3).

TABLE 17.3 Complications of liver transplantation according to time after transplant

First week	Primary graft non-function (1–2 days)
	Bile leaks—post-surgical
	Renal—acute kidney injury, calcineurin inhibitor (CNI) toxicity
	Pulmonary—pulmonary embolus, pneumonia
	CNS—seizures, headache, cerebrovascular accident
1–4 weeks	Acute cellular rejection (from 5 to 10 days)
	Cholestasis—Dug induced, ischaemic
	Hepatic artery thrombosis
5–12 weeks	Cytomegalovirus (CMV) hepatitis
	Acute cellular rejection
	Biliary complications—Ischaemic strictures, anastomotic stricture
	Hepatic artery thrombosis
	Hepatitis C recurrence
12 weeks to 6 months	Acute cellular rejection
	Biliary complications—Ischaemic strictures, anastomotic stricture
	Hepatitis B recurrence
	Epstein-Barr hepatitis
	Drug-related hepatitis
> 6 months	Ductopenic rejection
	EBV hepatitis
	Portal vein thrombosis
	Disease recurrence (HBV, HCV, tumours)

Primary Graft Non-function

Primary graft non-function occurs in 5% of LT and is associated with severe graft dysfunction manifested by hepatic coma, coagulopathy, jaundice, hypoglycaemia, renal dysfunction, lactic acidosis and hemodynamic instability. It is mainly related to a long cold and warm ischemia times and graft steatosis.

Acute Cellular Rejection (ACR)

ACR occurs in virtually all patients but is usually mild as the liver is considered a privileged organ with a higher resistance to immunological attack. Immunosuppression is usually started on the first post-operative day of liver transplant with methylprednisolone, in addition to oral immunosuppressants, most usually the calcineurin inhibitor tacrolimus. In patients with pre-existing renal dysfunction the use of renal sparing agents such as basiliximab is used early post-transplant to avoid the need for early exposure to Tacrolimus which can be nephrotoxic.

Acute or hepatocellular rejection requiring treatment escalation occurs usually after 5–20 days after LT in around 20% of patients. Clinical signs are non-specific and liver function tests lack specificity for the diagnosis (although a flare in ALT >100 IU/L, AST >100 IU/L, rising ALP or eosinophilia might be suggestive), so liver biopsy is mandatory for the diagnosis. The histological picture is the classic triad of portal inflammation, bile duct injury mediated by lymphocytes and venous endothelialitis. Increasing immunosuppression usually with high dose corticosteroids is the cornerstone of treatment and is effective in 90% of patients. In case of non-response further doses of corticosteroids or lymphocyte depleting antibodies may be needed to avoid chronic rejection and the need for re-transplantation.

Chronic or ductopenic rejection occurs in 2–5% of LT and is characterized by progressive loss of bile ducts and a cholestatic liver function tests. Liver biopsy is also needed for diagnosis and depicts loss of interlobular and septal bile ducts in 50% of the portal tracts. Chronic rejection is usually irreversible. Notably, only <2% of grafts are now lost due to chronic rejection.

Post-transplantation Infections

Roughly 60% of LT experience an infection, a major cause of morbidity and mortality after LT. Infections that occur during the first month after LT are nosocomial infections related to surgery, including pneumonia, wound sepsis, liver abscess and biliary sepsis. In contrast, opportunist infections, such as CMV, and reactivation of latent infections occur 2–6 months after LT when the immunosuppression is its peak.

The infection prophylaxis protocols used in most transplant centres reflect this vulnerability to infection and include: surgical antibiotic prophylaxis, anti-viral agents against CMV and HSV, co-trimoxazole for Pneumocystis jirovecii (6–12 months) and fluconazole against Candida.

CMV infection is the most important opportunist infection. Risk factors are CMV positive donor in a CMV negative recipient, past acute rejection and intense immunosuppression. Patients present with a mononucleosis-like syndrome and the bone marrow, gastrointestinal tract, retina and liver may be involved. In some centres routine prophylaxis with oral valganciclovir is effective; however, there is concern with the emergence of resistant strains. Another strategy is to regularly determine CMV viraemia and start therapy if persistent or increasing viraemia occurs or when disease develops. Intravenous ganciclovir is reserved for patients with severe infections.

Vascular Complications

A routine US Doppler is performed in all transplanted patients on the first post-operative day to assess vascular anastomoses patency. Hepatic artery thrombosis has an incidence of 1–7% and presents with graft dysfunction. Less commonly, it may be silent and present days to weeks later with ischaemic biliary lesions (ischaemic cholangiopathy) or recurrent bacteraemia and liver abscess. A Doppler ultrasound and/or CT scan is diagnostic. Therapeutic options include re-intervention and revascularization or re-transplantation. A hepatic artery stenosis results from anastomosis narrowing or kinking. A Doppler ultrasound will confirm the diagnosis and repair is surgical (if early in the post-operative course) or by angioplasty.

Reported portal vein thrombosis incidence is heterogeneous varying from 2.1% to 26%. It may present with graft dysfunction or ascites and bleeding due to portal hypertension. Surgical revision and thrombectomy may save the graft. If not, re-transplantation is necessary.

Biliary Complications

Post-surgical bile leaks are rare, occurring in 5% of LT. When they occur early (<30 days) they may present with localized/generalized peritonitis and/or biliary output from the drains. ERCP and plastic stent placement is the usual treatment; however, re-operation and surgical revision may be necessary. Anastomotic extrahepatic bile duct strictures have an incidence of 4–9% and usually present months after LT with intermittent fever, slow increase of bilirubin and an increase in alkaline phosphatase. It may be related to surgical technique, hepatic arterial problems and bile leaks. Magnetic resonance cholangiography allows the diagnosis. Treatment involves ERCP with balloon dilatation and/or plastic biliary stent placement which may need to be repeated. Resistant strictures may lead to the need for surgical biliary reconstruction. Ischaemic cholangiopathy results from progressive and indolent ischaemic damage of the bile ducts and resulting ischaemic strictures. Risk factors for this type of injury are AB0 incompatibility, prolonged cold ischemia time, hepatic artery thrombosis, rejection and DCD donors. Patients present with pruritus and cholestasis, as well as recurrent cholangitis. Magnetic resonance cholangiography is useful to identify the typical beaded appearance produced by the intrahepatic strictures and narrowing of the donor common hepatic duct. ERCP with balloon dilatation or stenting may improve cholestasis and treat cholangitis if a dominant stenosis is identified. Hepato-jejunostomy or re-transplantation is the definitive treatment.

Long-Term Follow-Up

De novo malignancies and cardiovascular diseases are the major causes of death in the long-term largely due to the lifelong immunosuppression. In addition, disease recurrence in the graft should be monitored. The prevalence of metabolic syndrome is 50–60% in LT patients and there is a significant risk of cardiovascular events with an incidence of 10% at 5 years and 25% at 10 years. A regular assessment of cardiovascular risk and treatment of modifiable factors relating to obesity, diabetes mellitus, hypertension and dyslipidaemia are of paramount importance.

After LT there is an increased risk of malignancy, with reported incidences of 3–26% according to follow-up duration. Skin cancer, particularly non-melanoma, is the most frequent de novo cancer in this group and risk factors include: older age, chronic sun exposure and a prior history of skin cancer. Patients with a history of alcohol abuse and smoking are at increased risk of oesophageal, oropharyngeal-laryngeal and lung cancers. Lymphoproliferative disorders are also a concern, particularly in patients with positive EBV serology and under aggressive immunosuppression combinations. The tumour presents in lymph nodes or the graft and should be suspected in patients with fever, weight loss and night sweats even in the absence of lymphadenopathy since it can affect the graft. Treatment involves reducing immunosuppression. Systemic chemotherapy may improve survival and treatment with rituximab has improved prognosis. Finally, patients with

PSC and inflammatory bowel disease have an increased risk of colorectal cancer and should undergo an annual colonoscopy. Annual cancer screening protocols should be implemented to address these issues and advice given with regard to smoking cessation, sun avoidance, use of sun blocks and optimizing doses of immunosuppression.

Prognosis

Re-transplantation is necessary in 7–10% of patients due to graft loss. The main indications can be divided into early (e.g. primary graft non-function and hepatic artery thrombosis) and late (e.g. ischaemic cholangiopathy, ductopenic and recurrence of primary liver disease).

At 1 year after LT survival rates vary between 71% for ALF and 95% for elective indications. Ten years following LT survival is 48% for patients transplanted for malignant tumours and around 70% in patients transplanted for chronic liver disease, benign tumours and metabolic diseases.

Overall quality of life after LT is good in the majority of patients who return to normal social, familial and work activities. The advent of LT has been a major advance in the treatment of advanced liver disease and has revolutionized the survival prospects for these patients who would otherwise have been consigned to a premature death. The pioneering work of the surgeons, physicians and scientists who enabled this breakthrough must not be underestimated. Nevertheless, the burden of lifelong immunosuppression and their side effects can have an impact and should be sought in the clinic.

Case Study Answers

1. **Should this patient be referred for liver transplantation based on the severity of his liver disease?**

    In this case we have a patient with NASH cirrhosis who had three admissions for chronic encephalopathy despite medical therapy. An EEG supported the diagnosis of chronic hepatic encephalopathy and a head CT ruled out structural neurological disease. For this reason, although his UKELD score was <49, the patient was referred for LT since he fulfilled the criteria for a variant syndrome.

2. **What aspects of the patient's medical history should be examined closely during transplant assessment?**

   The history of portal vein thrombosis (PVT) should be clarified. If it is an acute event and the patient is to be listed for LT, anticoagulation should be started. Conversely, PVT is not a contraindication, but is an important feature that will also impact the type of transplant surgery performed. An anastomosis between the donor portal vein and the recipient confluence of superior mesenteric vein or the use of a venous graft from the donor are possible options.

   The second factor to consider is the diagnosis of NASH cirrhosis that is usually associated with obesity, diabetes or metabolic syndrome. In this setting, a thorough cardiovascular assessment should include a cardiopulmonary exercise test to exclude ischaemic heart disease.

   Finally, the increased creatinine suggests the existence of renal dysfunction that should be investigated, with diabetic nephropathy considered in the differential diagnosis as this may be progressive after transplantation and may influence the choice and timing of the immunosuppressant regimen over the perioperative and early post-transplant period.

3. **Is the patients age a barrier to receiving a liver transplant?**

   Age is currently not a contraindication and the patient should be referred. However listing will depend on the pre-transplant evaluation and multidisciplinary team assessment of the individual case.

Bibliography

1. Starzl TE, Marchioro TL, Vonkaulla KN, Hermann G, Brittain RS, Waddell WR. Homotransplantation of the liver in humans. Surg Gynecol Obstet. 1963;117:659–76. PMID: 14100514; PMCID: PMC2634660.

2. Adam R, Karam V, Delvart V, O'Grady J, Mirza D, Klempnauer J, Castaing D, Neuhaus P, Jamieson N, Salizzoni M, Pollard S, Lerut J, Paul A, Garcia-Valdecasas JC, Rodríguez FS, Burroughs A. All contributing centers (www.eltr.org); European Liver and Intestine Transplant Association (ELITA). Evolution of indications and results of liver transplantation in Europe. A report from the European Liver Transplant Registry (ELTR). J Hepatol. 2012;57(3):675–88. https://doi.org/10.1016/j.jhep.2012.04.015. Epub 2012 May 16. PMID: 22609307.

3. Neuberger J, James O. Guidelines for selection of patients for liver transplantation in the era of donor-organ shortage. Lancet. 1999;354(9190):1636–9. https://doi.org/10.1016/S0140-6736(99)90002-8. PMID: 10560692.

4. Tschuor C, Ferrarese A, Kuemmerli C, Dutkowski P, Burra P, Clavien PA, Liver Allocation Study Group. Allocation of liver grafts worldwide—is there a best system? J Hepatol. 2019;71(4):707–18. https://doi.org/10.1016/j.jhep.2019.05.025. Epub 2019 Jun 12. PMID: 31199941.

5. Mergental H, Laing RW, Kirkham AJ, Perera MTPR, Boteon YL, Attard J, Barton D, Curbishley S, Wilkhu M, Neil DAH, Hübscher SG, Muiesan P, Isaac JR, Roberts KJ, Abradelo M, Schlegel A, Ferguson J, Cilliers H, Bion J, Adams DH, Morris C, Friend PJ, Yap C, Afford SC, Mirza DF. Transplantation of discarded livers following viability testing with normothermic machine perfusion. Nat Commun. 2020;11(1):2939. https://doi.org/10.1038/s41467-020-16251-3. PMID: 32546694; PMCID: PMC7298000.

6. ELTR. http://www.eltr.org/Overall-indication-and-results.html. Accessed 17 Oct 2021.

7. Mazzaferro V, Regalia E, Doci R, Andreola S, Pulvirenti A, Bozzetti F, Montalto F, Ammatuna M, Morabito A, Gennari L. Liver transplantation for the treatment of small hepatocellular carcinomas in patients with cirrhosis. N Engl J Med. 1996;334(11):693–9. https://doi.org/10.1056/NEJM199603143341104. PMID: 8594428.

8. Duvoux C, Roudot-Thoraval F, Decaens T, Pessione F, Badran H, Piardi T, Francoz C, Compagnon P, Vanlemmens C, Dumortier J, Dharancy S, Gugenheim J, Bernard PH, Adam R, Radenne S, Muscari F, Conti F, Hardwigsen J, Pageaux GP, Chazouillères O, Salame E, Hilleret MN, Lebray P, Abergel A, Debette-Gratien M, Kluger MD, Mallat A, Azoulay D, Cherqui D, Liver Transplantation French Study Group. Liver transplantation for hepatocellular carcinoma: a model including α-fetoprotein

improves the performance of Milan criteria. Gastroenterology. 2012;143(4):986–94.e3; quiz e14–5. https://doi.org/10.1053/j.gastro.2012.05.052. Epub 2012 Jun 29. PMID: 22750200.

9. Mathurin P, Moreno C, Samuel D, Dumortier J, Salleron J, Durand F, Castel H, Duhamel A, Pageaux GP, Leroy V, Dharancy S, Louvet A, Boleslawski E, Lucidi V, Gustot T, Francoz C, Letoublon C, Castaing D, Belghiti J, Donckier V, Pruvot FR, Duclos-Vallée JC. Early liver transplantation for severe alcoholic hepatitis. N Engl J Med. 2011;365(19):1790–800. https://doi.org/10.1056/NEJMoa1105703. PMID: 22070476.

10. Lee BP, Mehta N, Platt L, Gurakar A, Rice JP, Lucey MR, Im GY, Therapondos G, Han H, Victor DW, Fix OK, Dinges L, Dronamraju D, Hsu C, Voigt MD, Rinella ME, Maddur H, Eswaran S, Hause J, Foley D, Ghobrial RM, Dodge JL, Li Z, Terrault NA. Outcomes of early liver transplantation for patients with severe alcoholic hepatitis. Gastroenterology. 2018;155(2):422–30.e1. https://doi.org/10.1053/j.gastro.2018.04.009. Epub 2018 Apr 12. PMID: 29655837; PMCID: PMC6460480.

Chapter 18
The Hepatological Curiosities

Charmaine Matthews and Tim Cross

Key Learning Points
- One must always try to remember the rarer causes of liver disease when appropriate.
- Discussion with or referral to a specialist centre is advised.
- Isolated hyperbilirubinaemia is most commonly due to Gilbert's disease or haemolytic disease.
- Amyloidosis is a multi-system disease with a number of causes. Liver transplantation is a treatment for some patients.
- Schistosomiasis should be remembered in patients (particularly with portal hypertension) returning from endemic regions.
- Sarcoidosis must be considered in at-risk groups, particularly in the presence of respiratory problems, hypercalcaemia and an infiltrative blood picture.
- Wilson's disease should be considered in younger patients with liver abnormalities, particularly in the face of psychiatric or neurological symptoms and signs.

C. Matthews · T. Cross (✉)
Royal Liverpool University Hospital, Liverpool, UK
e-mail: tim.cross@liverpoolft.nhs.uk

© Springer Nature Switzerland AG 2022   381
T. Cross (ed.), *Liver Disease in Clinical Practice*, In Clinical
Practice, https://doi.org/10.1007/978-3-031-10012-3_18

Questions

1. Which of the following statements are true of these rare liver diseases?

   (a) Wilson's disease is characterised by a failure to excrete iron?
   (b) Kayser-Fleischer rings and a very low caeruloplasmin (<0.1 g/L) are diagnostic of Wilsons disease?
   (c) Urinary copper excretion is low?
   (d) The penicillamine challenge test is recommended in adults?
   (e) Trientine is an effective treatment?

2. Which of the following statements are true?

   (a) Alagille's disease often improves as the patient gets older?
   (b) Patients may have a flattened nose and pointed chin?
   (c) There are defects in the JAG1 gene?
   (d) Hepatic sarcoidosis often presents with cholestatic liver function tests?
   (e) BRIC is caused by a defect in the caused by mutations in the *ATP8B1* gene (18q21)?

Familial Non-haemolytic Hyperbilirubinaemias

See Table 18.1.

Gilbert's Syndrome

Background

A genetic disorder causing a deficiency of the glucuronyl transferase enzyme required for conjugation in the liver causing an isolated unconjugated hyperbilirubinaemia. Characterised by periods of jaundice, precipitated by illness, starvation and alcohol excess [1–3].

TABLE 18.1 The familial non-haemolytic hyperbilirubinaemias

Type	Diagnosis and treatment
Unconjugated	
Haemolysis	Splenomegaly, blood film, reticulocyte count, coombs test, lactate dehydrogenase, haptoglobin
Gilbert's syndrome	Jaundice mild (normally <70 μol/L). Affects up to 5% population. Familial. Bilirubin but other liver enzymes normal. Bilirubin elevated with fasting. Normal liver biopsy. DNA analysis
	No specific treatment needed
Crigler-Najjar Syndrome (glucuronyl transferase deficiency)	
Type I	No conjugative enzyme in liver. No phenobarbitone response, gene expression analysis, risk of kernicterus
	Liver transplantation may be needed
Type II	Absent or deficient conjugative enzyme in liver
	Liver biochemistry improves in response to phenobarbitone
Conjugated	
Dubin-Johnson syndrome	Black liver biopsy
	Secondary rise in BSP test
Rotor type	Normal liver biopsy. Raised urinary coproporphyrin
	BSP test no uptake
Other causes of hyperpigmentation	Carotenaemia, melanosis, haemochromatosis, hypo-adrenalism

BSB bromosulphalein

Diagnosis

Split bilirubin demonstrates an unconjugated (indirect) hyperbilirubinaemia. FBC, LDH, reticulocyte count and haptoglobin should be checked to ensure not caused by haemolysis.

Treatment

No treatment required. To prevent future episodes, avoid periods of starvation and consume alcohol within recommended limits.

Prognosis

No deleterious consequences and is associated with a normal life expectancy.

Alagille Syndrome

Background

Syndromic paucity of intrahepatic bile ducts [1]. A genetic condition related to the deletion on the short arm of chromosome 20 on jagged 1 (JAG1) gene which encodes Notch 2. Patients have chronic intrahepatic cholestasis. Patients have a characteristic triangular face with a flattened nose and a pointed chin (Fig. 18.1).

Diagnosis

Clinical manifestations include hepatosplenomegaly, short distal phalanges, butterfly vertebrae, retinal pigmentation, renal abnormalities and peripheral pulmonary arterial stenosis. A genetic test is available to substantiate the diagnosis.

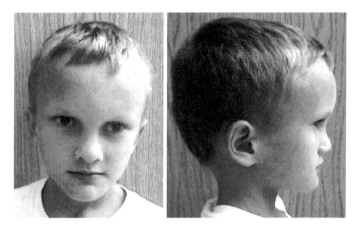

FIGURE 18.1 Characteristic facies of Alagille syndrome [8]

Liver biopsy shows scanty interlobular bile ducts. Portal fibrosis is not a feature so cirrhosis and portal hypertension do not develop.

Treatment

No treatment needed, tends to improve with time.

Prognosis

Patient survives into adult life but there can be growth and mental retardation. Hepatocellular carcinoma has been observed, but additional factors can be contributory to this.

Caroli Disease

Background

This is characterised by non-obstructive saccular or fusiform dilatation of the intrahepatic bile ducts. This can be associated with stone formation and recurrent cholangitis. *Caroli syndrome* is associated with congenital hepatic fibrosis [1, 2]. Renal disease is commonly observed in both variants including renal tubular ectasia, autosomal recessive and autosomal dominant forms of polycystic kidney disease.

Diagnosis

Patients may present with complications due to recurrent biliary sepsis or with variceal bleeding from portal hypertension. Kidneys may be palpable. Liver biochemistry is often normal with only modest elevations in bilirubin, aminotransferases and alkaline phosphatase, being seen. USS, CT and MRCP are useful to demonstrate the biliary tree abnormalities.

Mutations in polycystic kidney and hepatic disease 1 gene (PKHD1) have been seen in autosomal recessive polycystic kidney disease.

Liver histology may be normal or show features consistent with chronic cholangitis. In congenital hepatic fibrosis (CHF), ductal plate malformations are observed.

Prognosis and Treatment

Cholangitis is treated with antibiotics. Bile duct stones are removed endoscopically. There is an increased risk of cholangiocarcinoma, and portal hypertension can be seen in CHF which is managed as previously described (see 'portal hypertension' chapter). Liver transplant may be required for recurrent sepsis, and TIPs may be needed for complications of portal hypertensive bleeding. Renal dialysis or renal transplantation may be needed for some patients with end-stage renal failure.

Benign Recurrent Intrahepatic Cholestasis (BRIC) and Progressive Familial Intrahepatic Cholestasis (PFIC)

Background

This is a hereditary liver disorder characterised by intermittent episodes of intrahepatic cholestasis. Two forms of BRIC are described (BRIC1 and BRIC2). Both BRIC1 and BRIC2 are inherited in an autosomal recessive manner [4]. The prevalence of BRIC is unknown. BRIC is now believed to belong to a clinical spectrum of intrahepatic cholestatic disorders that ranges from the mild intermittent attacks in BRIC to the severe, chronic and progressive cholestasis seen in progressive familial intrahepatic cholestasis (PFIC).

BRIC1 is allelic to PFIC1 (see this term) and is caused by mutations in the *ATP8B1* gene (18q21) encoding a P-type ATPase expressed at the canalicular membrane of hepatocytes as well as in other epithelia. BRIC2 is allelic to PFIC2 (see this term) and is caused by mutations in the *ABCB11* gene (2q24) encoding the liver-specific bile salt export pump (BSEP). The disease-causing mutations in BRIC are generally missense mutations.

BRIC1 can display extra-hepatic features such as hearing loss, pancreatitis and diarrhoea. Cholelithiasis is a common manifestation of BRIC2. Patients with BRIC2 have a risk of hepatobiliary malignancy.

PFIC exists in three forms: PFIC1, PFIC2 and PFIC3. Disease may present in childhood or early adulthood. Other problems may be associated with PFIC1 (deafness, short stature, pancreatic disease, diarrhoea).

Diagnosis

Patients present with episodes of pruritus and jaundice. Manifestations include fatigue, loss of appetite, dark urine and pale stools. Hepatomegaly is a common finding. Between episodes patients show no symptoms and the interval between attacks varies from months to years. The factors triggering attacks are not entirely known but may include viral infections, pregnancy and the oral contraceptive pill.

Diagnosis is based on the clinical history (at least 2–3 episodes of cholestasis), serum biochemistry (low to normal serum gamma GT activity and cholesterol, elevated serum total bile acids and high levels of conjugated bilirubin during episodes), cholangiography (showing normal intra- and extrahepatic bile ducts), liver histology (revealing intrahepatic cholestasis with normal liver structure) and immuno-histochemical analysis (absent or reduced BSEP staining in majority of BRIC2 patients). Molecular genetic testing confirms the diagnosis and discriminates between subtypes.

Treatment

Management is mainly symptomatic: rifampicin and cholestyramine can be used to reduce pruritus and to induce remission of a cholestatic episode in some patients. Plasmapheresis/MARS (molecular adsorbents recirculation system) has also been shown to be of benefit in some cases. For individuals that are unresponsive to medical therapy, endoscopic nasobiliary drainage is generally effective. Partial external biliary diversion is also used to improve quality of life and prevent disease progression. Liver transplantation may eventually be indicated for patients with frequent and severe episodes.

Prognosis

The prognosis is generally good with a tendency for a reduction in the frequency of attacks with age. However, progression from BRIC to PFIC and cirrhosis has been reported.

PFIC may develop cirrhosis, HCC (especially PFIC2) and may require liver transplantation.

Amyloidosis

Background

Amyloidosis describes a group of conditions characterised by the extra-cellular deposition of amyloid protein [3]. There are different subtypes with varying presentations:

• AL amyloidosis or primary amyloidosis

• Fibril: Monoclonal immunoglobulin light chain

• This subtype is caused by an abnormality of the plasma cell which leads to folding of immunoglobulin light chains. It is the most common form in the developed world. It can affect liver, heart, kidney or nerves.
• AA amyloidosis or secondary amyloidosis
• Fibril: Serum amyloid A
• Usually secondary to a chronic inflammatory condition such as rheumatoid arthritis or familial Mediterranean fever (FMF). Most commonly affects kidneys, liver, spleen.
• FMF is a genetic disorder causing chronic inflammation. It manifests as recurrent fever, pleurisy and sterile synovitis. It is more commonly seen in Armenian, Turkish, Middle-eastern and certain Jewish populations.
• ATTR amyloidosis

• Fibril: Transthyretin

• This is a hereditary form of amyloidosis secondary to abnormal transthyretin protein formed in the liver. It can affect the eyes, adrenals, heart, spleen and nerves.

Diagnosis

Blood and urine tests can be useful in the work up for potential consequences, e.g. impaired renal function, proteinuria.

Histology: Amyloid shows apple green birefringence on polarisation of Congo red staining.

Amyloid is deposited in the columns of liver cells and the sinusoidal walls in the space of Disse.

Biopsy of abdominal fat.

Rectal biopsy.

Liver biopsy is associated with haemorrhage in up to 5% of cases.

Treatment

AL—chemotherapy/immunomodulators
AA—treat underlying inflammatory condition
FMF—colchicine
ATTR—liver transplant

Prognosis

Dependent on subtype. Historically AL amyloidosis patients have done the worst. Patients with amyloid must be referred to the local/national amyloid centre for evaluation and management.

Sarcoidosis

Background

Sarcoidosis is a chronic systemic disorder of unknown aetiology. Hepatic involvement is seen in 60–90% of cases. Organ dysfunction occurs as a result of inflammation and fibrosis development. Granulomas are seen around the portal tracts without caseation (Fig. 18.2) [1, 3]. A list of conditions causing hepatic granulomas is shown in Table 18.2.

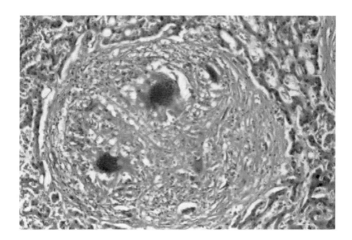

FIGURE 18.2 Fibrosing epithelioid granuloma with giant cells from a liver biopsy in a patient with sarcoidosis [9]

TABLE 18.2 Causes of hepatic granulomas

Disease	Diagnostic tests
AIDS	AIDS defining illnesses, HIV positivity, HIV RNA CD4 count
Berylliosis	Industrial exposure; agglutinin titre
Brucellosis	Blood culture, agglutinin titre
Drug reaction	Clinical history
Histoplasmosis	Chest X-ray, history, complement fixation
Infectious mononucleosis	Blood film, lymphopenias, monospot test, EBV IgM
Leprosy	Skin testing
Lymphoma	Staging CT, lymph node biopsy, LDH
Sarcoidosis	Serum ACE, chest X-ray, CT, broncho-alveolar lavage
Syphilis	Treponemal haemagglutination (TPHA), VDRL
Tuberculosis	History, chest X-ray, CT findings, culture sputum and/or urine, quantiferon test, acid fast bacilli detection in sputum, histology

AIDS Acquired Immunodeficiency Syndrome, *EBV* Epstein-Barr Virus, *LDH* lactate dehydrogenase, *CT* computer tomography, *VDRL* venereal disease research laboratory

Diagnosis

Many patients are asymptomatic. The condition is more common in young black people. Among Caucasians women over 40 years are more commonly affected. Typically patients have an elevated alkaline phosphatase with slight elevation in IgG. Aminotransferase levels may be increased. Chest radiograph, CT chest, spirometry and serum ACE (elevated) levels may help. Splenomegaly may not always mean portal hypertension in this setting. There may be intrahepatic cholestasis.

Treatment and Prognosis

No treatment may be necessary. There has been some use of ursodeoxycholic acid and corticosteroids, but their use is controversial. Decompensated liver disease should be managed in the usual way and patients with end-stage liver disease may benefit from liver transplantation. Prognosis is related to the severity of the underlying lung and liver disease.

Budd-Chiari Syndrome

Background

Budd-Chiari syndrome is caused by occlusion of the hepatic veins either by thrombus or due to mechanical narrowing of these veins. It classically presents with the triad of hepatomegaly, ascites and pain. The disease is rare and can be asymptomatic or present as fulminant hepatic failure. Patients can present with mild liver function derangement, but they can also have jaundice and if there is either chronic or acute liver failure patients may have hepatic encephalopathy [1, 3].

The causes of Budd-Chiari syndrome include diseases associated with thrombus formation (primary Budd-Chiari syndrome) including polycythaemia rubra vera, pregnancy, post-partum, malignancy, thrombophilic disorders (protein C and protein S deficiency, paroxysmal nocturnal haemoglobin-uria, lupus anticoagulant, factor V Leiden deficiency).

Secondary Budd-Chiari syndrome is characterised by extrinsic compression on the hepatic veins, but can also be associated with other conditions including congenital venous webs and stenosis of the inferior vena-cava.

Diagnosis

Diagnosis is made on Doppler ultrasound to assess patency of portal and hepatic veins. Further imaging with dual-phase CT of the liver to assess the hepatic vessels or liver magnetic resonance venography may be required.

If doubt persists hepatic venography and liver biopsy may be required to fully delineate the anatomy and decide the best approach.

A thrombophilia screen is recommended along with a test for the *JAK2* mutation.

Treatment

Treatment may be conservative with control of ascites and thrombus with a combination of diuretics and anti-coagulants. However, further intervention is often required. If thrombus is relatively new, transjugular intrahepatic porto-systemic shunting (TIPS) may be beneficial. There is some description of thrombolysis in this setting but it is not standard practice. If there is a mechanical obstruction or congenital abnormality, stenting of the affected vessel may be sufficient. Liver transplantation is now seldom used, but may be reserved for patients presenting with fulminant hepatic failure.

Prognosis

This depends on the cause of the Budd-Chiari and may be determined by factors associated with poor survival in liver disease as well as risk factors for thrombophilia that may lead to acute leukaemias (e.g. JAK2 mutation).

Hepato-pulmonary Syndrome

Background

The triad of liver disease, arterial hypoxaemia and intrapulmonary vascular dilatation has defined an entity commonly referred to as the hepato-pulmonary syndrome (HPS). With an estimated prevalence of 4–47%, it is a complication of chronic liver disease associated with portal hypertension (with or without cirrhosis) [5].

Diagnosis

Patients usually present with features of chronic liver disease but dyspnoea may be the main presenting symptom.

More characteristic features noted in HPS are:

- *Platypnoea* defined as increase in dyspnoea whilst sat upright/relieved by recumbency.
- *Orthodeoxia* defined by decrease in the arterial oxygen tension (by more than 4 mmHg [0.5 kPa]) or arterial oxyhaemoglobin desaturation (by more than 5%) when the patient moves from a supine to an upright position and vice versa.

Specific diagnostic criteria for hepato-pulmonary syndrome:
- Chronic liver disease.
- PaO_2 < 70 mmHg or alveolar–arterial oxygen gradient >20 mmHg.
- Intrapulmonary vascular dilatations.

Investigations

Contrast enhanced echocardiography or bubble echocardiography.
  Nuclear scanning to assess lung perfusion.

Treatment

No established medical management other than symptomatic management with oxygen therapy. Liver transplantation may result in complete resolution of this syndrome.

Porto-pulmonary Hypertension

Background

Porto-pulmonary hypertension (PPH) is considered present when pulmonary arterial hypertension (PAH) exists in a patient who has co-existing portal hypertension, and no alternative cause of the PAH exists (e.g. collagen vascular disease, congenital heart disease, or certain drugs). The aetiology is related to a complex association among the hyperdynamic, high flow circulatory state, excess central volume and non-embolic pulmonary vasoconstriction/obliteration [5, 6].

Diagnosis

Patients present with features of both portal and pulmonary hypertension. The most common presenting pulmonary symptoms were dyspnoea on exertion, syncope, chest pain, fatigue, haemoptysis and orthopnoea.
  The specific diagnostic criteria for porto-pulmonary hypertension must include the presence of the following:

1. Portal hypertension
2. Mean pulmonary artery pressure (MPAP) >25 mmHg
3. Capillary wedge pressure (PCWP) <15 mmHg
4. Pulmonary vascular resistance (PVR) >120 dynes s cm^{-5}

Screening tests: Chest radiography, electrocardiography and most importantly, transthoracic Doppler echocardiography to estimate pulmonary artery systolic pressure.

Right heart catheterisation is necessary to confirm the diagnosis of PAH and estimate its severity. Hepatic venous wedge pressure should also be measured during catheterisation to determine the severity of portal hypertension if porto-pulmonary hypertension is suspected.

Treatment

Treatment options are mainly derived from those used to treat idiopathic pulmonary hypertension (IPH). Current treatments include:

1. Epoprostenol, Bosentan, Ambrisentan, Sildenafil, Iloprost (prostacyclin analogue) are some of the drugs shown to improve haemodynamics and exercise performance; as a result, they are often considered as a bridge to liver transplantation.
2. Liver transplantation: Variable outcomes reported with increased intra- and perioperative mortality. For patients with severe PPH (MPAP >50 mmHg operative mortality from liver transplant was 100%, between 35 and 50 mmHg mortality 50% and <35 mmHg, perioperative mortality was 0%).

It is recommended that treatments are only commenced by clinicians experienced in managing porto-pulmonary hypertension.

Schistosomiasis

Background

Schistosomiasis (bilharzia) is an infection caused by a parasitic flatworm that is often released by freshwater snails [1, 3].

The parasite is found throughout Africa, but also lives in parts of South America, the Caribbean, the Middle East and Asia. It is associated with acute and chronic forms of disease.

The common variants of parasite include: schistosoma mansoni (found in South America, Caribbean, Africa and the Middle East); schistosoma haematobium (Africa and the Middle East); schistosoma japonicum found in the Far East), whilst schistosoma mekongi and schistosoma intercalatum are found locally in Southeast Asia and central West Africa, respectively.

Diagnosis

Clinical manifestations include the following:

Intestinal Schistosomiasis: Egg formation pre-sinusoidally can lead to portal hypertension and varices. (These should be managed as discussed in an earlier chapter.)

As the damage is pre-sinusoidal there is no cirrhosis. Hepatosplenomegaly can be observed.

Dermatitis: Swimmers itch.

Katayama fever: Acute schistosomiasis occurring weeks or months after the initial infection. It is associated with fever, lethargy, cutaneous bumps with an urticarial rash, liver and spleen enlargement and bronchospasm.

Chronic disease: This occurs due to chronic inflammation caused by the egg deposition in tissue. The eggs secrete proteolytic enzymes causing an eosinophilic reaction in the tissue in which they are found, e.g. brain, liver, intestines, bladder, etc.

- Bladder cancer is associated with schistosoma haematobium.
- Uro-genital lesions have been believed to increase the risk of HIV infection in some parts of Africa.
- Cerebral granulomatous disease has been linked with seizures, together with transverse myelitis and flaccid paralysis.

FAST-ELISA: This method is good for mansoni and haematobium (both sensitivity >95%), but less good for japonicum (sensitivity 50%).

Laboratory testing.

Immuno-blot techniques.

Treatment

The best treatment would be disease avoidance with improved access to clean water and sanitation and elimination of the water dwelling snails. In the event of infection, treatment with Praziquantel or Oxamniquine is recommended. Annual treatment with a single dose of Praziquantel may be needed.

Wilson's Disease

Background

Wilson's disease is an inherited disorder with defective biliary excretion of copper due to mutations on the ATP7B gene on chromosome 13, which encodes a copper transporting P-type ATPase [7]. The gene frequency is 1:90–150 and incidence (with neurological symptoms) 1 in 30,000.

The development of disease is caused by accumulation of copper in affected organs and tissues. Most cases present between the ages of 5 and 35 years, but the disease can present at any age. The disease can present in a variety of ways including: neuro-psychiatric disturbance, haemolysis, ataxia, subtle biochemical change, cirrhosis and acute liver failure. Less common manifestations include gigantism, renal abnormalities, cardiomyopathy, hypoparathyroidism, pancreatitis and infertility.

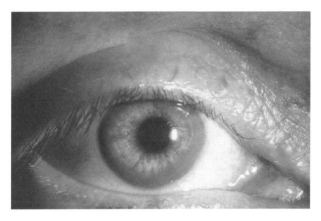

FIGURE 18.3 Kayser-Fleischer ring in Wilson's disease from [9]

Diagnosis

A combination of Kayser-Fleischer rings (Fig. 18.3) and a very low caeruloplasmin (<0.1 g/L) is sufficient to make the diagnosis.

The following investigations may aid diagnosis:

Biochemistry: A low alkaline phosphatase and elevated bilirubin (associated with Coombs negative haemolysis) are suggestive. In acute liver failure caused by Wilson's disease, a combination of both an alkaline phosphate/bilirubin elevation ratio of <4 and an AST:ALT ratio >2.2 gives a diagnostic sensitivity and specificity of 100%.

Serum Caeruloplasmin: Normally <0.1 g/L in Wilsons (beware acute phase response pushing value up and acaeruloplasminaemia).

Serum copper: A high or normal copper level in the face of a low caeruloplasmin suggests increase in copper not bound to caeruloplasmin (non-caeruloplasmin bound copper). The non-caeruloplasmin bound copper can be calculated thus:

Non caeruloplasmin bound copper

$$= \frac{\text{Total serum copper}(\mu g / L)}{\text{Serum copper}(\mu mol / L) \times 63.5} - \frac{\text{Caeruloplasmin bound copper}(\mu g / L)}{3.15 \times \text{caeruloplasmin}(mg / L)}$$

In most untreated patients levels are greater than 200 µg/L.

Some authorities use it to measure adherence to treatment rather than for diagnosis.

Urinary Copper excretion > 1.6 µmol/24 h (100 µg/24 h)— Diagnostic of Wilsons.

The penicillamine challenge test is not recommended in adults.

Hepatic Parenchymal Copper Concentration

Hepatic copper content >4 µmol/g dry weight is diagnostic of Wilsons disease (levels >1.2 µmol/g) are suggestive in the face of other supporting factors.

Liver histology can show a range of features including features suggestive of NAFLD, NASH and autoimmune hepatitis (Fig. 18.4). Other features include glycogenated nuclei in hepatocytes and focal hepatocellular necrosis. Approximately 50% of patients are cirrhotic at the time of diagnosis.

Genetic testing: Analysis of the ATP7B gene is advised for patients with a provisional diagnosis of Wilsons disease, for confirmation and to allow for screening of family members.

The diagnostic scoring system proposed for Wilson's disease is shown in Table 18.3.

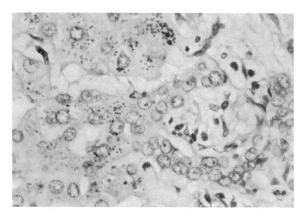

Figure 18.4 Cirrhosis in Wilsons disease. Numerous copper deposits in periportal liver epithelia (Rhodanine stain) [9]

TABLE 18.3 Scoring system for Wilson's disease (From 8th International Meeting on Wilsons disease, Leipzig 2001)

Typical clinical symptoms and signs	Points
Kayser-Fleischer rings	
Present	2
Neurological symptoms	
Severe	2
Mild	1
Serum caeruloplasmin	
0.1–0.2 g/L	1
<0.1 g/L	2
Coombs negative haemolysis	
Present	1
Liver copper (no cholestasis)	
>×5 upper limit of normal	2
0.8–4 μmol/L	1
Normal (<0.8 μmol/g)	−1
Rhodanine-positive granules	1
Urinary copper (no acute hepatitis)	
1–2× upper limit of normal	1
>2× upper limit of normal	2
Normal but >5× upper limit after D penicillamine	2
Mutation analysis	
Detected on both chromosomes	4
On 1 chromosome	1

Total score: ≥4 diagnosis established, 3 Diagnosis possible, ≤2 diagnosis unlikely

Treatment

All cases should be investigated and treatment commenced by clinicians with experience in managing Wilsons disease.

D-penicillamine: 750–1500 mg/day in two to three doses. Must be given with pyridoxine (25–50 mg/day).

Effective treatment and compliance determined by urinary copper excretion 2 days after cessation of treatment. Ideal range should be ≤1.6 µol/24 h. Urinary copper excretion should be 3–8 µmol/24 h on treatment (can be as high as 16 µmol/24 h when starting treatment).

Side effects: Fever, cutaneous eruptions, proteinuria, lupus like syndrome, elastosis perforans serpiginosa, pemphigoid, pemphigus, lichen planus, polymyositis and myasthenia gravis.

Trientine: 900–2700 mg/day in two to three divided doses.

Treatment with iron should be avoided.

Side effects: sideroblastic anaemia, lupus like syndrome.

Ammonium tetrathiomolybdate: Not commercially available.

Zinc: 150 mg/day. Do not take with food.

Side effects: Gastric irritation, immunosuppressant effects, elevations in serum lipase and amylase.

Other therapies: Curcumin and vitamin E may have roles in treatment but as of yet these are undefined.

Liver transplantation: Necessary for acute liver failure and decompensated cirrhosis.

Prognosis

If untreated the disease is fatal. With chelation therapy and liver transplantation, prolonged survival is more commonly observed.

Answers to Questions
1. Which of the following statements are true of these rare liver diseases?

   (a) Wilson's disease is characterised by a failure to excrete iron? False — copper

   (b) Kayser-Fleischer rings and a very low caeruloplasmin (<0.1 g/L) are diagnostic of Wilsons disease? True

   (c) Urinary copper excretion is low? **False high copper excretion > 1.6 μmol/24 h (100 μg/24 h) — diagnostic of Wilsons**

   (d) The penicillamine challenge test is recommended in adults? False

   (e) Trientine is an effective treatment? **True**

2. Which of the following statements are true?

   (a) Alagille's disease often improves as the patient gets older? **True**

   (b) Patients may have a flattened nose and pointed chin? **True**

   (c) There are defects in the JAG1 gene? **True**

   (d) Hepatic sarcoidosis often presents with cholestatic liver function tests? **True**

   (e) BRIC is caused by a defect in the caused by mutations in the *ATP8B1* gene (18q21)? **True**

References

1. Sherlock S, Dooley J. The liver in infancy and childhood. Diseases of the liver and biliary system. 11th ed. Blackwell Publishing Ltd.; 2002.
2. Suchy FJ. Anatomy, histology, embryology, developmental anomalies, and paediatric disorders of the biliary tract. In: Feldman M, Friedman LS, Brandt LJ, editors. Sleisenger and Fordtran's gastrointestinal and liver diseases. Saunders; 2016.
3. Bacon BR, O'Grady JG, Di Bisceglie AM, Lake JR. Comprehensive clinical hepatology. 2nd ed. Elsevier Mosby; 2006.
4. Houwen RHJ, Van der Woerd W. http://www.orpha.net/consor/cgi-bin/OC_Exp.php?Expert=65682.
5. Rodríguez-Roisin R, Krowka MJ. Hepatopulmonary syndrome—a liver-induced lung vascular disorder. N Engl J Med. 2008;358:2378–87.
6. Krowka MJ, Plevak DJ, Findlay JY, Rosen CB, Wiesner RH, Krom RA. Pulmonary hemodynamics and perioperative cardiopulmonary-related mortality in patients with portopul-

monary hypertension undergoing liver transplantation. Liver Transpl. 2000;6:443–50.

7. European Association for Study of Liver. EASL clinical practice guidelines: Wilson's disease. J Hepatol. 2012;56:671–85.

8. Russo P, Ruchelli ED, Piccoli DA, editors. Pathology of pediatric gastrointestinal and liver disease. Berlin: Springer; 2014.

9. Kuntz E, Kuntz H-D. Hepatology textbook and atlas-history • Morphology biochemistry • Diagnostics clinic • Therapy. Berlin: Springer; 2008.

Index

A

A1AT, *see* Alpha-1-antitrypsin
    (A1AT)
Abdominal US, 6
ACLF, *see* Acute-on-chronic liver
    failure (ACLF)
Acute cellular rejection (ACR),
    373–374
Acute fatty liver of pregnancy
    (AFLP), 279–280
Acute hepatic porphyrias
    management, 293
    types, 292–293
Acute intermittent porphyria
    (AIP), 292–293
Acute kidney injury, 30
Acute liver failure (ALF), 20, 47
    cardiovascular support, 28
    case study, 19–20, 33
    causes, 20–23
    classification, 20
    coagulopathy management,
        29–30
    definition, 20
    ECLS, 32
    epidemiology, 23
    initial resuscitation and
        referral, 26–27
    liver transplantation, 31–32,
        357, 361
    metabolic support, 30
    microbiological, 31

    neurological support,
        28–29
    non-paracetamol-associated,
        362–363
    plasma exchange, 32
    prognosis, 24–25
    renal support, 30
    respiratory support, 27
Acute-on-chronic liver failure
    (ACLF), 59–60
    case study, 57–59, 76–77
    definition, 59–60
    intrahepatic microcirculatory
        dysfunction, 64
    pathogenesis, 61–66
        adrenal dysfunction, 65–66
        cardiac dysfunction, 64
        circulatory dysfunction,
            63–64
        "the gut-liver immune
            axis," 63
        renal failure, 64–65
    and prognostication models,
        60–61
    systemic circulatory
        dysfunction, 63–64
Adaptive and innate immune
    systems, 226
Adrenal failure, 74
AIH, *see* Autoimmune hepatitis
    (AIH)
Alagille's syndrome, 384–385

© Springer Nature Switzerland AG 2022   405
T. Cross (ed.), *Liver Disease in Clinical Practice*, In Clinical
Practice, https://doi.org/10.1007/978-3-031-10012-3

Alanine aminotransferase
        (ALT), 7, 134
    autoimmune hepatitis, 212
    CHB, 158, 160–162
Albumin, 13
Alcoholic hepatitis, 71–72
Alkaline phosphatase (ALP), 7, 9,
        10, 15, 266
    causes of, 9
    investigation, algorithm for,
        10
Alpha-1-antitrypsin (A1AT)
    clinical presentation, 296–297
    deficiency, 295–300
    diagnosis, 297–298
    genetics and epidemiology,
        296
    overview, 295–296
    treatment, 298–300
Alpha-fetoprotein (AFP), 15,
        266, 342, 349
Alternative macrophages, 226
Amyloidosis
    classification, 389
    diagnosis, 389–390
    treatment and prognosis, 390
Anti-mitochondrial antibodies
        (AMA), 202
Anti-smooth muscle antibody
        (ASMA), 202
Anti-soluble liver antigen/
        liver-pancreas (SLA/
        LP) antibodies, 202
Ascites
    causes of, 69
    diagnostic paracentesis, 68
    empirical guide for
        management, 70
Aspartate aminotransferase
        (AST), 7
Aspartate transaminase
        (AST), 158
Atriopulmonary connection
        (APC), 309
Autoimmune hepatitis (AIH),
        277–278

aetiology, 199–200
case history, 196–197, 218–220
clinical features, 200–201
diagnosis, 198, 201
    biochemical activities,
        201–202
    immunological, 202–204
differential diagnosis, 206–207
epidemiology, 198–199
investigations, 208–209
liver transplantation, 215
management, 209–210
medication side effects, 213
outcome and prognosis,
        214–215
overlap syndromes, 216
    PBC-AIH overlap,
        216–217
    PSC-AIH overlap,
        217–218
pathogenesis, 197, 199–200
pathology, 204–206
patients selection, 210–211
pharmacological treatment,
        211–212
scoring systems, 207–208
stage of pregnancy, 215–216
treatment cessation, 214–215
treatment response, 214
Autoimmune pancreatitis type-1,
        225, 226
Azathioprine, 212
    IgG4-RD, 240

B
"Balanced coagulopathy," 29
Barcelona Clinic Liver Cancer
        (BCLC) staging
        system, 332
BCS, see Budd–Chiari syndrome
        (BCS)
Benign recurrent intrahepatic
        cholestasis (BRIC)
    diagnosis, 387–388
    prognosis, 388

treatment, 388
types, 387
Beta blocker therapy, 100
Bilharzia, *see* Schistosomiasis
Bilirubin, 9–12
Bland cholestasis, 45
Boston Consensus
    Histopathological
    Criteria, 234
BRIC, *see* Benign recurrent
    intrahepatic cholestasis
    (BRIC)
British Society of
    Gastroenterology
    (BSG) guidance, 5
Budd–Chiari syndrome (BCS)
    causes, 392–393
    diagnosis, 393
    pregnancy and thrombosis,
        280
    prognosis, 393–394
    treatment, 393
Budesonide, 212

C
Camden and Islington NAFLD
    Pathway, 138
Cardiac transplant, 320–321
Cardiorenal dysfunction, 65
Carolis' disease, 385–386
    characteristics, 385–386
    diagnosis, 386
    prognosis and treatment, 386
Cascade screening approach, 252
CD4+ cytotoxic lymphocytes
    (CTLs), 226
CFLD, *see* Cystic fibrosis liver
    disease (CFLD)
CHB, *see* Chronic hepatitis B
    (CHB)
Checkpoint inhibitor-induced
    liver injury (ChILI), 46
Cholestatic DILI, 45
Chronic disease, 397
Chronic hepatitis B (CHB), 151

biomarkers, 167–168
epidemiology, 153–154
HCC surveillance, 168–169
infection
    management, 162–164
    phases of, 160–162
management, 162–164
patient selection, 164–165
preventative measures
    diagnosis and disease
        workup, 155–158
    immunisation, 154–155
    screening, 154
See also Hepatitis B virus
    (HBV)
Chronic hepatitis C (CHC)
    antiviral therapy, 186
    case study, 178–179, 192–193
    DAAs, 187–192
    extrahepatic manifestations,
        183–184
    genotype 1, 181
    infection, 180
    interferon, 186
    investigation, 184–186
    management, 186–192
    mode of viral transmission,
        180
    presentation, 183–184
    sexual and vertical
        transmission, 180–181
    viral replication, 180
Chronic liver disease
    liver fibrosis, 13–14
    during pregnancy, 13–14
Cirrhosis, 13
    bacterial infections, 72–73
    frailty (*see* Frailty)
    hepatic inflammation in, 63
    NAFLD, 145
    nonpregnancy-related liver
        diseases, 274–276
    patients with, 63
    portal hypertension, 86–88
    sarcopenia (*see* Sarcopenia)
Cirrhotic cardiomyopathy, 64

Clinical remission, 214
Coagulopathy, 29–30
Computed tomography (CT), 117–119
　pregnancy, 274
Congenital erythropoietic porphyria (CEP), 294
Contrast-enhanced CT and MRI, 317
Controlled attenuation parameter (CAP), 135
Cross-over syndrome, 216
　See also Autoimmune hepatitis (AIH)
Crystalloids, 28
Cyclophosphamide plus corticosteroids IgG4-RD, 240
C282Y homozygosity, 249
Cystic fibrosis liver disease (CFLD), 300–304
　investigations, 302
　overview, 300–301
　treatment, 303–304
Cystic fibrosis transmembrane regulator (CFTR), 300
Cytomegalovirus (CMV) infection, 372
Cytotoxic T lymphocyte-associated protein 4 inhibitor (anti-CTLA-4), 46

D
DAAs, *see* Directly acting antiviral agents (DAAs)
Dane particle, 159
Decompensation, 59
　adrenal failure, 74
　alcoholic hepatitis, 71–72
　ascites, 68–70
　case study, 57–59, 76–77
　coagulopathy, 74–75
　decision making algorithm, 67
　hepatic encephalopathy, 71

hepatorenal syndrome, 73–74
　infections and sepsis, 72–73
　management, 66, 67
　renal failure, 73–74
　variceal haemorrhage, 66, 68
Dermatitis, 397
Diffusion-weighted imaging (DWI), 317
Directly acting antiviral agents (DAAs), 187–192
Donation after circulatory death (DCD), 368
Drug-induced autoimmune hepatitis, 45–46
Drug-induced liver injury (DILI), 4–5
　case study, 37–38, 53–55
　causality assessment, 46–47
　clinical diagnosis
　　algorithm, 48–49
　　liver biopsy, 50–51
　　pharmacogenetic testing, 51–52
　　time to onset, 48
　definitions, 42
　incidence, 39
　management, 52–53
　pathogenesis, 40–42
　patterns of
　　cholestatic, 45
　　drugs, 42–44
　　hepatocellular, 45
　phenotypes
　　ChILI, 46
　　drug-induced autoimmune hepatitis, 45–46
　risk factors, 40
　severity, 47

E
Eastern Cooperative Oncology Group (ECOG) performance status, 110
Elastography, 317–318
Encephalopathy, hepatic, 71
Endoscopic band ligation, 93, 95

Enhanced liver fibrosis (ELF™) test, 136
Erythropoietic porphyria (EPP), 294
Exercise programs, 119
Extra-corporeal liver support (ECLS) system, 32

F
Familial non-haemolytic hyperbilirubinaemias, 382, 383
Farnesoid X receptor (FXR) agonist, 144
FAST-ELISA, 398
Ferritin light chain *(FTL)* gene, 255
Ferroportin, 254–256
Ferroportin *(SLC40A1)* gene, 255
FIB-4, 135, 136, 146
FibroScan, 139
    See also Non-invasive liver elastography
FibroScan®, 136
Fibrosis
    identification and staging, 139–140
    liver biopsy, 139–140
    non-invasive markers, 135–139
    scoring systems, 135–137
    transient elastography, 136, 138–139
    See also Non-alcoholic fatty liver disease (NAFLD)
Fluid resuscitation, 28
Focal nodular hyperplasia (FNH), 317
Fontan-associated liver disease (FALD)
    biochemical markers, 315–316
    cardiac transplant, 320–321
    circulation, 310–311
    clinical presentation, 311–313
    definition, 310
    diagnosing cirrhosis, 313–315
    elastography, 317–318
    evaluation, 309–310
    hepatocellular carcinoma, 319–320
    imaging in, 314
    multiple composite scoring systems, 316
    portal hypertension, 318–319
    radiological imaging, 316–317
    recommended therapeutic approaches, 322–323
    screening, 321–322
    timescale of events, 311
Fontan circulation, 310–311
Frailty, 106–108, 121–122
    definition, 107–108
    FFI, 113–115
    interventions, 119
    KPS scores, 110–113
    LFI, 116–117
    mortality risk, 109–110
    pathophysiology, 108–109
Fried frailty index (FFI), 113–115

G
Gastric varices, 101
Gastroesophageal varices (GOV), 88–89, 101
Genome-wide association study (GWAS), 199
Gilbert's disease
    cause, 382–383
    diagnosis, 384
    prognosis and treatment, 384
Glucagon-like peptide-1 receptor agonists (GLP-1 RAs), 142

H
HAMP gene mutations, 255
HBV, *see* Hepatitis B virus (HBV)
HELLP syndrome, 269–271

Hepatic encephalopathy
(HE), 71
Hepatic haemorrhage and
rupture, 274
Hepatic venous pressure gradient
(HVPG), 318
Hepatitis, alcoholic, 71–72
Hepatitis B core antibody
(anti-HBc), 155
Hepatitis B core related antigen
(HbcrAg), 168
Hepatitis B e-Antigen (HbeAg)
negative, 164, 166
Hepatitis B e-Antigen (HbeAg)
positive, 164, 165
Hepatitis B surface antigen
(HBsAg), 153, 155, 276
Hepatitis B virus (HBV)
cirrhotic populations, 166
diagnosis and disease workup,
155–158
future therapies, 169
immunosuppressive agents,
166–167
infection, in pregnancy,
276–277
management, 162–164
NUCs, 163
Peg-IFN, 163–164
natural history and
immunology
acute infection, 160
phases of chronic
infection, 160–162
patient selection, 164–165
pregnancy, 167
transmission, 154
virology, 159–160
Hepatitis C virus (HCV), see
Chronic hepatitis C
(CHC)
Hepatitis E virus (HEV),
279–280
Hepatitis type C and delta
(HDV), 158
Hepatoadrenal dysfunction,
65–66

Hepatocellular carcinoma
(HCC), 246
case study, 328–329
current treatment modalities,
332–337
development, 297
diagnosis, 330–332
existing therapies
improvement, 343–345
FALD, 319–320
liver transplantation, 363
management
delisting patients, 342
liver transplantation, as
salvage therapy,
341–342
role of downstage, 339–340
waiting list, treatment,
340–341
new drugs and new targets,
293
screening and surveillance,
337–339
sorafenib, 347–348
systemic therapy, 345–347
Hepatocellular drug-induced
liver injury, 45
Hepatological curiosities
Alagille's syndrome, 384–385
alpha-1 antitrypsin deficiency,
295–300
BRIC
diagnosis, 387–388
prognosis, 388
treatment, 388
types, 387
Budd–Chiari syndrome
causes, 392–393
diagnosis, 393
prognosis, 393–394
treatment, 393
Carolis' disease, 385–386
Gilbert's disease
cause, 382–383
diagnosis, 384
treatment and prognosis,
384

HPS
   definition, 394
   diagnosis, 394
   diagnostic criteria, 394
   investigations, 395
   treatment, 395
   porphyria (*see* Porphyria)
PPH
   aetiology, 395
   diagnosis, 395–396
   treatment, 396
   sarcoidosis
      causes, 390–391
      diagnosis, 392
      treatment and prognosis,
         392
   schistosomiasis
      causes, 396–397
      diagnosis, 397–398
      treatment, 398
   Wilson's disease
      diagnosis, 399–400
      hepatic parenchymal
         copper concentration,
         400–401
      incidence, 398
      prognosis, 402–403
      Scoring system for,
         400–401
      treatment, 402
      urinary copper excretion,
         400
Hepatopulmonary syndrome
   (HPS)
   definition, 394
   diagnosis, 394
   diagnostic criteria, 394
   investigations, 395
   treatment, 395
Hepatorenal syndrome (HRS)
   alternative therapeutic agents,
      74
   classification, 73
   complex category, 65
   definition, 65
   pathophysiology, 65
   sepsis, 73

Hepcidin, 255, 256
Hereditary haemochromatosis
   (HH)
   case history, 245–246, 257
   clinical background, 246–247
   diagnosis, 246, 250–252
   disease expression, 248–250
   iron pathophysiology,
      247–248
   non-HFE haemochromatosis,
      254–257
   treatment, 252–254
Herpes simplex virus (HSV), 280
HFE gene, 247
HISORt criteria, 234
HJV gene mutations, 255
HPS, *see* Hepatopulmonary
      syndrome (HPS)
Human leukocyte antigen
   (HLA), 199
   alleles, 40, 41
Hyperbilirubinaemia, 11
   causes of, 11
   familial non-haemolytic, 382,
      383
Hyperemesis gravidarum (HG),
   267
Hypoglycaemia, 30
Hypovolaemia, 28

I
Idiopathic autoimmune hepatitis
   (AIH), 46, 50, 52
IgG4-related cholecystitis, 225,
   226
IgG4-related hepato-pancreato-
      biliary disease
   case history, 241–243
   definitions, 226
   demographics and clinical
      presentation, 229
   diagnosis, 233–237
   disease associations, 228–229
   disease monitoring, 237–238
   disease phenotypes, 225–226
   epidemiology, 227–228

IgG4-related hepato-pancreato-
        biliary disease (*cont.*)
    histopathological
        characteristics, 232–233
    induction treatment, 238–239
    laboratory parameters,
        229–230
    maintenance treatment, 224,
        239–240
    management, 238
    outcome, 240
    pathophysiology, 226–227
    radiological features, 230–231
    systemic and organ-specific
        criteria, 224
IgG4-related hepatopathy, 225,
        226
IgG4-related pancreatitis, 225,
        226
IgG4-related sclerosing
        cholangitis, 225, 226
Inherited systemic iron overload,
        254
Interface hepatitis, 204
Interferon, 186
International Autoimmune
        Hepatitis Group
        (IAIHG), 207
Intestinal schistosomiasis, 397
Intracranial hypertension, 28
Intracranial pressure (ICP),
        28–29
Intrahepatic cholestasis of
        pregnancy (ICP),
        267–269
Intrahepatic microcirculatory
        dysfunction, 64
Iron overload, 255
Isolated gastric varices (IGV) 1
        and 2, 101

J
Japanese International
        Consensus Diagnostic
        Criteria (type I and II
        AIP), 234

Juvenile haemochromatosis (JH),
        254

K
Karnofsky Performance Status
        (KPS) scores, 110–113
Katayama fever, 397

L
Lactate, 28
Lichen planus, 184
Liver
    anatomy, 2
    biopsy, 50–51
        AIH, 204
        role, 139–140
    deranged liver function tests
        alcohol, 3
        drug-induced liver injury,
            4–5
        metabolic factors, 4
        viral hepatitis, 4
    fibrosis, 13–14
    immunologic functions, 3
    metabolic functions, 2–3
    potential liver disease, 5–6
Liver biopsy, 250
Liver cirrhosis, 319
Liver frailty index (LFI), 116–117
Liver function tests (LFTs), 5
    case study, 1–2, 16–17
    hepatocellular damage
        alkaline phosphatase, 7, 9,
            10
        bilirubin, 9–12
        isolated GGT elevation, 9
        serum aminotransferases,
            7–8
    synthetic function
        albumin, 13
        platelets, 13
        prothrombin time, 12
Liver graft allocation, 368–369
Liver stiffness measurement
        (LSM), 136

Liver transplantation (LT),
        31–32, 320–321, 356
    autoimmune hepatitis, 215
    case-study, 356
    contraindications, 378
    long-term follow-up, 376–377
    patient selection
        contraindications,
            364–366
        indications, 357–358
        malignant liver disease,
            363–364
        prognostic scoring systems,
            358–363
        super-urgent, 361–363
    post-transplant care
        ACR, 373–374
        biliary complications, 372
        complications, 372
        primary graft nonfunction,
            373
        vascular complications,
            372
    pregnancy, 278–279
    pre-transplant assessment
        cardiopulmonary, 366–367
        imaging, 367
        liver graft allocation,
            368–369
        nutritional, 367–368
        renal dysfunction, 367
    prognosis, 377
    as salvage therapy, 341–342
    surgery, 369–371

M
Magnetic resonance (MR)
        imaging, 338
Major histocompatibility
        complex molecules
        (MHC), 41
Malignant liver disease, 363–364
MELD, *see* Model of end-stage
        liver disease (MELD)

MELD-XI score, 316
Memory B cells, 226
Metabolic syndrome
    interventions for, 142–144
    prevalence, 376
Metformin, 142
Milan criteria, 334
Model of end-stage liver disease
        (MELD), 108, 117
    liver transplantation, 359
    nonpregnancy-related liver
        diseases, 359
Modified King's College
        Criteria (KCC), 24–25
Multiple composite scoring
        systems, 316
Multiple single-nucleotide
        polymorphisms, 226
Mycophenolate plus
        corticosteroids,
        IgG4-RD, 240

N
N-acetylcysteine, 26
NAFLD fibrosis score (NFS),
        135–137, 146
Nitric oxide (NO), 87
Non-alcoholic fatty liver disease
        (NAFLD)
    blood tests, 134
    case study, 128, 145–147
    cause of, 129
    clinical history and
        examination, 133–134
    diagnosis, 133, 139
    fibrosis
        identification and staging,
            139–140
        liver biopsy, 139–140
        non-invasive markers,
            135–139
        scoring systems, 135–137
        transient elastography,
            136, 138–139

Non-alcoholic fatty liver disease
(NAFLD) (*cont.*)
  imaging techniques, 135
  management, 140–145
    cirrhosis monitor, 145
    liver-specific agents, 144
    liver transplantation, 145
    multidisciplinary
      approach, 145
    weight loss and lifestyle
      modification, 141–142
  medication, 142–144
  natural history, 132–133
  pathophysiology, 131
  progression, 132
  terminology used in, 128–131
Non-invasive liver elastography,
  302
Nonpregnancy-related liver
  diseases
  cirrhosis and portal
    hypertension, 274–276
  HBV infection, 276–277
Non-selective beta blockers
  (NSBB), 92, 93
Noradrenaline, 28
Nottingham liver disease
  stratification pathway,
  139
NS5A, 187
NS5B, 187
Nucleos(t)ide analogues (NUCs),
  163

O
Oesophageal varices, band
  ligation of, 98
Online Mendelian Inheritance in
  Man (OMIM)
  classification, 254
Optimise Fontan circulation,
  321–322
Orphan liver disease
  A1AT
    clinical presentation,
      296–297

deficiency, 288
diagnosis, 297–298
genetics and epidemiology,
  296
overview, 295–296
treatment, 298–300
porphyria
  case study, 290–291
  classification, 292–295
  haem biosynthesis
    pathway, 291
Orthotopic heart transplantation
  (OHT), 320
Overlap syndromes, 216
  See also Autoimmune
    hepatitis (AIH)

P
Parenchymal liver screen, 6
Pegylated-interferon (Peg-IFN),
  163–164
Peripheral anti-neutrophilic
  cytoplasm (p-ANCA),
  202
Peripheral helper (Tph)
  cells, 226
"Physiologic reserve," 108, 109
Pi gene, 296
Plasma exchange, 32
Plasmapheresis, 32
Platelet dysfunction, 75
Platelets, 13
Polyclonal
  hypergammaglob-
    ulinaemia, 229
Porphyria
  case study, 290–291
  classification, 292–295
  haem biosynthesis pathway,
    291
Porphyria cutanea tarda (PCT),
  293
Portal hypertension, 318–319
  case study, 82–84
  to cirrhosis, 86–88
  classification, 84–86

nonpregnancy-related liver
    diseases, 274–276
pathophysiology, 84–91
varices (*see also* Varices, portal
    hypertension)
    development, 88–89
    diagnosis, 89–90
    manifestations, 89
    surveillance, 90–91
    treatment, 91–101
Portopulmonary
        hypertension(PPH)
    aetiology, 395
    diagnosis, 395–396
    treatment, 396
Positive end expiratory pressure
        (PEEP), 27
Prednisolone, 211
Pre-eclampsia, 269–271
Pregnancy, 13–14
    acute viral infections and,
        279–280
    AFLP, 271–273
    autoimmune hepatitis, 277–278
    case study, 262, 281–282
    classification, 254
    clinical characteristics of, 279
    gallstones, 281
    HBV infection, 276–277
    hepatic haemorrhage and
        rupture, 274
    hyperemesis gravidarum, 267
    ICP, 267–269
    liver transplantation, 278–279
    physiology in, 266–267
    pre-eclampsia, 269–271
    and thrombosis, 280
Primary biliary cholangitis/
        cirrhosis (PBC), 216
Primary sclerosing cholangitis
        (PSC), 216
Programmed cell death 1
        inhibitor (anti-PD-1), 46
Progressive familial intrahepatic
        cholestasis (PFIC), *see*
        Benign recurrent

intrahepatic cholestasis
    (BRIC)
Prophylaxis, portal hypertension,
    100
Protease inhibitor, 190
Prothrombin time (INR), 75

R
Radiological imaging, 316–317
Radiological markers, 17
Remission, 214, 239
Renal dysfunction, 367
Renal failure, 73–74
Renal vasoconstrictor/vasodilator
        imbalance, 65
Renin-angiotensin-aldosterone
        systems, activation, 65
Retroperitoneal fibrosis, 228
Rituximab therapy, 240
Roussel Uclaf Causality
        Assessment Method
        (RUCAM), 46–47

S
Sarcoidosis
    causes, 390–391
    diagnosis, 392
    treatment and prognosis, 392
Sarcopenia, 106–108, 121–122
    CT muscle mass measurement,
        117–119
    definition, 107–108
    interventions, 119
    KPS scores, 110–113
    mortality risk, 109–110
    pathophysiology, 108–109
Schistosomiasis
    causes, 396–397
    diagnosis, 397–398
    treatment, 398
Scientific Registry of Transplant
        Recipients (SRTR), 110
Sepsis, 72–73
Serological markers, 17

SERPINA1 gene, 296
Serum aminotransferases, 7–8
Serum-ascites albumin gradient
    (SAAG), 69
Serum copper, 399
Serum markers, 315
Sodium-glucose co-transporter 2
    (SGLT-2), 143
Sofosbuvir, 187
Sorafenib, 347–348
Spontaneous bacterial peritonitis
    (SBP), 69
Statin, 143–144
Sympathetic nervous (SNS),
    activation, 65
Systemic circulatory dysfunction,
    63–64
Systemic venous hypertension,
    311

T
T follicular helper (Tfh), 226
Thrombin elastography (TEG),
    75
Thrombocytopaenia, 30, 315
Thrombosis, 280
Total cavopulmonary connection
    (TCPC), 309
Transarterial radioembolisation
    (TARE), 334
Transferrin receptor 2 (TfR2)
    mutations (type 3), 255
Transjugular intrahepatic
    portosystemic shunts
    (TIPSS), 99–101
Two-tiered risk stratification
    algorithm, 138
Type 4 haemochromatosis, 255

U
UK Revised Criteria, 24–25
Ultrasound, 317
United Kingdom Model for
    End-Stage Liver
    Disease (UKELD),
    359–361

United Network for Organ
    Sharing (UNOS), 110,
    113
Ursodeoxycholic acid (UDCA),
    217

V
Variceal haemorrhage, 66, 68
Varices, portal hypertension
    development, 88–89
    diagnosis, 89–90
    manifestations, 89
    surveillance, 90–91
    treatment
        endoscopic variceal
            ligation, 98–99
        failure of first-line therapy,
            99
        gastric varices, 101
        medical therapy, 97–98
        non-selective beta
            blockade, 92, 93
        prevent development,
            91–92
        prophylactic, 92–95
        secondary prophylaxis,
            100–101
        TIPSS placement, 99–101
        variceal haemorrhage,
            95–97
VAST score, 316
Venesection, 252
Viral hepatitis, 4
Vitamin E, 144

W
Wilson's disease
    diagnosis, 399–400
    hepatic parenchymal copper
        concentration, 400–401
    incidence, 398
    prognosis, 402–403
    scoring system for, 400–401
    treatment, 402
    urinary copper excretion, 400

Printed in the United States
by Baker & Taylor Publisher Services